PRAISE FOR *PERFECT BALANCE:*

"With this book, physicians and patients alike now have the opportunity to learn about the exciting new approach that Dr. Greene offers for lifelong improvements in women's health, and patients have the means to become partners with their health care providers. *Perfect Balance* is a remarkable achievement and a breakthrough in thinking and medical practice that should enable thousands of doctors and millions of women to bring meaningful improvements to their overall health and enjoyment of life."

>—David Feldman, M.D., associate clinical professor of obstetrics and gynecology, University of California, San Francisco–Fresno

"At last, cutting-edge knowledge that brings doctor and patient together. Every doctor who takes care of women and women of every age need this book."

>—Ricki Pollycove, M.D., M.H.S.,
>Fellow of the American College of Ob-Gyn

"This book is sure to be a guiding light for women everywhere. It will empower women to become educated consumers who will then be better equipped to navigate the many different medical specialists and myriad of treatment options available today. Dr. Robert Greene offers clear solutions to the problems that many women face, from the teenage years well into mid-life. This book will help women with illness prevention and it will also show them how to successfully advocate for themselves should an illness occur."

>—Dr. Jeanne Leventhal Alexander, founder and president of the
>Alexander Foundation for Women's Health

"This is for women everywhere whose doctors told them, 'It's all in your head.' Ladies, share this book with your doctors and make sure they read it from cover to cover."

>—Ann Louise Gittleman, Ph.D., author of the *New York Times*
>bestseller *Before the Change* and *The Fat Flush Plan*

Dr. Robert Greene's
Breakthrough Program for Finding
the Lifelong Hormonal Health
You *Deserve*

Perfect
Balance

ROBERT A. GREENE, M.D., AND LEAH FELDON

Clarkson Potter/Publishers
New York

Copyright © 2005 by Robert A. Greene and Leah Feldon

All rights reserved.

Published by Clarkson Potter/Publishers, an imprint of the Crown Publishing Group, a division of Random House, Inc., New York.
www.clarksonpotter.com

CLARKSON N. POTTER is a trademark and POTTER and colophon are registered trademarks of Random House, Inc.

Printed in the United States of America

Design by Jennifer K. Beal

Library of Congress Cataloging-in-Publication Data

Greene, Robert A.
Perfect balance : Dr. Robert Greene's breakthrough program for finding the lifelong hormonal health you deserve / Robert A. Greene and Leah Feldon.
Includes bibliographical references.
1. Endocrine gynecology—Popular works. 2. Women—Health and hygiene—Popular works.
3. Hormones—Popular works. I. Feldon, Leah, 1944– II. Title.
RG159.G74   2005
618.1—dc22   2004021076

ISBN 1-4000-5136-3

10 9 8 7 6 5 4 3 2 1

First Edition

To Morgan
You keep me balanced!

ACKNOWLEDGMENTS

Perfect Balance will profoundly change the way health care is offered to women. However, it wouldn't have been possible to create such revolutionary change without an enthusiastic band of visionaries who made it possible. I'd like to introduce you to each of the people who truly deserve your gratitude; without them, this book would have remained my private fantasy.

First and foremost, my wife and life partner, Morgan Pritchard. She is not only the source of my passion, but the one that harnesses it and keeps me focused. Ever since I first began discussing this project with her, it was her encouragement that kept me going.

A special thanks goes to my eloquent writing partner, Leah Feldon. Though we came together as a blind date, I'm delighted with the creative relationship that has blossomed. She is a friend and an ally as well as a true collaborator who has been instrumental in conceptualizing and articulating my message. Leah's insights and talent put life into this text.

My ever enthusiastic agent, Stedman Mays, of Scribblers House Literary Agency: You not only embraced this project, but helped foster and expand it into something even bigger than I had imagined. I look forward to a long and exciting relationship.

Natalie Kaire, a brilliant and gifted editor with a unique blend of patience, dedication, and a keen attention to details—and this project had many of them. Don't ever stop asking "Why?" This wouldn't be the book it is without you.

To all the wonderful people at Clarkson Potter and the Crown Publishing Group, I owe you my most sincere gratitude for enthusiastically embracing this project. Jenny Frost, your support was a driving force in this work. Lauren Shakely and Pam Krauss, your oversight throughout this project has been invaluable; it's clear that you've earned the respect of all who work with you. Annetta Hanna, thanks for your initial guidance. Phillip Patrick, you've created the groundwork for unprecedented success. I am grateful for your marketing vision and appreciation of the importance of this book. Tina Constable, Tammy Blake, and Penny Simon, you're a talented PR team. Your advice, enthusiasm, and planning have been phenomenal. Sona Vogel, whose skill and precision polished the final manuscript—thank you.

Special thanks to Suzanne Somers for sharing her experience so openly. You've empowered countless women to seek out individualized solutions and personal fulfillment. And your sense of humor has truly given the "seven dwarfs" new meaning.

Without the hard work of a truly dedicated bunch at my office, I could never have found the time to complete this work. I am especially indebted to Lori Thomas and Lisa Hawley for helping create an environment where women can go for answers. Judith Crabtree, WHC-NP, a colleague with a winning smile and a caring demeanor capable of reassuring everyone that meets her. Rea McFadden, our dietician, provided nutritional information that was helpful in creating the charts and tables in chapter 4. Mare Deutcher, you are a delight. Thank you for reading and rereading with tireless enthusiasm. You've made major life changes to join me on this quest, and I'm grateful for so many reasons. To the many patients who entrust us with their care, we appreciate each and every one of you. You honor us with your confidence—a precious gift that we cherish.

A work of this nature requires dedicated library support to provide the references necessary to support my suggestions. For that invaluable service, I thank Billie White and her dedicated team at Mercy Medical Center's library. Your efforts are solidified throughout this work.

My one regret is that my mentor, Dr. Oscar Kletzky, didn't live to see this work come to fruition. He set me on this path with the first brain-imaging study we performed together. I wish he were here to see how far this path has taken me and the many women it has benefited.

Finally, my heartfelt thanks to my mother and father, Ferne and Jerry Greene, for making all this possible.

—Robert Greene

My thanks and great appreciation to all those involved in this worthy project: First, of course, to the amazing Doctor Greene, an extraordinary physician, a true woman's advocate, and now a dear friend, for inviting me to share in his empowering vision. It's been a real pleasure. As always, special thanks to my old friend and superagent, Stedman Mays of Scribblers House, for his brilliance, insight, and for always providing a good laugh when needed. Undying gratitude to Natalie Kaire, our mega-talented editor for her cut-to-the-chase, spot-on editing, indefatigable spirit, and steady guiding hand—this book wouldn't be what it is without her. Thanks, too, to the rest of the terrific team at Clarkson Potter/Crown, mentioned above, who have been incredibly enthusiastic and supportive throughout, and to Sona Vogel for her terrific copy editing in the final stretch. My love and very very special thanks to my husband, Adam Mitchell, for his love, understanding, and support through some very long work-intensive days and months (I'm back!), and to the rest of my family and good friends who have been there for me—especially Eda and Steven Baruch and Jonathan Kahan, who have gone beyond the call of duty to help me realize my dreams. And Mom—another one here for you.

—Leah Feldon

CONTENTS

PREFACE

Our patients are beset with a deluge of conflicting information from incomplete studies to inaccurate reporting. *Perfect Balance* is one of those rare works that is able to communicate current concepts in evidence-based medicine to patients and professionals alike. Much of the confusion regarding menopause and women's health care that has ensued in recent years has been the result of unqualified individuals espousing ridiculous, and sometimes dangerous, approaches to these difficult and complex clinical issues. It is refreshing (and about time) to have a well-respected and internationally-recognized physician such as Dr. Robert Greene to address these difficult clinical issues. This book should be required reading for all women as well as their health care providers!

—Lee P. Shulman, M.D., F.A.C.M.G., F.A.C.O.G.

The Northwestern Memorial Hospital Distinguished Physician and Professor of Obstetrics and Gynecology

Chief, Division of Reproductive Genetics

Medical Director, Graduate Program in Genetic Counseling

Codirector, National Ovarian Cancer Early Detection Program at Northwestern Feinberg School of Medicine, Northwestern University, Chicago, IL

Perfect
Balance

INTRODUCTION

When it comes to how you feel, hormonal balance is everything, and no woman is immune. When you have just the right amount of one hormone in proportion to the others, you feel that you're at your peak—energetic, optimistic, mentally sharp, sexy, and vital. When your balance is off, when you have too much of one or too little of another, you feel less well—moody, lethargic, forgetful, uncomfortable, maybe even sick.

This book is about getting the balance right—finding your Perfect Balance and feeling the best you can.

Millions of women of all ages experience symptoms of hormonal imbalance on a day-to-day basis. My medical practice, in fact, is a microcosm of generational challenges. At one point last year, I was treating practically an entire family. The first patient, Jane, was an eighteen-year-old with severe depression, who had been referred to me by her psychiatrist. Her fifty-six-year-old mother was so impressed with Jane's progress that she made an appointment to see me for help with her menopause-related sleep and cognitive problems. Then she brought along her youngest daughter, a sixteen-year-old suffering from unexplained weight gain. Finally, her thirty-eight-year-old stepdaughter flew in from out of town for help with sexual dysfunction and infertility. All these women had very different problems that required different interventions, but all their problems were due to hormonal imbalance—and all, I'm happy to say, were dramatically improved once their hormone equilibrium was restored.

As a practicing OB/GYN and hormone specialist, I treat women like Jane and her family every day, and with unparalleled success. One of the reasons I'm able to relieve their symptoms and help them achieve excellent overall health—often when other doctors cannot—is my other field of expertise, brain science. My unusual combination of medical specialties, which grants me an insider's knowledge of cutting-edge brain-related hormone studies and treatments, allows me to formulate *individual* solutions targeted for *specific* problems.

The unfortunate truth is that while good health care providers try their best to stay on top of the latest developments, modern medicine is excruciatingly specialized, and the most significant information in one medical field can take years to reach another—and still longer before it gets put to practical use. That's why the intricate interaction between your brain and your hormones, a crucial factor in terms of how you feel, is still not being fully addressed by the mainstream medical community and why it is seldom factored into treatments and diagnosis. One of my goals here is to bring you up to speed on this hugely important link and show you how to use it to feel better and be healthier.

Your brain controls your personality, moods, sexuality, perceptions, cognition, and senses—in short, everything that's *you*. And since nothing alters your brain's chemistry more profoundly than hormones, keeping them balanced enables your brain and entire system to function at its peak and helps you avoid problems related to premenstrual syndrome (PMS)—mood swings, depression, anxiety, irritability, bloating, and fatigue—not to mention the hot flashes, forgetfulness, low libido, moodiness, sexual dysfunction, and insomnia that menopausal women frequently endure.

This essential hormone-brain link became clear to me during one of my research projects earlier in my career. Through the use of brain-imagining techniques, I discovered that estrogen depletion reduces blood flow to the brain, which in turn can cause forgetfulness, slow thought processing, reduced mental clarity, and other common conditions. I also found that when a woman is having a hot flash, her brain blood flow is reduced even further. In chapter 2, we'll talk more about these fascinating breakthrough studies and the huge implications they have in terms of your health. Let me just say here that these findings are revolutionary. They have scientifically confirmed what you and most other women have felt intuitively for ages—that the moods, memory lapses, and cognitive and energy dips that you feel at various times of the month and during periods of hormonal transition, such as menopause, are *not* imaginary. They are, in fact, very real and tied very closely to hormonal imbalance. Even more important, my findings mean you and every woman can actually improve and alleviate these kinds of conditions by establishing healthy hormonal balance—and, in so doing, can ward off serious potential problems like dementia that often occur later in life.

FINDING YOUR PERFECT BALANCE

In *Perfect Balance,* I've transposed my findings and other cutting-edge scientific research into a solid, easy-to-follow, evidence-based program that gives you the tools to achieve symptom-free hormone balance and excellent overall health—now and in the future. I've also provided you with all the information and basic knowledge you need to be a strong advocate for your own health care. Considering the state of medical management today, you must be fully informed so that you can participate in your own health care and make smart personal decisions. Even if you have an excellent doctor, most clinicians these days are forced to spend less and less time with each patient if they want to meet their overhead, and the limit of six to eight minutes per patient currently being encouraged by insurance companies is not sufficient time for any doctor to see the breadth of a problem, formulate a plan, and discuss the nuances of that plan with a patient.

Hormones are an extremely confusing issue today for any woman considering hormone supplementation or replacement, whether it's for contraception, symptom management, disease prevention, menopause, or simply to feel better. I've had patients come to me in tears because they felt positively horrible after they stopped their hormone replacement therapy but were afraid to resume their treatment because of alleged health consequences.

THE WOMEN'S HEALTH INITIATIVE STUDIES

There's no doubt that much of this fear and confusion was (and is) fueled by the media. The media thrives on sensational headlines—especially when reporting on complicated medical issues. The termination of the first arm of the Women's Health Initiative (WHI) study in 2002 is a perfect case in point. The study's focus was the potential correlation between hormone therapy and the risk of breast cancer and other health problems like heart disease. When they closed the study prematurely (ostensibly because of health risks to the participants), the WHI reported that women taking Prempro (a combination estrogen/progestin therapy) faced a 26 percent increased risk of developing breast cancer. These were scary—but misleading—figures. As it turns out, the reported 26 percent increase was a gross exaggeration and has no meaning in the real world since it doesn't factor in the average, or *baseline,* risk. The baseline risk for developing cancer around the time of menopause is 2 percent. A 26 percent increase of a 2 percent risk means that the risk of developing breast cancer around menopause is only 2.5 percent. (Actual math: 26 percent of 2 percent.) That's a very minimal increase in real-life terms—and that's the way the story should have been reported.

The heart disease aspect of this arm of the WHI study was misleading for a different reason. The study (whose participants were mostly Caucasian women who started on hormones at the average age of sixty-five) concluded that if you start combination hormone therapy at sixty-five years of age—which is many years *after* most women's bodies stop producing hormones—your risk of heart disease will increase slightly. But what caused the slight increase—being estrogen deficient for more than 15 years or taking the combination hormone replacement for 5.2 years? That was unclear. The kicker is that two months after the study conclusions were published, we found out that 30 percent of the women in the study were obese and about 25 percent were tobacco users. Were these the women who had an increase in heart disease? And how do the study's statistics apply to you? If you're a slim, fifty-year-old black or Asian woman who doesn't smoke, probably not much. Finally, when the WHI closed down the arm of the study looking at menopausal women taking estrogen only (as opposed to the estrogen/progestin combo) and finalized their analyses, they found that women had about a 25 percent *lower risk* of developing breast cancer. And they didn't find any increased risk of heart disease. These updated results were also published—albeit with considerably less fanfare. But by then most women were so scared that they didn't want to consider hormone therapy anyway.

Perhaps the most distressing thing to me about these kinds of studies is that they don't consider how you feel; they focus only on disease prevention or treatment. The WHI study participants were symptom-free—that is, they didn't feel any symptoms of hormonal imbalance. (That, in fact, was a requirement for women enrolling in the study.) So there was no way to determine if hormone therapy improved or worsened their symptoms—they didn't have any. How they felt was simply not a factor. But certainly quality of life is a huge issue. It is for my patients, and I'm sure it is for you, too.

THE PERFECT BALANCE APPROACH

Am I advocating hormone therapy? No . . . and yes. I'm advocating symptom-free hormonal balance—Perfect Balance—and if it takes prescription hormone therapy to achieve that, I believe it should definitely be considered (and we'll be discussing the best, safest, and most appropriate therapies for your specific symptoms in the second half of the book). But often you can improve or alleviate common symptoms of hormonal imbalance—the mood swings, bloating, hot flashes, sleep disorders, low libido, memory problems, migraines, and other disturbances so many of you experience—through changes in your diet, exercise, and lifestyle habits or alternative approaches such as mind-centering techniques, vitamins, or herbs. That should always be the first line of defense. My feeling is if you can solve your problem naturally, there's no reason to go the hormone therapy route.

The Perfect Balance program is designed with that firmly in mind. It helps you pinpoint your hormonal imbalances and correct them, first through a diet and lifestyle program and then, if necessary, through cutting-edge hormonal replacement therapies targeted to your particular complaints.

Because there's such a huge array of hormone supplement formulations, brands, and delivery systems on the market (patches, pills, vaginal rings, creams, injections, and so on), I've devised a Perfect Balance Hormone BioSystem™ that will make it easy for you and your physician to sort through the myriad therapeutic options and choose those that will best help equalize your imbalances and meet your other needs and goals. My BioSystem categorizes viable hormone therapies into five groups: *BioIdentical* hormones—those that are so close to what your body produces that even your brain can't tell the difference; *BioSimilar* hormones—formulations that are similar but not identical to your hormones and offer some distinct advantages; *BioLimited* hormones, which are designed to replicate some functions of your own hormones while deliberately limiting the functions of others; *BioUnknowns*—phytoestrogens like soy, flax, and some herbs that are under investigation and act in ways that are still unknown; and *BioAntagonists,* which effectively turn off your natural hormones and are used to control or prevent diseases like breast

BIOIDENTICAL: Hormone preparations (estradiol, testosterone, or progesterone) chemically identical to the ones produced naturally by your body. Available only by prescription and typically used to supplement hormones that your body isn't producing in sufficient quantities. Manufactured from plant extracts (yam or soy beans) in single hormone formulations that can be applied to the skin as a patch, cream, or gel; inserted into the vagina as a cream, tablet, or ring; or swallowed in the form of a tablet or capsule.

BIOSIMILAR: Hormone preparations that closely resemble your own hormones but are modified to offer some benefit that Bioldentical hormones can't, such as their ability to be combined with another hormone in one convenient preparation. Dosage is somewhat less flexible than Bioldenticals. Typically used for contraception (as birth control pills—estrogen/progestin combinations) and menopausal hormone therapy; also require a prescription from a health care provider.

BIOLIMITED: Prescription drugs that are designed to mimic a limited number of hormone functions. Typically used to promote pregnancy (the fertility drug clomiphene) or to treat medical conditions like cancer (tamoxifen). Available as pills, injections, and in devices such as IUDs or pellets/capsules that are implanted under the skin.

BIOANTAGONIST: Drugs used to reduce hormone production or block a hormone's action altogether. Typically prescribed to treat premature puberty, excessive hair growth, endometriosis, uterine fibroids, and hormone-sensitive cancers. Available as tablets, nasal sprays, injections, or implantable devices. Should be used on a short-term basis only to reduce the risk of any adverse effects.

BIOUNKNOWN: Herbs, supplements, and new drugs currently under investigation that can produce a hormone-like effect and don't fit any of the other categories. They may ultimately prove to be safer than some existing hormone preparations, but at this point, since there is no certainty as to how they work, there is also a chance they might prove to be harmful.

BIOMUTAGEN: Toxins used in food products as preservatives, in household items to kill insects or weeds, and present in the environment as various forms of pollutants. Should be avoided since they can cause symptoms such as uterine bleeding and hot flashes, as well as serious problems like infertility, miscarriage, birth defects, and even cancer.

cancer. And I'll introduce you to *BioMutagens,* the toxic chemicals in the environment that disrupt your hormones, cause imbalances, and should absolutely be avoided.

THE PERFECT BALANCE PHILOSOPHY

If there's one thing I've learned from all my research and clinical experience, it's that hormones are not a one-size-fits-all issue. Every woman's hormonal balance, imbalances, and symptoms are different. That's why no conscientious health care provider or study should ever suggest that *all* women should be on hormone therapy or all women shouldn't, or that the same course of therapy will work for every woman. What works for your neighbor or sister won't necessarily work for you.

My philosophy is simple: Listen to your body. We now know that hormonally induced symptoms are not just annoyances, but warning signs, red flags sent up by your brain to get your attention—to alert you to hormonal imbalance. Frequently the severity of your symptoms—the depression, anxiety, hot flashes and night sweats, insomnia, agitations, fatigue or aches, or even the worsening of "normal" pains—correlates with the severity and importance of the hormonal imbalance. If the imbalance is minor, your symptoms are usually subtle—sort of like a whisper from your brain. If the imbalance is more severe, your symptoms become more intense—more a roar than a whisper. Your decisions regarding hormone treatment should be based on your *individual* symptoms, your "hormonal whispers." They're the best determination of hormonal imbalance—more accurate than blood tests or study reports. If you have symptoms, they are happening for a reason and shouldn't be ignored. My goal here is to help you learn how to interpret those signals from your brain, get to the root of the problem, and correct the imbalance. While the discomforts of hormone imbalance may not indicate a serious disease, they can have a huge impact on how you feel day to day, and correcting them now could even prevent trouble ahead.

FEELING YOUR BEST

The Perfect Balance program is about feeling your best. It shows you how to correlate your symptoms with specific types of hormonal imbalance—to be able both to understand the problem and to fix it. In the following chapters, I'll take you step by step through all things hormonal. I'll show you how and why you feel the way you do in all the stages of your life as your hormones shift and resettle. Most important, I'll show you how to interpret the some-times quiet, coded signals your brain sends about your hormonal balance, so that you can attend to those whispers before they turn into shouts. As the Per-fect Balance program guides you into optimal hormonal balance, it provides you with the high quality of life and long-term vitality that you deserve—no matter what your age.

PART ONE

HORMONES: A NEW VISION

CHAPTER ONE

THE HORMONE REVOLUTION

Hormones are essentially chemicals secreted in tiny amounts by various glands and tissues in our body that circulate in the bloodstream and ultimately control numerous body functions that occur in cells and organs. While some have been much maligned for turning strong career women into weepy marshmallows and spunky teenagers into monosyllabic sulkers, they are hardly just the troublemakers they're made out to be. Hormones are, in fact, absolutely essential. They tell us when we need to eat, sleep, drink, warm up, even when to have sex. They strengthen our bones, alert us to danger, and help keep our bodies and brains vital and fully functional—and that's just for beginners. Hormones, in short, are crucial to our very existence. They are the ultimate coordinators, keeping all our bodily parts and functions regulated and directed toward the same purpose—whether that purpose is as basic as eating or as complicated as reproduction.

But powerful as they are, hormones don't act on their own. They are in effect handmaidens of the brain, which is the commander in chief of all body operations. As hormones surge through our bloodstream, they're delivering instructions, generated mainly by our brain, to cells in various sites in our body. (They also deliver information *from* cells *to* the brain.) They are the brain's major intercommunication system for transmitting essential information from cells in one part of the body to cells in another. And there are a lot of them flowing through our body at any given time—we currently know of more than two hundred hormones, and we are constantly discovering more. Within the last ten years, scientists have discovered at least nineteen hormones that help establish and manage appetite and weight alone. And we've uncovered a few other surprises that have turned our old concept of hormones upside down and inside out.

NEW FINDINGS

We used to think that hormones were produced only by nine endocrine glands—the thyroid, parathyroid, pancreas, adrenals (2), gonads (2: ovaries and testes), pituitary, and pineal—and that the hormones these glands produced each had only one function. The ovaries and the testes, for example, were thought to be involved solely in reproduction; the adrenals were meant to regulate stress; the pituitary monitored growth; and so on. But over the last decade, we've discovered that hormones are not only produced by the endocrine system, but are, in fact, secreted by other parts of our body, as well. Hormones are released by the stomach, skin, bones, white blood cells, even our extra belly fat—in fact, almost every part of the body can produce some hormones. That makes for a lot of chemical messages running through our body and a lot of hormonal interaction. Contrary to old-school thinking, no hormone is an entity unto itself. Each one impacts the others, and that mutuality plays a huge role in the way you feel on a day-to-day basis. There are four major hormone groups in terms of function and what they do for you, and even though they cross over into other territories, these categories are their home ground:

SEX HORMONES (estrogen, testosterone, and progesterone) are the big guns—the hugely important hormones produced by your ovaries that we'll be focusing on throughout the book. As a woman, the levels of your sex hormones shift more frequently and more dramatically than most of your other hormones, creating a delicate balancing act with one another and with every other hormone in your body. We've always known that the sex hormones influence reproductive status and define gender, but we've only recently discovered that they are much more all-encompassing than had been previously considered. The powerful effects of estrogen on the brain; the rather limited abilities of progesterone in areas other than the uterus; and testosterone's ability to help build muscle, regulate sexuality, and act as a building block of estrogen coalesce to form a fragile relation-ship that has a tremendous impact on your mental, physical, and emo-tional well-being. Sex hormones are, in fact, largely responsible for establishing and maintaining a considerable part of adult functioning.

THE METABOLIC HORMONES (AKA ENERGY HORMONES): This group, which targets all metabolic processes and monitors and regulates our physiology, includes the thyroid hormones, insulin, growth hormone (GH), and many others. Their job is to regulate how we use our calories—the ones from our most recent meal as well as the ones we've stored as fat. They decide if we need to store our calories, use them to build more tissue, or burn them to keep warm. And they ensure our health and survival by monitoring our need for energy.

REGULATORY HORMONES: These hormones (aldosterone, melatonin, parathyroid hormone, and others) help us maintain body temperature, reg-ulate the amount of urine we produce, adjust to changes in time zones, and monitor the amount of oxygen in our blood. They're the hormones that control how we function in environments ranging from frozen mountain peaks to sweltering deserts. When they're out of balance, they can cause bloating, insomnia, fatigue, sweats, and more.

STRESS HORMONES: which include cortisol, epinephrine, and norephi-nephrine, among others, are produced mainly in the brain and adrenal glands and serve as our body's alert system. They fire up when something is threatening our health or survival (this includes our need for food and water, temperature stability, and general well-being). When stress hor-mone levels are *briefly* elevated, they promote memory formation, moti-vation, and energy production. When they're *chronically* elevated, on the other hand—a situation that's increasingly common in our fast-paced, multitasking world—they can become toxic and adversely affect our emo-tional state, memory, and even sleep patterns.

HORMONE EQUILIBRIUM

All these hormones operate in your system like a finely balanced mobile. Just as every part of a mobile is interconnected and shifts when one section moves, each of your hormones is interrelated to the others, and a shift in the level of one will invariably affect the level of another, as well as the overall balance of your system. There's a constant breeze moving the mobile pieces, too—the environment. (Toxic chemicals in our food, water, and air can disrupt the nat-ural rhythm of our hormones.) When your personal "hormonal mobile" is well balanced, you feel your best and your health flourishes. When the pieces are tilting too much one way or the other, you get symptoms of hormonal imbalance like sexual dysfunction, mood and sleep disorders, and cognitive problems. And when the mobile is severely askew, serious problems, disorders, and diseases are likely to set in.

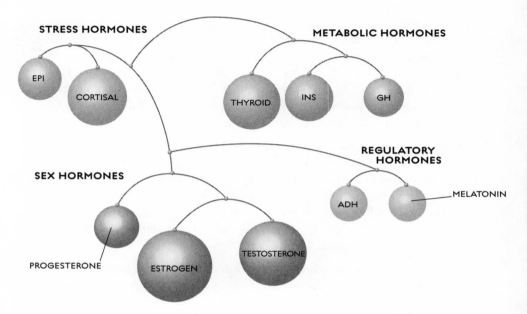

THE INTRICATE INTERWEAVING OF HORMONES

The sex hormones are in the center of a woman's hormone mobile because they play the central role in her hormone balance. Aside from their role in reproduction, they provide key functions within each of the other hormone categories. Testosterone, for example, fulfills an energy hormone role by stimulating muscle growth, which helps a woman's body burn more calories. And when estrogen levels are high, they can promote fluid retention, even though fluid balance is technically a regulatory hormone function. It's these kinds of crossovers that make sex hormones so powerful and their balance so vitally important. And because these interhormonal relationships are hugely variable and complex, sex hormone imbalances can manifest as symptoms that may appear to have nothing at all to do with the sex hormones themselves. Estrogen, progesterone, and testosterone play multifaceted roles in mood status (anxiety and depression), temperature changes (hot flashes and night sweats), appetite (cravings), sleep (insomnia), and other regulatory functions.

A good example of one abnormal hormone level causing an imbalance with others is *polycystic ovarian syndrome (PCOS)*, a common disorder (it affects at least one in ten reproductive-age women) that's usually caused by an abnormally high level of the hormone insulin. Typical symptoms of PCOS are weight gain, acne, excess hair growth, and irregular menstrual cycles. The latest evidence suggests that the high insulin levels actually cause the ovaries to produce excessive testosterone. Once the insulin problem is treated, the other hormonal imbalances often self-correct without additional treatment.

Another classic example of hormone interdependence is when one hormone prevents the message of another hormone from getting properly delivered to the brain. This block deprives you of a particular hormone and triggers an imbalance. Too much estrone (the "bad" estrogen), for instance, can block estradiol (the symptom-relieving "good" estrogen) from entering a cell, effectively producing symptoms of estradiol depletion like hot flashes (more about that on page 225). When hormones multitask successfully, all systems run smoothly. It's only when they fail—when your body has exhausted its ability

CASE IN POINT

Karen, twenty-eight years old, first came to see me seeking a solution to infertility. She had stopped using contraceptives about six years earlier, and she and her husband, John, had been trying unsuccessfully to have a baby for about two years. She had never gotten a clear diagnosis when she'd sought other medical advice and had repeatedly gone through fertility therapy at considerable cost with no results. During our consultation, I learned that her periods were very irregular and that she had been gaining weight despite frequent and rigorous workouts. Karen also said she felt tired, was worried about an increase in hair growth on her upper lip and chin, and had been experiencing irregular menstrual cycles ever since she stopped taking birth control pills. At that point I had a pretty clear idea of the problem, especially when blood tests confirmed that she had a very high level of insulin in her blood. I told Karen that correcting her insulin imbalance would not only help her become pregnant, but also lower her risk of miscarriage and improve her health. Both she and her husband were surprised at that diagnosis! Karen had polycystic ovarian syndrome (PCOS). We discussed the options, then set the plan into motion. Karen started on dietary and lifestyle changes to help stabilize her insulin and stress hormone levels. Although there was some definite improvement, it wasn't enough to correct the severe insulin imbalances, so I started Karen on Glucophage (generic name metformin), a drug traditionally given to people with diabetes. Within a few months, Karen began losing weight—and trusting me more. By the eleventh month of her program, she had lost twenty pounds and became pregnant. About eight months later, she happily delivered a healthy boy. No fertility treatment was necessary.

to increase production of a diminished hormone or convert enough of one hormone into another—that your brain sends you a warning sign in the form of a symptom. Those "whispers" are hormonal messages transmitted by the brain to let you know that you've got a hormonal imbalance—and that you should do something about it.

We actually experience minor brain-hormone alerts on a daily basis. Take perspiration, for example. When it's hot, a reflex initiates perspiration to produce a cooling effect. That in turn results in bodily water loss. Since your health is dependent on maintaining a balance between water and temperature, if you perspire excessively, your brain, which is always monitoring water loss, initiates action to reduce the risk of dehydration. It sends a hormonal message in the form of *antidiuretic hormone (ADH)* to your kidneys to slow urine production, which reduces water loss. If you keep sweating, another alert is eventually triggered—thirst. That, of course, motivates you to drink and replace the lost fluid. Drinking means you listened to the whisper and took action. Your brain acknowledges your response by quieting that whisper.

The bottom line is this: When all your hormones are in sync and in balance with themselves and other hormones, you feel your best—you think more clearly, move more fluidly, and have more energy. When they're not, you can experience all sorts of problems, some profound, others that manifest more as a general malaise. You may not feel horrible or sick, but you just don't feel great. Unfortunately, because subtle symptoms of hormonal imbalance are hard to articulate or even consciously acknowledge, many imbalances go unrecognized and untreated. Learning how to recognize symptoms of imbalance and alleviate them is one of the goals of this book. Let's start by taking a closer look at each of the sex hormones and examining just how they're able to exert such a powerful influence on your life.

THE SEX HORMONES

Your sex hormones (*estrogen, testosterone,* and *progesterone*) are produced mainly in your ovaries and to a lesser degree in other organs and tissues, such as your adrenal glands and body fat. From a chemical standpoint, they're steroid hormones, which means they're produced at a slow, regular rate, have a more lingering effect on their target organs, and are oil-soluble. (More about the importance of that in a minute.) Sex hormones are also built from one another—that is, by simply binding to the right enzymes, one hormone can become another. That's an important aspect, because it's what makes it possible for one sex hormone to be converted into another, which helps them remain balanced and allows cells to function even when the levels of a particular hormone are low. Your brain constantly monitors your hormone levels and sends a signal to convert one hormone to another when it decides the conversion is necessary.

ESTROGEN: MOST VALUABLE PLAYER

Estrogen is actually a group of three hormones: *estradiol* (which you produce in your reproductive years), *estriol* (which is produced only during pregnancy), and *estrone* (the dominant estrogen of menopause). Of the three, estradiol is by far the most important because of its sweeping effects on your brain and body. It's the one that most people are referring to when they talk about estrogen per se, and the only estrogen that impacts your brain. (Throughout the book I will be referring to estradiol whenever I use the term *estrogen*.)

ESTRADIOL: THE "GOOD" ESTROGEN

Although estradiol is produced in the smallest amounts of all the sex hormones, it fulfills more functions in your system than any other hormone. It controls, monitors, or modifies well over 300 bodily needs—that's ten times more tasks than those of most other hormones! The only other hormone that comes even close in terms of importance is testosterone—and it contributes to only about 110 functions. Estradiol (which is produced solely in your ovaries) promotes neuron growth and causes positive mood changes, healthy sexual lubrication, and normal sleep patterns. It hardens bones, dilates blood vessels, and keeps your skin wrinkle resistant. In addition, it improves your sense of smell, keeps your hearing sharp, and helps you maintain your balance and coordination. In short, it has a huge effect on your brain and entire well-being.

One of the truly momentous effects of estradiol is that it slows brain aging by stimulating nerve growth, functioning, and healing. And it's one of the most powerful antioxidants that the body produces—twice as potent as vitamins E and C combined. In fact, we now think that one of the reasons women age more rapidly after the onset of menopause is that they lose the antioxidant properties of estradiol (see page 50). Estradiol's antioxidant abilities allow it to diminish the production of cell-damaging free radicals, which are essentially unstable molecules that accelerate the aging process; increase the risk of heart attack, stroke, and blood clots in the legs (deep vein thrombosis); and contribute to dementia and other brain diseases.

HORMONES AND RECEPTORS

As I've noted, hormones travel through the bloodstream carrying instructions from the brain to cells throughout your body. The instructions are essentially orders for the specific cells to institute some sort of physiological change—to create a protein, secrete an enzyme, or grow in size. To assure that the message is not delivered to just any cell, the designated cell (or cells) has receptors that allow the hormone to enter and deliver its message. Once the hormone is in the cell, the receptor interprets the message, acts upon the instructions (which often sets off other physiological changes in the body), and usually sends a message back to the brain that the mission has been accomplished. So the receptor is an important part of the brain-hormone connection. No receptor, no connection, no interaction with the brain (although there are a few exceptions).

One of the major discoveries of the last decade is that a hormone's potency—that is, its ability to effect changes in the body—is largely dependent on its interactions with these kinds of receptors. It's the receptors (or lack of them) that allow sex hormones to cause major changes in cells in some parts of the body (parts that have receptors) while having no effect whatsoever in other parts (parts that don't have receptors). That means not all hormones in any given category have the same benefits—or the same risks—in all parts of the body. It's why, for instance, progesterone can stop cell growth in the uterus lining and promote cell growth in the breasts. This is one of the reasons you hear so many clashing opinions in the ongoing hormone and estrogen therapy controversy. Many people simply don't understand that estrogen can have different effects in different parts of the body.

ESTRONE: THE "BAD" ESTROGEN

Although it's relatively harmless in normal quantities, large amounts of estrone in your body can inhibit the abilities of estradiol. The excess estrone effectively blocks estradiol from binding to the cell receptors and renders the estradiol ineffective. This deprives the brain—and you—of estradiol's formidable benefits. (When one hormone crowds out another like this, it's referred to as a *competitive inhibitor.*) Obesity-related symptoms such as blood clots, heat intolerance, and sweating are often a result not so much of estradiol deficiency as of an imbalance caused by too much estrone preventing estradiol from doing its job. Because excess quantities of estrone stimulate the liver, it can also cause gallstones, and because it promotes ongoing endometrial cell division, it increases the risk of vaginal bleeding and endometrial cancers.

Estrone is associated largely with menopause and is often the dominant estrogen in obese women. This is because estrone is made primarily by fat cells, and in aging women the fat cells continue to produce this weak estrogen long after the ovaries stop making estradiol. Because estrone doesn't have nearly the potency of estradiol, it can't help much in terms of relieving brain-related hormonal symptoms like hot flashes, mood disorders, and sexual dysfunction. In truth, estrone's only major value is that it can be converted into estradiol.

ESTRIOL: THE ESTROGEN OF PREGNANCY

Estriol is the least potent and certainly the most limited of the estrogens. Its activity as an estrogen is about a thousand times *less* useful than estradiol. That's because the only time it circulates in your body is during pregnancy. Estriol is, in effect, a waste product; it's your body's way of getting rid of some of the excess estradiol you produce during pregnancy. (Pregnancy is the only time you actually produce excess amounts of estradiol; most of the time it's too little, not too much, that's the problem.) The excess estradiol is actually converted into estriol in the placenta (the barrier that, among other things, separates a mother's blood from her developing baby), then excreted out of the body in urine. So estriol doesn't participate naturally in hormone balance. The only known function of this hormone is to promote blood flow to the uterus during pregnancy (which is, of course, important only during gestation) and to help an expectant mother get rid of unneeded estradiol and other excess hormones produced by the fetus.

MEN AND ESTROGEN

Men make estradiol, too (actually even more than women do at certain times in their cycle and postpartum). It's just that men also produce much more testosterone, so the balance is different. Many studies over the last few years indicate that men's continued production of estradiol—they produce it well into their seventies, while women stop estradiol production at menopause—helps protect them from age-related brain diseases like Alzheimer's. In fact, a typical sixty-five-year-old man has about five times more estradiol than a sixty-five-year-old woman who's not on estrogen therapy! When women opt not to take estrogen therapy, their risk of developing Alzheimer's is three to five times higher than that of men.

TESTOSTERONE AND OTHER ANDROGENS

Most people think of testosterone as a male sex hormone. And of course men do produce it in relatively high quantities, but women produce it, too, and it actually plays a hugely important role in your life. Testosterone impacts your libido, stamina, mood, and even self-confidence. Some of the more common

TOTAL TESTOSTERONE VS. FREE TESTOSTERONE: THE IMPORTANCE OF CARRIER PROTEINS

The difference between your *total testosterone* level and your *free testosterone* level is a factor often overlooked in treating symptoms of low testosterone, and it can make a big impact in the diagnosis and treatment of various hormone problems.

As I mentioned, testosterone (like estrogen and progesterone) is an oil-soluble steroid hormone—and that's an important factor. Because our blood is composed primarily of water, and water and oil don't mix, steroid hormones can't travel through the bloodstream on their own. They have to hook up with *carrier proteins,* which transport them through the bloodstream and prevent them from coalescing into oil slicks that would create major problems for the heart. The snag? Carrier proteins also bind the hormones in a way that limits their ability to *exit* the bloodstream and enter the cell. To actually enter a cell, the steroid hormones must be released from the carrier. It's rather like a swimmer leaving a raft and swimming to shore. Once the hormones are released and they reach a cell, they can easily enter the oil-based cell membrane and deliver their message. The carrier protein is then free to pick up another steroid hormone and start again. If you have an excess amount of carrier proteins, they can bind up *too much* hormone, leaving less of that hormone available (or "free") to enter your cells and go to work.

That's why the measurement of your total testosterone level doesn't truly reflect your chances of experiencing symptoms of testosterone imbalance. If some of the testosterone is still bound to the carrier protein, it's there, but it's bound up and ineffectual. And that's why it's the free testosterone level that really counts. That's the measurement of how much testosterone is free from its carrier protein and able to enter the cell, deliver its message, and effect changes. The ability of birth control pills to reduce acne is a perfect example of how this works. The pills change the ratio of *free* to *total* testosterone. The estrogen in the pill *increases* production of the sex hormone–binding carrier protein, which in turn keeps more testosterone bound up and leaves less free to enter cells. Less active testosterone means less acne-producing oil in the skin. This, of course, is a double-edged sword, since less free testosterone in your system may improve skin, but it can also reduce libido.

symptoms associated with low levels of testosterone are sexual dysfunction (decreased sexual desire, response, or sensitivity), hair loss, fatigue, depression, and hot flashes.

Testosterone is one of a group of sex hormones referred to as *androgens*. Testosterone is the primary androgen you produce and the one that most influences your daily life. It stimulates muscle growth and strengthens bones and so plays an important role in maintaining healthy weight, stamina, and energy and staving off osteoporosis. Unlike estrogen and progesterone, which you produce in more or less equal amounts until you flirt with menopause, your testosterone level decreases every year after you pass your twentieth birthday. By the time you reach forty, you're producing only half the amount of testosterone that you did at twenty—and then it continues to decline.

The other androgens, *andro* (androstenedione) and *DHEA* (dihydroepiandrosterone), can be converted into testosterone but are of little conse-

CASE IN POINT

Mary, age fifty-two, had had a hysterectomy because of continual and severe pelvic pain and heavy vaginal bleeding. While the surgery had been necessary, I had advised against the removal of both ovaries. Mary had nonetheless decided to have her ovaries removed. Postsurgery, she had initially done very well. She had continued her estrogen replacement regimen (an estradiol patch worn on her hip) and had experienced only minor problems with sleep and mild hot flashes. Her real problems became more noticeable when she returned to work and realized that she was having significant problems with both short-term memory and math, obviously vital abilities for a high-functioning career woman. And she was also suffering from sexual dysfunction. Mary had tried working with her family practitioner to correct her hormone imbalance, but all attempts either failed to improve her symptoms or created new ones. Finally, they had agreed she should come to me to see what I could recommend. The problem was immediately clear to me. As I had warned, with her ovaries gone, Mary was no longer producing any testosterone, and while some women might not feel the effect, Mary certainly was. We needed to reestablish the correct estrogen-testosterone combination to relieve her symptoms. Her plan involved a slightly higher-dose Bioldentical estradiol patch combined with a gel of micronized Bioldentical testosterone that she rubbed into her skin each evening. She also started on a hormonally balanced diet, with healthy protein early in the day (for improved cognition) and healthy Hormone Power Carbs (see page 72) for her evening meal; and she started a regular exercise program. After four months, her memory problems disappeared, her libido returned, and she says now that she feels better than she did ten years ago.

quence as far as providing any symptom-relieving benefits in their original state. They essentially help maintain balance by acting as building blocks from which new estrogens and testosterone are created—that is, when more estrogen or testosterone is needed, these serve as the chemical foundation for that production. (There is no serious evidence that supports using DHEA or andro in supplement form, despite any advertisements you may see. In fact, if you were to take them, they would more likely create a hormone imbalance than help in any way.)

PROGESTERONE: THE HORMONE OF PREGNANCY

Progesterone is produced by your body only for reproductive purposes. (When you hear someone speak of a "progestogen" or "progestin," the reference is to a synthetic hormone that is part of a contraceptive device or menopausal treatment.) Progesterone is produced in the ovaries, right at the site of egg release—the corpus luteum. Basically, if you don't ovulate (release an egg), you don't produce progesterone. That's why this sex hormone is produced only by women of reproductive age. Once you stop ovulating at menopause, you no longer produce progesterone. The main function of progesterone is to transform the uterine lining so that it is receptive for embryo implantation. If this happens and a pregnancy develops, the placenta takes over the production of progesterone so the uterus—the muscle that contains a pregnancy—can relax and stretch to accommodate a growing fetus. When progesterone levels are high, as they are during pregnancy and even at various times in your cycle, the progesterone relaxes the muscles not only in the uterus, but in all other parts of the body, leading to symptoms like fatigue and constipation. The high levels of progesterone that occur naturally just after ovulation each month cause some of the common symptoms of PMS—mood swings, lethargy, depression, anxiety, and so on.

All three major sex hormones, estrogen, testosterone, and progesterone, are now manufactured and prescribed for replacement, supplementation, or contraception or to treat diseases and illnesses. I'll be giving you the lowdown on all the various types and formulations, including the newest BioIdentical hormones, starting in chapter 7 with the Perfect Balance Hormone BioSystem and throughout the second half of the book as we pinpoint the best alternative and hormone solutions for your specific imbalances. But first, to truly understand how these new hormone therapies work, and to get fully in tune with the tremendous impact your own hormones have in your daily life, let's take a close look at the hormone-brain connection . . . and just what it means to you.

CHAPTER TWO

THE HORMONE-
BRAIN CONNECTION

Our brain is the seat of our very existence. It controls our awareness, perceptions, thought processes, and creativity. It's also the core of our memory and monitors the environment through our senses of sight, smell, taste, sound, and touch. It signals our body when we need food and water and even alerts the body when we're satisfied sexually by triggering the orgasm. As we saw in the last chapter, the brain depends heavily on hormones to thrive and accomplish all these tasks. And therein lies a major difference between women and men. Since the hormonal makeup of men and women are very different, so are the effects of hormones on their brains. That's a big part of why women function differently from men, why their conditions are unique, and why treatments for those conditions need to be tailored specifically to meet their needs. Let's take a closer look at how it works.

BRAIN STRUCTURE

On the surface, most human brains look fairly similar. They're a rather gelatinous bumpy mass, weigh in at about three pounds, and are composed of about a hundred billion neurons and ten times that amount of supporting cells. Aside from the fact that the male brain tends to be about 10 percent larger, you really can't tell by examining any specific aspects of a brain whether it's male or female—which is why it's taken scientists so long to recognize the differences between the two. We now know that men and women are essentially "wired" differently. While our brain cells are the same, they're connected and intertwined in different ways, and hormones, as we'll see in a minute, play a big role in guiding the intricate construction.

The major structural difference is that while the male brain has many more neurons (brain cells), the female brain has many more nerve connections *per neuron.* That's what levels the playing field in terms of our cognitive

BRAIN BASICS

Our brain, spinal cord, and peripheral nerves make up what's called *the nervous system.* This system, an amazing treelike structure, is devoted to data monitoring and controlling all aspects of our health. Neurons, the basic informational cells of the brain, gather electrical signals through *dendrites,* which resemble the roots of a tree. These signals are sent to the nerve's trunklike body, which directs the signals up and outward to other nerves through branchlike structures called *axons.* The unique pattern of these connections forms the networks that come to represent our unique memories and thus makes each individual nerve irreplaceable. Like a tree, each nerve grows and changes over time. A nerve's ability to continually change and adapt (known as its *plasticity*) allows us to create more memory storage, generate spontaneous thoughts, and solve problems in unique and original ways throughout our lives.

Neurons, like other cells in our body, die from time to time. To keep us from losing information when a neuron dies, the brain forms networks from groups of neurons. These networks, like small brain forests, create a redundancy of stored information and offer a multitude of alternative ways to access it. The average neuron in an adult brain has about 50,000 connections with other neurons; larger neurons can have as many as 120,000 connections. At the connection points, nerves communicate through the release of chemical signals called *neurotransmitters,* which alert the next nerve to incoming information. They tell the receiving cell to pass the electrical signal along, suppress it, or modify it in some other way.

abilities. This greater number of nerve connections makes it easier for women to use several areas of their brain simultaneously when solving a problem, while men use more neurons in fewer regions to solve the same problem. Both do equally well in solving problems, but the setup makes for some essential physiological differences.

The biggest one is the amount of energy your brain needs to function well. Both the male and female brain function internally by creating minute chemical and electrical signals, which requires an incredible amount of energy. But as a woman, your brain needs even more energy than a man's. Because you use more regions of your brain in almost any given task, and use more nerve connections to access those regions, your brain is more *metabolically active* than your male counterpart's. That creates the need for a higher brain blood flow. Since your brain works harder to access more areas, it needs more nutrients and oxygen—and those life essentials are delivered through the blood.

NEUROTRANSMITTERS

Neurotransmitters are chemicals that carry messages from one nerve connection to the next, and more nerve connections call for more neurotransmitters. That's another reason a woman's brain needs more calories and oxygen than a man's: It produces more neurotransmitters.

Neurotransmitters are essentially the way our nerves communicate with one another—and they're terribly important to our day-to-day life. *Dopamine,* one of the key neurotransmitters, promotes pleasure, attentiveness, and motivation. It may also be one of the key secrets behind chocolate's popularity— chocolate promotes the release of this exhilarating elixir, as do cocaine, gambling, and other less benign addictions. Many of the other neurotransmitters are feel-good chemicals, too: *Serotonin* puts you in a positive mood, keeps you serene and optimistic, and attaches a positive feeling to memories. *Norepinephrine* heightens mood and mental alertness. (Too little norepinephrine makes you feel lethargic; too much makes you anxious.) *Acetylcholine* promotes memory, attention, and learning. *Glutamate* helps you retain information longer by converting short-term memory to long-term memory. *Endorphins (enkephalins),* the brain's natural morphines, can reduce pain and promote a euphoric feeling. And *gamma-aminobutyric acid (GABA)* helps you sleep and wards off anxiety.

SEX HORMONE IMPACT ON KEY NEUROTRANSMITTERS

Sex hormones—especially estrogen—greatly improve neurotransmitter signaling, the way your nerves communicate with one another, and that in turn has a tremendous influence on the way you feel. Here's how:

SEROTONIN: Estradiol causes your body to produce more of this feel-good neurotransmitter, which helps improve your mood and provokes feelings of contentment.

DOPAMINE: Both estradiol and testosterone increase dopamine production. More dopamine means a more intense feeling of gratification whenever you achieve a goal, be it an orgasm, salary raise, or satisfaction of a craving.

NOREPINEPHRINE: Estradiol enhances both the production of norepinephrine and the sensitivity of the nerves that receive it. That makes you feel more alert, less fatigued, and much more energetic.

ACETYLCHOLINE: Estradiol (and converted testosterone) boosts the production of the acetylcholine transmitter, which helps improve memory formation and recall. (Drugs used to treat Alzheimer's also increase the sensitivity of the acetylcholine receptors.)

GABA: GABA helps you fall asleep and keeps nerves from firing too rapidly (a condition that can induce anxiety, panic, or even seizures). Estradiol helps guarantee that this neurotransmitter is released at the appropriate times. Progesterone, on the other hand, mimics GABA, which decreases a nerve's sensitivity to other incoming signals. That's why high levels of progesterone make you lethargic and tired. (Sleeping pills also work by mimicking GABA.)

ENDORPHINS: These are our body's natural "pain relievers." Estradiol amplifies the endorphin response, which gives you a greater tolerance to pain and increased sensitivity to pleasure. Too little can actually keep you from producing the winning combination of neurotransmitters needed to achieve an orgasm.

Your brain relies on about twenty other neurotransmitters to function, but current imaging studies have not yet determined if or how those neurotransmitters are impacted by hormones.

THE BRAIN-BLOOD FLOW EFFECT: LANDMARK RESEARCH

One of estrogen's most important roles when it comes to brain functioning is promoting greater blood flow to the brain so that this all-important organ gets all the calories and oxygen it needs to grow, thrive, and operate at peak performance. Essentially, estradiol dilates the blood vessels to and within the brain. Without sufficient supplies of estradiol, less blood can be delivered to the brain, and it can't function as efficiently, which can result in forgetfulness, depression, sexual dysfunction, and even clumsiness.

This brain–blood flow effect was a big part of my early neurological research, and it provided some of the first clues that women who are estrogen deficient have reduced brain blood flow. In my research, I used SPECT imaging (single photon emission computed tomography) to determine the brain-related physiology of menopausal symptoms—specifically to measure changes in the brain during hot flashes. SPECT imaging allowed me to actually see what was happening inside the brain as hot flashes were occurring. Since the brain can't store calories the way muscle can, it needs a steady source of nutrients, which it gets through regular, steady blood flow. That nutrient-rich blood flow is directed toward whichever areas of the brain are actively working at any particular time. Whether you're dreaming, walking, reading, talking, or meditating, your brain increases blood flow to the specific brain regions necessary to support that activity. Those blood flow changes are measured by SPECT.

One of the major goals of this study was to learn more about verbal and short-term memory problems—both very common around menopause and, to a lesser degree, during particular times in the menstrual cycle, and both associated with a drop in estrogen. (Some of my patients jokingly refer to these memory lapses as the "whachamacallit syndrome"—as in, "Can you pass me the . . . uh, whachamacallit?" If you've ever had the feeling that a word is right on the tip of your tongue but you can't access it, or forgotten a name or telephone number three seconds after you've heard it, or lost your point in the middle of a pithy conversation, you've had a whachamacallit moment. While these kinds of cognitive lapses are certainly not a disease, they can be disconcerting—especially if you're giving a keynote speech, introducing a visiting dignitary, or winding up a high-powered board meeting.)

The study's findings were remarkable. As the scans revealed, not only was brain blood flow markedly reduced in the estrogen-deficient subjects—

particularly in the left temporal and parietal regions, where short-term and verbal memory are generated—but during a hot flash there was a further and even more dramatic reduction of blood flow to the brain. This was a true breakthrough. Moreover, the findings indicated that estrogen replacement therapy prevented hot flashes, normalized brain flow, and improved memory.

This research was the first positive proof that estrogen loss creates measurable changes in brain physiology and the first to confirm the vital interconnection between the sex hormones and the brain. And as it provided an explanation for the verbal and short-term memory problems associated with menopause, it was instrumental in establishing estrogen's vital role in terms of brain health. (Aside from cognitive issues, these findings linking estrogen and brain blood flow are critically important in terms of overall brain health, since when there isn't enough blood to provide the brain with the calories and oxygen it needs, the production of damaging free radicals increases and can lead to possible irreversible neuron damage.)

Another research study I was involved in showed that women who had more hot flashes actually produced more free radicals in proportion to the frequency and intensity of their hot flashes. This is hugely important, not just in terms of your brain health, but with respect to your overall health and well-being. Aside from the damage free radicals cause in the brain, they can render cholesterol more likely to stick to blood vessels; and excessive amounts of free radicals can irreversibly damage cell DNA—even turning it into a seed for a cancerous tumor.

With SPECT and the newer imaging techniques, such as MRI (magnetic resonance imaging) and PET (positron-emission tomography) scans, we've discovered the astonishing array of other effects hormones can have on your physiology through their impact on the brain. We've seen how estrogen and testosterone affect smell, hearing, balance and coordination, emotions, and sensitivity to pain; how estrogen loss can negatively impact memory; and how testosterone influences mood, libido, energy level, self-confidence, and motivation. And we can now objectively quantify previously immeasurable feelings and emotions as we look into the brain and see what biological changes occur when we're happy, anxious, angry, hungry, in love, and in lust. Our ability to visibly track the neurochemical changes that create these subjective experiences not only validates the human experience, but removes the stigma from psychiatric illness as it provides insights for new treatment options.

THE ANATOMY OF THE BRAIN-HORMONE CONNECTION

Our brain is able to assess every pain and itch, monitor the vital functions of our internal organs, control the movement of our limbs, generate thoughts, interpret and integrate all sensations from all our senses, regulate our heart rate, monitor our need for water, oversee calories, and adjust our temperature—all simultaneously and at unimaginable speeds. The brain can do so much with such efficiency because of the way it's organized. Brain-mapping studies have given us an amazing new understanding of which regions of the brain handle all these diverse functions. This illustration and the following list show you some of the most hormonally sensitive regions in of the brain, the ones that have a considerable impact on your day-to-day life.

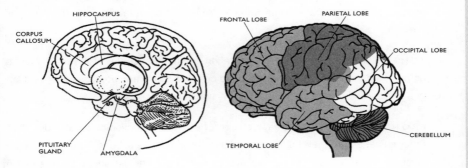

HYPOTHALAMUS: The interpretation and processing center for hormones, as well as the command center that sends out hormonal messages to the rest of your body. It integrates the incoming hormonal messages with thought centers of your brain (cerebral cortex, occipital cortex, and so forth) and guides your thoughts and actions based on the messages. It's also the seat of your most basic drives, like hunger, thirst, sleep, and arousal.

PITUITARY GLAND: Monitors the blood for incoming hormonal signals and serves as the dispatcher for the messages from the hypothalamus. The pituitary is rather like a hormone release center—when the hypothalamus decides a particular hormone is needed, it signals the pituitary to release it.

AMYGDALA: The seat of rage, anger, passion, and many other basic emotions, and the most rapid and direct link between your brain and your environment—there is no filtering or editing by the thinking brain until the signal moves past this region. The amygdala helps integrate emotion and behavior, allowing you to interact appropriately with other people. When estrogen is low, the frontal lobe of the brain that controls emotions is not able to override the amygdala as effectively, which can result in impulsive behavior driven by instinct.

CEREBELLUM: Regulates balance and coordination by integrating space orientation and movement. When estrogen and testosterone levels are low, processing in this region slows and you can't respond as quickly—a contributing factor in falls and hip-related fractures among older women.

CEREBRAL CORTEX: The thin sheet of nerve cells that covers the brain's surface, where emotions, memory, sensory input, and muscular movements are initiated. Your active decision to move starts here. Of the many hormonal influences in this area, one of the most notable is that when estrogen is low, short-term memory lapses occur.

PARIETAL LOBE: The area of the brain where the sensory input for pain is processed and integrated with emotion. When estrogen levels are high, your pain threshold is higher.

TEMPORAL LOBE: The communication and hearing center of the brain. Most of us form and interpret our native language on the left side and process music and languages learned after puberty on the right side.

FRONTAL LOBE: The area in charge of executive functioning skills—your ability to formulate a plan, then follow through and solve a problem. Long-term low estrogen levels diminish this skill (a decline that is one of the earliest and scariest signs of aging). Women also experience diminished functioning in this part of the brain during low estrogen postpartum months, leaving them feeling slightly disoriented and scattered—a condition some call "baby brain."

OCCIPITAL LOBE: The vision center in the back of your brain. Though this seems the least sensitive to sex hormones, the nerves of the retina, the area of the eye that collects and sends information to this brain region, is very sensitive to estrogen. (Women who take estrogen in menopause are at much lower risk of macular degeneration, the leading form of age-related blindness.)

CORPUS CALLOSUM: The informational bridge between the right and the left sides of the brain (anatomically larger in women than men) that makes it possible to efficiently use both sides of the brain simultaneously. It also augments creativity.

HIPPOCAMPUS: The data-organizing region of the brain. We temporarily store memory here until nerves can grow to store information.

HORMONES INFLUENCE
BRAIN-RELATED DISEASES

The male brain, of course, has all these regions, too. Since the male brain has more brain cells, it's more resistant to neuron loss. If a few cells get damaged, no problem; there are plenty more there. So men are less likely to develop Alzheimer's and other diseases caused by *generalized* loss of neurons. Women, on the other hand, tend to recover from *regionalized* brain injuries, such as strokes, better than men. If one area of the brain gets damaged, they can use their multiple connections (in their larger, more efficient corpus callosum) to access other regions of the brain—sort of like a backup system.

Hormones also influence the outcome and manifestations of brain-related illnesses in ways that are only now being defined. Symptoms of both multiple sclerosis and schizophrenia, for instance, ebb and flow with shifts in a woman's hormone levels. The following chart is a sampling of other brain-related disorders in which hormones make a difference.

Knowing whether or not you're more or less likely to get one of these disorders obviously doesn't help you much if you're suffering from one. But it does provide doctors with tremendous insights into optimizing specific treatment plans—and it might even keep you on your toes in terms of prevention.

DISEASE	FEMALE-TO-MALE OCCURRENCE RATE
Anorexia nervosa	13:1
Alzheimer's disease	3–5:1
Migraine headaches	3.5:1
Depression	3:1
Anxiety/panic disorder	3:1
Multiple sclerosis	3:1
Mental retardation	1:2.5
Autism	1:3
Schizophrenia	1:3
Dyslexia	1:3
Parkinson's disease	1:4
Tourette's syndrome	1:9

THE BRAIN-HORMONE-GENDER CONNECTION

The gender differences in the male and female brain start taking shape from the moment of conception. That's essentially when your sex is defined and you receive your genetic assignment—you are either a male (with XY chromosomes) or a female (with XX chromosomes).

The Y chromosome, which is responsible for determining male sex, has one primary gene (and multiple copies) whose only function is to create a testosterone-dominant hormonal equilibrium during the early stages of embryonic development. Testosterone elevations begin about the seventh week in pregnancy and continue until birth. From the thirty-fourth week until several weeks after delivery, a male baby's testosterone level is about *ten times higher* than a female baby's. In the absence of testosterone and these subsequent elevations, an embryo becomes female by default. In other words, it's the presence or absence of testosterone that establishes male or female characteristics during fetal development. These first several months of fetal brain development set the basic plan for how the structures of the brain are formed. It determines if the baby is more likely to have the larger number of neurons with fewer connections, as in the male-type brain, or fewer numbers of neurons with more connections, as in the typical female brain. These hormone-induced effects on the developing brain have irreversible lifelong effects on cognition and behavior.

HORMONES AND THE ADULT BRAIN

Studies on adult transsexuals have also provided some dramatic opportunities to confirm the effects of the hormone-brain connection on verbal skills and the plasticity of the adult brain. Several studies have shown that there are actually measurable changes in cognition when an adult goes through sexual reassignment. One well-designed study that tracked the verbal ability of a group of men going through sexual reassignment found that the subjects had better verbal skills after they had undergone the hormonal transition than before and that they were no longer as efficient in solving problems involving three-dimensional imagery or numerical challenges. This, in fact, was one of several studies that shocked the scientific world by demonstrating that the adult brain is still profoundly impacted by the hormonal milieu.

The hormonal influence on the brain isn't over once the brain is formed and gender is determined—far from it. Sex hormones and their activational effects continue to exert a powerful influence on the way the adult brain functions well into our golden years. (*Activational effects* refers to the way hormones can *activate,* or influence, a nerve's sensitivity to stimuli.) They can actually increase the likelihood that a nerve will transmit a signal—and that's exactly what estrogen does. In the adult brain, estrogen activates nerves, increasing their signal transmission. Imagine for a second that a neuron is like a track runner. Before a race begins, the starter calls out, "Runners, take your mark." At that signal, each runner gets ready so she can begin the race quicker and more efficiently. Estrogen has a similar effect upon neurons. It signals the neurons and primes them so that they're ready to act. Progesterone has an opposite effect. Rather than urging neurons into action, it slows them down and decreases the chance of a nerve successfully transmitting a signal.

The ability of estrogen to speed neural firing and make nerves more likely to send a signal, and progesterone's ability to decrease that likelihood, is

HORMONAL INFLUENCE ON SEXUAL ORIENTATION

This issue of gender identity and sexual orientation is actually one of the most fascinating to come out of the brain research of the last decade. It now seems indisputable that the relative balance of sex hormones we've been exposed to during brain development (as well as during puberty to a lesser degree), and the way those hormones organize nerve connections in the brain, creates fundamental effects that mold our gender identity and sexual orientation. Of course, culture, personal experience, and environment exert an influence, too, but hormones set the foundation. Mainstream science is increasingly leaning toward a biological explanation for sexual orientation and preference. Anatomical studies have found microscopic differences in the hypothalamus of same-sex-oriented men and women when compared with heterosexuals. It now seems far less likely that there's a "gay gene" and far more likely that sexual orientation is heavily influenced by hormonal impact during brain formation. Clearly this issue is not yet settled, but as the studies continue, I'm convinced there will eventually be good reason for people to feel empowered to accept that their sexual orientation is biologically driven.

important to you because it means that in most cases, estrogen improves your brain functioning and performance, while progesterone impedes it. That's why the relative amount of these hormones in your system affects your memory, mood, and level of alertness.

Since estrogen and progesterone levels change in relation to each other—one goes up while the other goes down—women often notice changes in their cognitive abilities within any given menstrual cycle. When progesterone levels are high, more signals to the brain are blocked, which often results in cognitive problems—some minor, others major. This opposing, ever shifting balance of estrogen and progesterone is, in fact, one of the activational influences that most differentiate women from men. Since the male hormone profile is more stable and lacks progesterone, men don't experience comparable fluctuations of brain functioning.

ESTROGEN HELPS THE BRAIN RESIST AGING

Sex hormones, especially estrogen, also contribute to neuron survival. Today, since women are living longer than ever before, the greatest challenge is remaining independent and unimpaired in later years. Estrogen dramatically improves the chances of meeting that challenge by slowing brain aging.

Estrogen's specific effects on longevity are under intense investigation, but we do know several things for sure: Neurons are irreplaceable, and keeping them healthy is vitally important; and estrogen is a major neuroprotectant. As we discussed, estrogen is a potent antioxidant and hot flash suppressor, minimizing neuron damage by reducing free radical production.

Testosterone has a positive effect on brain aging, too. It's been estimated that about 80 percent of the testosterone used by your brain is converted into estradiol, the "good" estrogen. (Since men also freely convert testosterone to estradiol, their higher testosterone levels provide them better protection against problems like Alzheimer's disease.) For men and women, testosterone is not only the key to how the brain forms, it also plays an important role in how well it ages.

VIVE LA DIFFÉRENCE: COGNITIVE DIFFERENCES BETWEEN WOMEN AND MEN

One of the most interesting issues regarding the brain-related differences between men and women is how they manifest themselves in our everyday life and influence the ways we see and interpret the world.

While modern brain imaging allows us to see precisely which areas of the brain are being used when a person is doing specific tasks, the way this information translates into practical differences can be subtle. Looking at the way men and women function within groups gives us real insight into how gender-specific cognitive patterns developed, and it's worth examining these differences.

While women tend to excel on verbal fluency tests and perceptual speed-related tasks, men generally outperform women on tests of mathematical reasoning and mental rotational skills. When shown a picture of an object, for example, men more accurately predict what the object would look like from other angles. Men also tend to navigate their way through mazes more effectively, perform better on feats of engineering and hand-to-eye coordination, and excel at perceptual tasks like being able to detect level horizontal planes. In turn, the female brain has other visual talents, such as identifying matching objects, tracking landmarks, and remembering visual tableaus. Women also have a better color vocabulary and better dexterity in small motor skill activities like fine jewelry work or embroidering. The combination of these tendencies makes women better crime witnesses—or so say police investigators. And it was certainly women's superior dexterity that made them the tool builders in ancient societies—a proclivity that is still displayed in today's primitive societies.

All these different propensities are most certainly a direct effect of how men's and women's brains are "wired" and a result of the hormones they're exposed to during development. Visual spatial abilities, for instance, are a testosterone-driven skill. And women's superior verbal and communication skills are most likely a result of brain organization. While a man might listen to a conversation strictly for content, a woman is hearing content but also picking up on visual and emotional overtones.

BRAIN AS TIMEKEEPER

One of the brain's least-appreciated and most important functions is timekeeping, and this, too, is linked intrinsically to hormones. Most of us are familiar with the concept of a biological clock—the idea that a woman's reproductive abilities wane as the clock ticks away. But in truth, your body is really regulated by another kind of clock, one that is run by your brain, not your ovaries.

The brain takes charge of your biological clock by integrating signals from the other parts of your body as well as your sense organs—especially your visual senses. Most of our bodily functions occur on a daily schedule that revolves around our sleep-wake cycle. Because humans have poor night vision, we've developed patterns that are most active during the day. And because we have relatively inferior auditory and olfactory senses compared with other animals, we receive cues that guide our sleep-wake cycles primarily through our visual system. It's important that your brain be in sync with your sleep-wake cycle so that it can effectively guide the release of hormonal signals to the rest of your body. Those signals are designed to coordinate your immune response, memory storage (long-term), even growth and metabolism. People who are chronically sleep deprived suffer memory loss, are susceptible to infections, and have a higher incidence of depression. There is also a tendency to gain weight because of a drop in growth hormone production.

Sex hormones and stress hormones are typically released on a *diurnal* (daytime) basis, which means estrogen and testosterone levels are at their highest points in the morning. Stress hormones, like cortisol and prolactin, are also usually elevated slightly in the morning. This morning cocktail, ordered by your brain and served up by your ovaries and adrenal glands, primes you to take on the day. The important thing to note here is that the timing of this morning burst of hormonal activity is controlled by your brain.

The brain is also in charge of your lifelong calendar and schedules the onset of puberty, the initiation of menopause, and your monthly menstrual cycle's egg release all through your reproductive years—all of which we'll discuss in the next chapter. This brain-run reproductive fertility scheduling is another of the key differences between the male and the female brain. Men's biological clock ticks at a very steady rate throughout their lives. It slows down a bit in old age, but it doesn't generate anywhere near the variances in sex hormone production that women experience each month and throughout their lives. The bottom line is that as a woman, your hormone-brain connection is much different from a man's, and that makes your hormonal journey unique—not just as member of the female sex, but also as an individual within that group. And as you're about to see, the journey is a fascinating one.

CHAPTER THREE

YOUR LIFELONG
HORMONAL
JOURNEY

Your hormones shift much more often and more dramatically than any man you know. While men go through gradual hormonal changes every decade or so, your hormone balance shifts substantially at least several times a month, and the changes you experience at certain junctures in your lifelong hormonal journey are profound. The symptoms, issues, and feelings these hormonal fluctuations create are unique to each woman. For some, the hormonal variations are hardly noticeable; for others, they're profound and create tremendous challenges. We'll be tackling specific challenges in our troubleshooting section, but first let's take a close look at the most important milestones of your hormonal journey, with an eye on their intimate link with your brain and the impact they have on your life at various junctures along the way.

Once you receive the XX chromosome that makes you female, develop in the testosterone-free fetal environment that helps "hardwire" your female brain, and enter the world, your true hormonal journey begins. And it begins with a big surge of estrogen. Immediately after birth, you experience a temporary spike in estrogen that lasts a few months. It is, in fact, much like the surge you'll experience later at puberty, but here it serves quite a different purpose. This postbirth rush of estrogen gives an additional boost to your brain development—and you certainly need it. While most other mammals are born with fully developed brains, humans' brains are only about 25 percent developed at birth. That means 75 percent of our brain growth and development takes place *after* delivery. After this initial mind-building burst of estrogen, levels decline slowly throughout your first year of life, and by the time you're twenty-four months, the estrogen is virtually undetectable.

AN INTERESTING NOTE

Boys don't get the extra hormonal push at birth—and they don't need it. Because of the testosterone present in their fetal environment, their brain development in utero is more advanced than that of females. So at birth, a baby boy's brain is actually more developed than a baby girl's. The female at-birth estrogen surge equalizes that discrepancy pretty quickly so that male and female brainpower is on par, but the setup does have some interesting consequences. One of the most significant is that because a greater part of a male's brain formation takes place in the womb, males are more susceptible to brain damage due to premature birth than females. That explains why rates of various learning disabilities are as much as 300 percent higher among boys. And it could account for the fact that premature female babies have a higher survival rate than males—the early estrogen surge may better facilitate completion of development.

CHILDHOOD

While hormones are dormant from age two to eight or nine, brain development certainly is not. In fact, it's under full steam. Imaging studies show that brain volume increases about 300 cc (cubic centimeters) between the ages of three months and ten years. That's a huge increase! This brain volume boost is kind of like a "memory upgrade" that prepares you for adulthood and mostly involves the size and number of neuron branches (dendrites) rather than the number of connections (synapses).

Like the sex hormones, the levels of metabolic hormones (insulin, thyroid hormone, and others) are traditionally stable during childhood. Unfortunately, however, that seems to be changing with our modern diet, which gives rise to childhood obesity and childhood diabetes. We're only beginning to learn how these elements will ultimately affect our kids, but many distressing findings point to a diet-induced hormone imbalance. There's some evidence that early metabolic changes increase the risk for cancer by making breast and other tissue susceptible to possible DNA damage. If the cells are already damaged before the onset of puberty, when they will grow and divide further, it would mean the surging hormones would be stimulating the growth of damaged cells—a known cause of cancer.

PUBERTY AND THE TEEN YEARS

The transition from puberty to adolescence is not so much a single identifiable event as a series of changes that begins when the brain detects the body is ready to enter the childbearing years. This is when the ovaries awaken from their dormant stage. The major trigger for this awakening is body fat. When the brain senses that the body has enough calories stored as fat to support reproduction—usually about 20 percent of body weight—it initiates an increase in the production of *luteinizing hormone (LH)*. This hormone production begins the transition from girl to woman.

The first physical changes of puberty—slight breast growth, followed by a serious spurt in height—are brought on by the nightly high pulses of growth hormone (GH) and the production of weak estrogens by fat cells. Sparse underarm and pubic hair begins to appear as the adrenal glands start producing androgens, a hormonal event referred to as *adrenarche*. As the nightly pulse frequencies of LH continue to increase, the ovaries produce more estrogen and testosterone, which causes an increase in breast size, fuller pubic hair, and further development of the vaginal opening. These cardinal hormonal events are referred to as *pubarche*. Finally, after two to four years of these bodily changes, *follicle-stimulating hormone (FSH)* and LH begin to follow their monthly-programmed changes resulting in *menarche*—the first menstrual cycle and the ability to become pregnant.

From a quality-of-life standpoint, these early teen years are anything but a smooth ride. Puberty is a time of real hormonal chaos. It takes time for the ovaries to establish their adult pattern, and as the brain attempts to initiate the programmed hormonal changes, the ovaries often respond unpredictably. Some months may bring extremely high hormone levels, prompting severe acne, bloating, and breast tenderness. During other months, ovulation might not occur at all, resulting in heavy bleeding and an emotional storm. And thanks to high testosterone levels with an assist from the adrenal glands, the first stirrings of sexual thoughts are realized. Muscles and bones also respond to this testosterone signal, making the body stronger and adjusting proportions, while putting an end to any further growth in height.

It's not surprising that during this transition, as a young girl's hormones and brain learn to communicate with each other, emotions can become extremely volatile. And when puberty starts early, navigating the emotional minefield can be even trickier. While the body of an eight- or nine-year-old might have an adultlike appearance, it will take time for the brain to match the body's maturity.

CASE IN POINT

When I first met Sarah, she had just turned sixteen and had been at a residential school for troubled teens for several months. Her parents had decided on boarding school after Sarah's high-risk behavior had nudged her off the honor roll and onto the police department's A-list of unruly teens. A psychiatrist had diagnosed Sarah as having a bipolar mood disorder but admitted she fell short of the official criteria for the disorder since she was so young. Sarah was on a mood stabilizer (Neurontin) and a medication for attention deficit hyperactivity disorder (Ritalin), but she wanted to quit because it made her extremely tired and caused her to gain weight. She was referred to me because in addition to all these problems, she hadn't had a menstrual cycle for about four months. By the time she came in, Sarah was overweight and had worsening acne. When she realized that I took her complaints seriously, we quickly established a rapport, and she listened with interest as I explained how hormonal imbalances often created a roller-coaster effect, triggering binge eating, anger, fatigue, and irregularities in her menstrual cycles. Eventually, I diagnosed her with polycystic ovarian syndrome, a condition characterized by erratic menstrual cycles, symptoms of excess testosterone, and insulin resistance. Over the course of six months, we stabilized her menstrual cycles and cleared up her skin with a birth control pill (Yasmin). I treated her insulin resistance with a diet that reduced simple sugars and increased fiber and protein, and I added a medication called Glucophage XR. Finally, I advised her psychiatrist to switch her from Neurontin to Topamax, since they were similar drugs but the latter was associated with weight loss. The transformation was dramatic. When her parents came to visit, they were thrilled to find the girl they had known before the hormonal chaos of puberty wreaked havoc on her life. Sarah was eventually able to stop taking the Ritalin, and I'm pleased to report that she was able to return home six months ahead of schedule. Needless to say, success stories like Sarah's are some of the most rewarding aspects of my practice.

One of the most exciting changes of adolescence in terms of the brain is the second wave of development, when there is about a 25 percent increase in the growth of neurons (including their branches, twigs, and connections) that begins around the onset of puberty and peaks when girls are about eleven years old and boys are about twelve. This brain growth spurt lasts for several years and explains the rapid upswing in intellectual potential we see in most youngsters during this transition into adulthood.

Once this growth wave is over and the "thinking brain" has reached its full size (in the late teens), the final changes in the maturing brain begin to take place; these are associated with insulation, or *myelinization.* Remember, neurons are like wires that rely on tiny electrical charges to transmit signals, so it makes sense that insulating these nerves improves the brain's efficiency. This insulation process is most active during the teen years and stabilizes in the mid-twenties. The resulting insulation, which shows up as "white matter" on neuroimaging, not only helps prevent short-circuiting, but also increases the speed at which the brain can fire its messages. Once this myelinization is complete, the brain is effectively hardwired. Though estrogen's role in this maturation of white and gray matter during the teen years is not yet fully confirmed, there's no doubt in my mind that the continued and consistent exposure to estrogen (and its potent activational effects) during this time is one of the main reasons girls tend to "mature" earlier.

This transitional period, while the brain is being myelinized and is bathed in cognition-promoting estrogen and testosterone, is one of the best times for learning, which is why good education during these adolescent years pays off down the road. If your interests in specific subjects—math, sciences, or the arts—are encouraged and explored during this period, there's a good chance they'll play a major role in your adult life. (In essence, the increased activity in those brain regions at this time promotes neuron growth there.) The bottom line: The intense brain-hormone connection during this period creates changes that influence you in later years.

THE MAJOR REPRODUCTIVE YEARS

From the late teens to the mid-thirties, most women feel their best and are in their prime in terms of health and fitness. These are the peak biological years and, in turn, the major reproductive years. Whether or not you decide to actually have children during these years, the important point is this:

Your hormones are going to stick to the biological script whether you do or not. A recurring theme in that script is your menstrual cycle, the pattern of monthly hormonal changes coordinated by your body and brain in preparation for ovulation and possible conception, and understanding its full scope is one of the keys to achieving excellent hormonal health. The following graph shows the dynamic relationship between estrogen, progesterone, and testosterone during a typical menstrual cycle.

SEX HORMONE BALANCE THROUGHOUT MENSTRUAL CYCLE

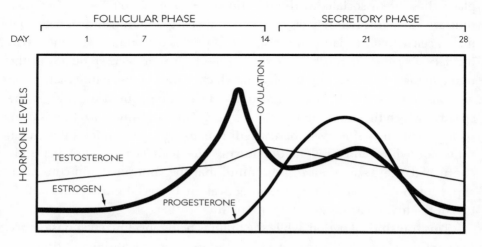

DAYS ONE THROUGH FOURTEEN

Day one through day fourteen of your twenty-eight-day cycle is called the *follicular phase,* since this is the time that the *follicles* (immature eggs) go through the final changes necessary for fertilization. During the first three to five days, your menstrual bleeding occurs. Near the end of your period, your brain sends your ovaries a message via FSH to begin secreting progressively higher levels of estrogen. While that's going on, your ovaries are also producing a fairly stable amount of testosterone and, most important, no opposing progesterone (see graph). That's a feel-good combination—you feel confident, sexy, and fit because of the testosterone; mentally alert and sharp thanks to the activational effect of the estrogen; and happy and content because of an elevation in serotonin and other neurotransmitters (provoked by the high estrogen levels)—and there's no mind-dulling, lethargy-producing progesterone to put a damper on it all. So this part of the cycle is generally a good one. As you approach day fourteen (ovulation), your brain works faster and more efficiently than at any other time of the month (in terms of both storing and retrieving information), and your athletic abilities peak. You experience a heightened sense of alertness, a more acute sense of smell, and an increase in sexual desire.

The high free testosterone level around ovulation increases libido, and, of course, having a healthy libido during your most fertile time increases the likelihood of reproduction. The high energy level and good mood that tend to prevail at this time make you more attractive in the eyes of a potential mate. And there's some evidence that your finely tuned olfactory senses help rev up your sensitivity to *pheromones* (airborne sexual attractants) given off by a potential mate. The bottom line: Your sex hormones are fully in sync with one another in optimizing your chances for conception. Ovulation brings an end to this feel-good period each month and triggers the next phase.

DAYS FIFTEEN THROUGH TWENTY-EIGHT

The second phase of the menstrual cycle (called the *secretory phase* because it involves the *secretion* of progesterone) is not as much fun. It starts after ovulation on about the fifteenth day of your cycle and continues until the onset of vaginal bleeding (approximately day twenty-eight). During this phase, your estrogen production drops to about 50 percent of what it was just before ovulation. It then begins a gradual ascent until day twenty-two of your cycle, when it reaches an even higher level than just before ovulation, but this time progesterone is in the picture to counter its feel-good effects.

Progesterone levels start a steady rise immediately after ovulation (day fifteen). The primary role of the progesterone is to get the uterine lining ready to support a pregnancy, but it produces some notable side effects. For one, it brings your usual temperature of 98.6 degrees Fahrenheit up to around 99.5 degrees, a

ASK DR. GREENE

Q: HOW DO BIRTH CONTROL PILLS WORK?

A: Birth control pills contain progestin (a synthetic form of progesterone) and estrogen. The progestin prevents both egg development and egg release so that you can't become pregnant. The estrogen is added to the formulation to block the negative side effects of the progestin (thus preventing vaginal dryness, slower cognition, fatigue, and depression). Essentially, the pill dramatically reduces production of your own estrogen, testosterone, and progesterone and defines a new state of balance.

43

sign many women use to identify the fertile window when conception is prime. But more important, the shift from estrogen dominance to progesterone dominance has profound effects on your brain. Remember, while estrogen stimulates your brain to work quicker and more efficiently, progesterone suppresses signal transmission in your brain, which can leave you feeling a bit sluggish and clumsy.

The upsurge in progesterone can also cause you to feel emotionally vulnerable and compromise your cognition. This can have quite an impact on women who rely on particular hormone-sensitive skills in certain careers. Verbal functions, for instance, are particularly affected by estrogen—it enhances your ability to communicate clearly and concisely. So if you're a chemist working alone in your lab, you might not notice a difference when your estrogen levels drop during this phase. But if you're a litigating attorney who counts on strong oratory skills to convince tough judges and juries, you'd be likely to notice the effects.

Testosterone also plays a big role during the secretory phase. In addition to estrogen and progesterone, you produce testosterone throughout your cycle. While total testosterone levels remain fairly constant during the whole cycle, the amount of testosterone that is actively able to influence you at any given time—the free testosterone—is influenced indirectly by your estrogen level.

As estrogen increases, it induces your liver to increase production of the carrier protein *sex hormone–binding globulin (SHBG)*. Typically, about 98 percent of your testosterone attaches to the SHBG, which leaves less than 2 percent available to your brain and muscles. But here's the really interesting part of this equation. The levels of SHBG rise slowly, lagging as much as seven days behind your estrogen rise. The SHBG carrier protein has the greatest impact on testosterone during this second phase of your cycle. And what it does is sink your free testosterone to

MIND-BOGGLING FACT

Just before ovulation, you can probably perform tongue-twisters about 10 percent better than during other times in your menstrual cycle. That's because the elevated levels of estrogen quicken your ability to process words, and both the estrogen and high testosterone levels help the muscles in your mouth to work more effectively.

the lowest level in your monthly cycle. That can present you with some challenges. You may experience a drop in energy level, a souring of mood, and even a reduction in math skills.

Late in this phase, around day twenty-two, as your estrogen levels peak and begin to fall, your testosterone levels rise again. Again, this is a somewhat delayed effect because of the fluctuations in your SHBG level. Unfortunately, it doesn't make for smooth sailing. This high testosterone–low estrogen combo results in oily skin (which is why so many women get preperiod pimples), irritability, and aggression. Behavioral variations are naturally trickier to pin down, but they make sense considering that men's normal high testosterone–low estrogen profile tends to make them aggressive. Finally, the higher testosterone level paired with low estrogen levels tends to optimize performance of skills that involve three-dimensional visualization. That actually could be a real plus if you're an engineer or architect—you may feel you're working at your peak at this time. But if you're a surgeon, computer whiz, or pianist, or do any other kind of work that

CYCLE CONTROL— ARTIFICIALLY INDUCED MENSTRUAL CYCLES

With the ease and availability of hormonal contraception like birth control pills, patches, and vaginal rings, a lot of women are choosing to limit menstrual cycles to four per year. It works safely and effectively simply by artificially readjusting your estrogen-to-progesterone balance. Each hormonal contraceptive (pill, patch, or ring) releases enough progesterone to prevent your brain from generating the LH signal necessary for an egg to be released, and it inhibits vaginal bleeding by stabilizing any further growth of the uterine lining. The only variation among the different kinds of hormone contraceptives is the amount of estrogen or the type of progesterone. Essentially they all produce similar results, but you might feel better on one formula or another depending on your personal makeup. The progesterone in one pill, for instance, might make you feel tired but have a calming effect on your slightly hyper sister. Many women feel the scheduling control gives them a new freedom, like enjoying a honeymoon without a period, as well as great hormone stability—fewer mood swings, bloating, irritability, and other common period-related symptoms. Cycle control is actually now considered one of the important noncontraceptive benefits of birth control pills, and even women who aren't sexually active are using hormone contraceptives for their other health benefits.

involves fine motor skills, you may feel like a bit of a klutz during this last part of the cycle. The prime time for your particular fine motor skills is at ovulation, when estrogen dominates.

THE LATE REPRODUCTIVE YEARS: LATE THIRTIES TO EARLY FIFTIES

The transition from the reproductive to postreproductive years starts at about your mid-thirties. This is when your fertility rate begins to decline and your hormonal patterns get increasingly chaotic and unpredictable—and for some women it can be a pretty bumpy ride. One month your body may produce too much estrogen; another month you might not produce progesterone at all. As a result, symptoms can vary wildly, from bloating, breast tenderness, and heavy bleeding one month to hot flashes and crying spells the next. Feelings and issues seemingly unrelated to hormones, like mood instability, unprovoked anger, unexplained weight gain, and miscommunication with others, may seem to spring up from nowhere. It can be a real challenge.

With a few exceptions, this "midlife" hormonal chaos—often referred to as *perimenopause* (literally "around menopause")—is remarkably similar to what you went through during puberty. During these years (unlike in puberty), testosterone levels get progressively lower, adding to feelings of vulnerability, fatigue, and diminished self-confidence. You've also got symptoms of estrogen withdrawal to deal with, and your stress hormones are most likely elevated, too, thanks to the pressures of everyday responsibilities. On the positive side, as an adult you have a fully formed frontal lobe in your brain, so at least impulse control is generally much less problematic this time around. Still, the disruption of quality of life from sex hormone imbalances can be devastating. Studies have shown that 50–85 percent of perimenopausal women experience symptoms like hot flashes, night sweats, mood swings, forgetfulness, fatigue, and sleep disturbances. Fortunately, as you'll see in the later chapters, there are viable solutions to all these problems.

During this transition, the time between menstrual periods typically becomes shorter at first (at the onset of perimenopause) and then shifts toward progressively longer time spans between periods. And there may be several months interspersed when you return to normal cycling. Like all things hormonal, there's a wide degree of variability in timing—some women may experience these inconsistent cycles much earlier or later than others. This unpredictability is a big part of the frustration felt by so many women during this time.

Your hormonal balance is more easily disrupted during these years than it was before. Anything that may have caused a minor hormone imbalance earlier in your journey, like tobacco use, poor nutritional habits, or severe stress, is now amplified. Smoking, for instance, accelerates ovarian aging by converting estrogens to mild *antiestrogens* (called *catecholestrogens*), which diminish the number and quality of fertile eggs. Even without these kinds of harmful disruptions, the likelihood of conceiving (without contraception) between the ages of forty and forty-four is about 10 percent a year. That rate drops to 2–3 percent per year between ages forty-five and forty-nine. This isn't to say you can't get pregnant. You still ovulate during these transitional years, just less consistently than during your peak fertility years. So there's still potential for pregnancy, and you still need to use contraception if you're not looking to conceive.

Although there are exceptions, usually by the time you're forty years old, your testosterone level is only about half of what it was when it peaked in your twenties. And by the time you reach fifty, it's halved again, leaving you with only 25 percent of the testosterone you had in your reproductive prime. Not surprisingly, the substantial drop in testosterone can have a heavy impact on your quality of life. Not only does it tend to diminish your libido, it also contributes to a loss of muscle mass. For most women, the rate of muscle loss averages about half a pound per year. This silent loss of muscle is one of the leading causes of age-related weight gain, since muscles use calories, and when there's no muscle to burn the calories, the calories are stored as fat.

As testosterone levels fall, it takes more effort to maintain your fitness level. As your muscles lose their fullness, they also lose the protein that gives you strength and the glycogen they store as their fuel supply. So as testosterone levels fall, you have to work harder to stay fit. If you don't, you'll notice a greater sense of fatigue, less strength, and more muscle aches when you do exert yourself. In essence, the bad habits you got away with in your teens, twenties, and early thirties when you had surging hormones to protect you tend to catch up with you as you approach forty.

As free testosterone levels continue to fluctuate along with estrogen levels, your degree of alertness may also be reduced. Aside from fatigue, that's one of the most common complaints women have during these transitional years. And then there's mood fluctuations. Testosterone and estrogen together tend to create the ultimate feel-good cocktail for women. Since you're used to enjoying that cocktail, you're likely to notice when it's not being served up. Testosterone has also been linked to a strong sense of self-confidence; when levels are lower, you feel less confident and more anxious. There's no doubt that the combination of low testosterone and fluctuating estrogen levels is a big contributor to the anxiety so many women feel during this time period.

There are a number of ways that hormonal changes in the late reproductive years affect a woman's sexuality. As estrogen and testosterone levels fall, the tissue that lines the vagina becomes thinner, drier, and more easily irritated, so that even with the best lubricant, intercourse can become uncomfortable, even painful. Lower estrogen levels make you more sensitive to pain sensations, diminish vaginal blood flow (which diminishes sexual arousal and lessens orgasmic response), and reduce the sensitivity of the clitoral area. So by the time you reach your late forties, your hormonal balance has shifted in ways that not only reduce libido, but decrease the likelihood that sex will be as enjoyable as it once was.

MENOPAUSE AND THE POSTREPRODUCTIVE YEARS: FIFTIES AND SIXTIES

Menopause, literally a permanent pause in *menses,* or your monthly cycle, marks an official end to your childbearing years—and the beginning of the rest of your life. Every woman reacts to this dramatic hormonal shift in her own way—both emotionally and physically. Many of my patients accept the change with open arms, eager to embrace the freedoms and wisdom that naturally come with age. Others dread the idea of aging and mourn their lost youth. Not surprisingly, menopause garners conflicting views in the medical community, too.

There are essentially two schools of thought on the subject. One believes that menopause is a natural occurrence and that women should approach the transition in a "natural way," with no medical help or interference. Proponents of this point of view say that menopause is not a disease, so it should not be treated as one. The opposing school of thought reflects the medical approach, which posits that the very real symptoms of an indisputable hormonal imbalance during this transition can greatly interfere with the quality of life and lead to health problems, so it's a good idea to take steps to correct the imbalance medically. I fall right in between these two schools: I feel hormonal imbalance is definitely *not* a disease but should certainly be addressed by those who experience uncomfortable symptoms. The bottom line is that the average American woman today lives well into her eighties. A century ago, most women barely made it into their fifties. So menopause, "natural" or not, was hardly a problem in previous years. If you really wanted to play devil's advocate, you could argue that it's not "natural" to use modern pharmaceuticals to help you live into your eighties. But however you see it, what *is* undeniably natural today are the inevitable hormonal imbalances you experience as you age.

From adolescence to menopause, your body produces sex hormones primarily to support reproductive functions. Now, without any fertile eggs left, it

COMMON SIGNS OF NATURAL AGING

ESTROGEN DEFICIENCY	TESTOSTERONE DEFICIENCY
Hot flashes	Decreased libido
Night sweats	Decreased lean body mass (loss of muscle)
Sleep disturbances	Abdominal weight gain
Depression	Depression
Anxiety	Decreased alertness
Decreased sexual responsiveness	Fatigue
Vaginal atrophy	Decreased motivation
Accelerated aging of the skin	Loss of self-confidence
Tooth loss	Decreased dreaming
Increased appetite and weight gain	Cognitive impairment
Forgetfulness and cognitive	Bone loss
impairment	Loss of pubic hair
Increased risk of Alzheimer's disease	Reduced strength
Bone loss	Brittle nails
Dry eyes	Dry skin
Increased craving for sweets	Clumsiness
Decreased muscle coordination	Breast tenderness and/or enlargement
Dizziness/vertigo	Reduced sexual response
Decreased sense of smell	
Hearing loss	
Heart palpitations and an altered stress	
response	

simply produces a much lower quantity of these hormones. Estradiol drops dramatically, and progesterone production stops altogether. That leaves you with more "bad" estrogen than "good" estrogen. (Remember, while estradiol is the reigning estrogen during the "feel good" years, estrone is the dominant estrogen during these postreproductive years.) And as we've discussed, estrone offers few brain benefits, is relatively ineffective as an antioxidant, and can actually act in opposition to the small amount of estradiol that you still produce, as well as decrease the free testosterone that often serves as a stand-in for estradiol in your brain. A high concentration of estrone can actually contribute to the discomfort you already feel because of the loss of estradiol. Although the higher estrone level helps protect your bones, it worsens brain-related symptoms of menopause like hot flashes, insomnia, mood changes, and forgetfulness.

Testosterone production can help with this somewhat, since your brain is able to convert testosterone to estradiol. Some women continue to produce enough testosterone during menopause to minimize typical discomforts. If you're among them, you may not have hot flashes and such, but you'd be more inclined to experience problems associated with your skin, like increased hair growth on your face and chest and more oil production on your scalp and face (because the skin is not as efficient as your brain at converting testosterone to estrogen). But whichever way your hormones lean, it's likely that you'll experience symptoms of some kind during this final shift in the hormone-brain equilibrium.

APPROACHING THE JOURNEY'S END: SEVENTIES AND BEYOND

Some women age very well—with lucid and curious minds, agile movements, and general good health; others look, act, and feel well beyond their years. There are, of course, many different factors involved in aging, among them genetics, diet, exercise, and lifestyle habits. But the most current evidence tells us that the key to the aging process is the production of free radicals and how our body reacts to them.

You naturally produce *free radicals* throughout your lifetime. They are essentially unstable oxygen molecules with an unpaired electron. In very basic terms, a free radical is looking to steal an electron from another molecule so that it can pair up with it and become stable. When it succeeds, the result is a process called *oxidation,* and it's just as damaging as the kind of oxidation that causes cars to rust when left outside too long. If the free radical steals an electron from a cell membrane, the oxidation causes cell damage (something to which the nerve cells in the brain are particularly vulnerable). If the electron is stolen from a protein in the cell, the protein can lose the ability to perform the vital function it was designed to perform, which is what happens in the brains of people with dementia. If an electron is stolen from your DNA, it can cause breaks in the strand and a subsequent mutation, which is what happens in the skin when you're exposed to too much sun over your lifetime and to the breast and colon if you consume too many calories on a regular basis. So free radicals can be quite dangerous.

On the other hand, we need some free radicals to help in digestion, to help our body fight off infections, and to stimulate cell growth and repair. The goal is not to eliminate free radicals altogether, but rather to harness them—and the body has its own way of doing that. It contains and neutralizes free radicals by producing or using *antioxidants*. Antioxidants mop up these charged sparks, absorbing their damaging potential. That's why it's important, especially as you age, to get lots of antioxidants in your diet—and to watch your hormonal balance. I've been involved in some truly fascinating medical research that's shown that estrogen not only works like an antioxidant, but also decreases the production of free radicals in the brain. Estradiol is able to gain access to any cell and be prepared for these electrical storms. *Estrogen actually slows brain aging.*

When we're young, any damage free radicals cause to proteins, cell membranes, or DNA is rapidly repaired. As we age, this damage occurs faster than we can repair it. So anything that promotes the rate of free radical damage— like an increase in its production or a decrease in our ability to prevent the damage—results in an acceleration of the aging process. The more sun exposure you get or the more cigarettes you smoke, for instance, the more free radicals you produce. Both activities increase skin damage—and hence skin aging. Though people have tried using various vitamin E creams to prevent skin damage, they're ineffective at minimizing wrinkles and other signs of aging. Estrogen, on the other hand, has a profound effect on preserving the youthful qualities in the skin. Here this multifunctional hormone not only absorbs free radicals, but also promotes collagen production and the normal moisture content of the skin. In other words, it helps keep your skin elastic and wrinkle-free.

Estrogen provides other important benefits in your postreproductive years. It has been shown to slow the age-related decline of fine motor skills thought to be the result of wear and tear on the neural membranes from free radical damage. To a degree, estrogen also counters weight gain after the onset of menopause. When brain functions degenerate with age, many women experience a reduction in their senses of smell and taste, which increases their cravings for sweets as compensation. A big "sweet tooth" can obviously lead to weight gain. Estrogen helps improve taste and smell sensations and thus takes the bite out of the sweet tooth.

So while getting older is inevitable, it can be a terrific ride. With balanced hormones, you have a very good chance of staying vital, sharp, healthy, and independent all through your golden years.

CHAPTER FOUR

EATING RIGHT FOR PERFECT BALANCE

We've all heard the expression "You are what you eat," and it couldn't be more true. What we eat and *don't* eat has a huge impact on our health and well-being. But one of the factors too often overlooked in the ongoing discussions of diet these days is the tremendous impact diet has on our hormones and brain. While some hormones are actually the driving force behind your food choices, others influence how you process and manage your calories. And poor food choices can easily cause a hormonal imbalance, just as smart choices can cure an imbalance.

The Perfect Balance diet plan considers all these aspects and creates a hormone equilibrium that keeps you optimally balanced. No matter what your age or hormonal status, the plan prevents diseases, keeps your body functioning at peak, establishes eating habits that will put you in good stead for the rest of your life, and minimizes fatigue, weight gain, bloating, and other hormone-induced problems. At its core, the plan is designed to work *with*, rather than *against*, your millennia-old hormonal programming.

Many of the hormones that regulate our appetite, digestion, and energy balance are the result of hundreds of thousands of years of natural selection. Those of us alive today are the progeny of humans who managed to survive times of food scarcity by slowing their metabolism and hoarding stored body fat. Our ancestors had about 250 genes and more than 40 hormones geared to establishing, protecting, and maintaining those emergency fat reserves, and as their genetic offspring, so do we. We are, in essence, hardwired to *resist* weight loss, and like our ancestors, we're also engineered to eat heartily when food is plentiful. Both were handy survival mechanisms as our forebears hunted and gathered on the plains, but they are a real handicap for us today, with double cheeseburgers and fries and cookies and ice cream around every corner.

Therein lies the crux of a good number of hormone imbalance problems—modern food and eating habits; old hormones. The omnipresence of supersize, "value priced," nutritionally bankrupt processed food and the constant barrage of advertising appealing to our ancient hormonally programmed appetites is gravely upsetting our hormonal balance. Our hormones and brain—indeed, our entire physiology—were designed to operate on the kinds of foods that were available to the earliest humans—unadulterated whole foods like grains, fruits, vegetables, nuts, legumes, seeds, and occasional eggs and meat. Our system operates best when we eat those foods; when we don't, we experience health problems. Obesity is one of the more obvious, but there are plenty of others: reproductive problems, sexual dysfunction, more severe PMS, migraine headaches, even cancer. You can improve many of these conditions and regain your hormone balance to a large degree simply by choosing foods that are compatible with your hormones rather than at odds with them. And you'll feel tremendously better while you're doing it.

THE HORMONE–BRAIN FOOD CONNECTION

Food is fuel. It gives us the energy (in the form of calories) to grow, move, think, digest, build muscle, and even maintain proper body temperature. When you take in food, your brain determines the best way to use those new calories based on your energy needs. When you were a child and still growing, your brain released growth hormone (GH) instructing the body to use food calories for growth. If you are cold, the brain raises the level of certain metabolic hormones, which instruct the body to use the incoming calories to generate heat. And if you're facing a stressor, your brain releases stress hormones to alert the body to use the caloric energy for fight or flight. So your brain, hormones, and diet form an intimate synchronistic triangle.

This relationship is especially important to you as a woman. Because of your biological role in reproduction and the tremendous calorie requirements involved in bearing a child, your brain regulates your daily calories to ensure that your fat stores are kept up. (And that's true whether you decide to have children or not.) It won't even initiate puberty until it senses you have enough caloric energy to support a healthy pregnancy—which is why girls in famine conditions start their cycles so much later than normal and why women with anorexia nervosa or other eating disorders often stop menstruating altogether. Their brain, sensing their inability to bear a healthy child safely, simply calls off the possibility of reproduction.

But while the brain has an appropriate response to food scarcity, it's ill-equipped to cope with an overabundance of food. That's the source of America's current obesity epidemic. Over 45 million people, including 31 percent of American women and about 20 percent of our children, now meet the standards for obesity. Sixty-five percent more are overweight. Obesity is a symptom of, and a contributor to, hormonal imbalance. It interferes with vital hormone functioning in almost every category. It causes insulin resistance and ultimately diabetes, creates an imbalance between the "good" and "bad" estrogen, interferes with thermoregulatory hormones, and initiates the production of new hormones that further perpetuate obesity.

FAT PRODUCES ITS OWN HORMONES

One of the most fascinating discoveries of the last decade is that fat actually produces its own hormones—we know of at least nineteen. This is a real revelation. Fat (also called *adipose tissue*) had always been thought to be a passive energy store—a place to bank calories for later use. The fact that fat cells not only store calories, but also affect our metabolism and appetite through their production of hormones makes weight control even more important. These hormones are not a problem if your weight is healthy, since you'll have very low levels of them, but the fatter you are, the more of these hormones you produce, and the more you experience deleterious health effects, such as slower blood flow, bone and joint strain, high blood sugar levels, and an increase in free radical production.

All of us—men and women—typically have around 45 billion fat cells by the time we reach adulthood. Each fat cell is capable of expanding to one thousand times its original size to accommodate calorie storage. Because the oily chemicals that make up fat cells are large molecules, fat serves as an excellent insulation—a handy adaptation since we don't have thick fur to help preserve our body heat like most other mammals. These fat cells are divided into two groups. The first, *subcutaneous fat cells,* are little calorie storage bins tucked conveniently beneath our skin to insulate our inner organs from varying environmental temperatures. The second group, *visceral fat cells,* are located primarily in the abdomen and provide calorie needs between meals and during various activities. These are the ones that produce hormones. These fat cells act rather like accountants. They inform your brain of the approximate number of calories you have in reserve by releasing hormones in proportion to their stored energy load. The more fat you have stored, the more hormones these fat cells release.

LEPTIN IMPACTS APPETITE AND TEMPERATURE

One of the key hormones released is *leptin*—derived from the Greek word *leptos,* meaning "thin." Leptin, discovered in 1994, changed our understanding of the role that fat cells play in our use of calories and led scientists to develop a whole new way of thinking about obesity. The discovery not only gave us more insight into the ongoing struggles many people have controlling their weight, but was also a clear validation for a good number of women, including many of my patients, who instinctively felt that their progressive weight gain was somehow related to a hormonal imbalance.

Leptin is produced by the *ob gene,* named in recognition of the high leptin levels typically associated with obesity. Leptin influences your brain's regulation of appetite and body temperature. You could think of it as the body's calorie release valve. Unlike many other hormones involved in digestion and absorption, leptin maintains a fairly stable level. It reacts to the number of calories you've stored as fat rather than to your individual meals.

As you gain weight and accumulate more visceral fat, you produce more leptin. Your brain's initial response to high leptin levels is to suppress your appetite. If you ignore this attempt and keep eating even though you're not really hungry, the brain turns up your body temperature to burn more calories. Unfortunately, if this happens enough times, your body soon gets used to its higher temperature, and as your weight gradually increases and leptin levels remains chronically elevated, your brain ultimately becomes desensitized to the "slowdown" alert. Eventually, the part of your brain that controls appetite (the *arcuate nucleus* of the hypothalamus region) interprets your elevated leptin level as normal. And that is the point of no return. From then on, if your leptin level starts to drop, your body goes into "survival" mode. In an effort to ward off calorie loss, your brain raises your appetite and lowers your metabolism. The result? You eat more and burn less fat.

So leptin, a genuine hero in our ancestors' ongoing battle for survival in lean times—a lower metabolism meant fewer calories were needed for survival, and an increased appetite encouraged a search for food—is now one of the major culprits in our unsuccessful attempts at weight loss. Once you've lost about 5–8 percent of your weight on a diet, your leptin levels decline noticeably. Your brain doesn't know the difference between conscious dieting and starving, so it prevents further weight loss by grinding your metabolism to a crawl. This so-called plateau effect is one of the major obstacles to successful weight loss.

Interestingly, we've found that leptin levels fluctuate during monthly menstrual cycles. They're higher during the second half after ovulation (secretory phase), when progesterone levels are at their highest. This could explain the rise in basal body temperature that marks your most fertile time. It also explains the cravings for "comfort foods" many women feel during the last seven to ten days of their cycle. Levels also remain high during pregnancy, contributing to typical increased appetite and the heat radiation so many women feel while pregnant.

Some of the temperature regulatory disturbances caused by leptin manifest themselves through a complex relationship with thyroid hormones. Recent studies have shown that leptin can enhance the heat-generating properties of thyroid hormone. While thyroid hormone determines how fast your engine is revving, leptin, like the accelerator in a car, determines whether or not you're burning more or less fuel. The two work together toward a common end point. So if you're obese and your leptin level is high, you'll probably feel warmer than normal-weight people in the room

SOMETHING YOU SHOULD KNOW

Ultralow levels of leptin, which are associated with low body fat, can add up to missed menstrual cycles. As the storage of fat decreases, so does the circulating level of leptin. So too little leptin can actually disrupt fertility—something to mention to your doctor if you think you might fit that bill.

with you. This explains why so many people with obesity complain of excessive perspiration, even though their thyroxine levels measure as normal.

ADIPONECTIN

Adiponectin, another major hormone produced by visceral fat cells, discourages your body from using stored fat as fuel and encourages you to eat more. Adiponectin is essentially a signal to your liver to slow down glucose production, which decreases your appetite. When your brain senses a drop in glucose, your appetite reawakens. This system helps maintain a stable glucose level between meals and keeps hunger at bay. If your brain senses you have *too much* glucose in your bloodstream, the adiponectin sends a "slowdown" message to your fat cells that causes them to stop breaking down fats and start conserving energy—and you begin to gain weight. So adiponectin is, in effect, one of the key hormones that slow metabolism. If you're overweight, your adiponectin levels remain chronically low, your metabolism slows, and your appetite becomes more persistent. One the other hand, when you follow the Perfect Balance plan, you'll produce less adiponectin, speed up your metabolism, decrease your appetite, and lose weight.

The main purpose of this important line of communication between the brain and fat stores is to meet your needs for energy between meals and to synchronize your calories with your activity level. When your heart and muscles need more fuel, as they do during exercise, for instance, your fat cells release stored calories, which are used by your muscles as an energy source. When you go to sleep, on the other hand, parasympathetic nerves become more active and you *store* all available calories. That's why it's not good to eat shortly before going to bed and why eating at night tends to pack on the pounds.

SLEEP-TIME TIP

Try not to eat meals within three hours of going to sleep. While you sleep, your brain triggers hormonal changes that promote calories to be stored in their long-term form (fats) rather than their short-term form (glycogen).

OTHER HORMONES INVOLVED IN FOOD CHOICES

About forty hormones exert their influence on appetite, metabolism, or behavior. Some do it on a short-term (immediate) basis— they're rather like hunger on/off switches, since they either promote appetite or signal satiation. Others, like leptin, help establish and maintain your weight over the long term through their effect on metabolism rather than their impact on individual meals. Obviously we can't get into all forty of these hormones here, so just a quick word on the major players.

GHRELIN, a "hunger hormone," was discovered only within the last several years. Secreted by your empty stomach directly into your bloodstream, it urges your brain to find something to eat. During a meal the levels of ghrelin promptly decline, which serves as feedback to your brain and prompts you to stop eating. But there's a bit of a snag with ghrelin that can sabotage weight loss plans. As you successfully lose weight on any given diet, you produce *higher* levels of ghrelin, which makes you hungrier and prompts you to find something to eat. This hormone is another of the key reasons most dieters fail to lose more than 5–10 percent of their total goal weight. Studies have shown that the more weight lost, the greater the *increase* in ghrelin levels, which leads to more persistent and intense hunger. (One of the reasons gastric bypass surgery typically reduces appetite is that the surgery causes food to bypass the key region of the stomach where ghrelin is normally secreted. When no food passes through it, there's about a 75 percent reduction in ghrelin, and levels stay low all the time. Less ghrelin, less hunger.)

PYY3-36, another interesting, newly discovered hormone, is released by your colon in response to food. Once it enters the bloodstream, it travels rapidly to your brain and decreases your appetite for up to twelve hours by directly inhibiting activity in the hunger center of your brain (the arcuate nucleus). Even though the effect of this hormone is rapid in onset, it's not released naturally by your body until food begins to reach the end of your small bowel. And that takes time—sometimes more than two hours, depending on what you ate. If you're a speedy eater, you're likely to take in too much food long before the PYY3-36 signal is able to do its job. Your body just doesn't have a chance to send the "stop" signal to your brain fast enough for you to lose your appetite before you feel "stuffed." Eating slowly is clearly the way to go, since it gets this hormone working for you.

THYROID HORMONE

Thyroid hormone is one of your most important fat-stabilizing hormones. It is, in effect, your power regulator. It determines whether your calories are used to fuel movement in your muscles or to generate heat. The thyroid hormone is like the transmission in a car: It determines how fast your engine (your metabolism) idles in neutral (at rest) and how fast you can move. Your brain determines whether it's necessary for the thyroid hormone to rev up your metabolism to warm you up or gear it down to reduce the wasting of calories.

If you're in a colder environment and need to warm up, your brain sends *thyroid-stimulating hormone (TSH),* which encourages your thyroid gland to release *thyroxine.* This is analogous to pressing the gas pedal and revving your engine while your car is in neutral. It makes your heart rate increase and encourages your muscles to generate heat. If this happens when you don't actually need the heat to warm up, you typically feel as though you're overheating and may become somewhat anxious and irritable. If it happens consistently, you'll start to lose weight. These are symptoms of *hyperthy-roidism*—too much thyroid hormone. If the situation isn't corrected, a person with this condition ends up burning fat- *and* muscle-stored calories. This makes the muscles (including the heart muscle) weak and atrophic and is part of the reason long-term hyperthyroidism is associated with heart failure.

In contrast, people with *hypothyroidism*—too little thyroid hormone—experience the opposite. They're generally cold, sluggish, and fatigued and gain weight for no apparent reason. Without enough thyroid hormone, they simply can't burn sufficient calories to keep the weight off or to stay comfortably warm in cold weather. It's as if they're stuck in first gear—moving slow, feeling little energy, and having trouble, like an old car with a tired engine struggling to get uphill. Because people with too little thyroid hormone can't really rev their engines effectively, their bodies can't react well to situations of changing temperature, exercise, and stress. That's why keeping thyroid hormone in balance is really important to your quality of life—and, of course, your weight.

The majority of us don't have hypothyroidism or hyperthyroidism, but we do feel the effects of thyroid hormone—especially those of us who overeat and don't exercise. When we eat, the calories we take in have to do something. About 10 percent of them are burned as we absorb and digest the food—just the act of digestion generates heat through a process called *diet-induced thermogenesis.* The rest of the calories are either converted to movement or stored as fat. And the ones that are stored generate more heat. So if you eat a lot and are more or less sedentary, chances are you're going to be hot a great deal of the time. That's one of the reasons exercise is so important to true hormonal balance.

INSULIN

Insulin, a hormone made in the pancreas (the large gland just behind the stomach), plays a vital role in nutritional and hormonal balance. Insulin's main job is to move glucose (blood sugar) out of our bloodstream and into muscle or fat cells, where it's stored for later use. Theoretically, every time we eat and our blood sugar starts to rise, our insulin level also rises so that it can get rid of the sugar in the bloodstream and nudge our blood sugar back to levels that are normal and healthy for the brain, kidneys, and the rest of our body. Bottom line: Your insulin level is dependent on when and what you eat. When the food you eat causes your blood sugar levels to be chronically high (and we'll discuss those foods in a minute), your insulin level also stays chronically high, since it's continually needed to move that sugar from your bloodstream into your cells. And when your body produces a lot of insulin on a steady basis, your fat cells become larger as they absorb more sugar from your bloodstream. As they grow, you need more insulin on a steady basis, creating a vicious cycle of chronic insulin elevation, a condition known as *insulin resistance.*

Calorie-dense diets (with food containing extremely high amounts of calories) cause insulin levels to remain higher longer, which causes too much sugar to be removed from the bloodstream too quickly, and results in the kind of abnormally low blood sugar levels that trigger fatigue and hunger. As you eat more to satisfy that hunger, you gain weight. Once you're overweight, your body needs higher amounts of insulin to stimulate your expanding and progressively more resistant fat cells. As you get fatter, the fat cells become more resistant to the insulin, and your body produces more of it to compensate, which makes you fatter still. Finally, the pancreas simply can't produce enough insulin to keep up, your blood sugar starts rising, and before you know it, you meet the criteria for adult-onset or type 2 diabetes.

Essentially, all of these hormones are part of a complex chemical interaction. Insulin and leptin actually change the way your body uses calories, depending on what is happening in your reproductive cycle. These two hormones are integrated by your brain in such a way that if the level of either becomes too high or too low, your brain will stop sending the LH signal to your ovaries, and you'll stop ovulating. So what you eat can definitely affect your monthly cycles, fertility, and other reproductive issues. If you're obese, the associated high leptin levels increase your risk of abnormal menstrual cycles by at least 25 percent, and the more you weigh, the higher your risk of menstrual problems.

SEX HORMONES AND DIET

Contrary to what you might have heard, estrogen does not cause weight gain. In fact, when estradiol levels are high (as they are in your reproductive years), you're actually *less* susceptible to insulin resistance, abdominal obesity, and

LITTLE-KNOWN FACT

Even if your weight and cycles are normal, your sensitivity to insulin is higher during the estrogen-dominant phase and diminished during the progesterone-dominant phase. So if you're trying to lose weight, your efforts will be more successful during the first two weeks in your cycle than the second two, when progesterone production begins and leptin levels start to rise.

diabetes than you are when levels of this "good" estrogen are low (as they are during your menopausal years). But if you're overweight, your fat cells will produce more estrone, the "bad" estrogen, and high levels of that estrogen can interfere with the ability of estradiol to improve many brain-related symptoms—including an overactive appetite. That's the only diet-estrogen connection, but it's a big one, because the imbalance between both kinds of estrogen brought on by dietary habits and choices can have a huge impact on your quality of life. It can make you feel tired, destroy your libido, make you constantly hot and sweaty, affect your ability to concentrate, and reduce your chances of getting pregnant if you're looking to conceive.

Testosterone also impacts your metabolism because it promotes a breakdown of fats that your body uses as fuel. So when your testosterone is low,

SLOW TIMES

Slow down! It takes people of normal weight about ten minutes after finishing a meal to feel fully satiated. Obese adults take at least twice as long. So stop *before* you think you're finished to give your brain a chance to catch up with your body. Eating too fast contributes to chronic overeating. Slow down to allow your hormones to signal your brain that you've started eating. You'll avoid that overstuffed feeling that often pops up thirty or so minutes after a meal.

there's less fat breakdown, and you burn calories less efficiently. The end result is an increase in fat combined with a reduction in muscle, bigger fat cells, and higher estrone levels. Progesterone also plays a significant role in metabolism, since it increases the production of fatty acids for storage in fat cells. So when progesterone peaks during the second half of your menstrual cycle, you produce more fat and are at higher risk for weight gain. Same thing if you're pregnant—the high progesterone levels help you hold on to calories so you have an adequate amount to share with your developing fetus.

Now that you're up to speed on some of the intricate—and unexpected—ways your brain, hormones, and diet are intricately linked, let's put theory to work for you in short-circuiting some of these hormonal reactions.

THE PERFECT BALANCE PROGRAM

The Perfect Balance diet plan reflects the *flexitarian* nutritional approach I've developed for my patients and use in my everyday practice. Being a flexitarian (flexible + vegetarian) is like being a "flexible vegetarian." It's making plant foods the foundation of your diet and supplementing with animal products—meat, fish, fowl, and dairy. Essentially, it's cutting back on your dependence on animal products—especially meat—but not eschewing them all together. Daily intake is at least 75 percent plant foods and no more than 25 percent animal foods. The Perfect Balance diet principles, two-week sample meal plan, and food pyramid will help you reach that mark naturally and easily.

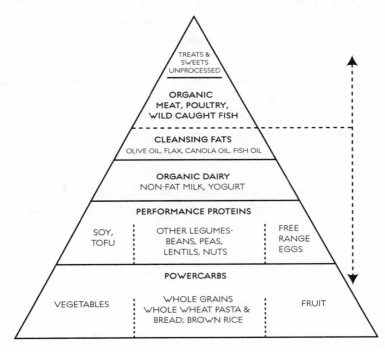

The Perfect Balance diet is based on the same kind of fresh, unprocessed foods that have helped hormones stay balanced over millennia—and these foods remain extremely hormone friendly today. Whole grains, fruits, vegetables, nuts, legumes, and seeds are rich in nutrients, low in calories, and naturally full of antioxidants and phytoestrogens. They incorporate a variety of ingredients, all in biologically appropriate proportions, so that a diverse selection of them automatically provides a diet rich in fiber, phytonutrients, and numerous absorbable vitamins and minerals, all interacting the way they were meant to in their natural form. Eating a variety of these whole foods minimizes your risk of creating a hormonal imbalance; helps prevent (or reverse) obesity; and can actually improve symptoms related to problems like sexual dysfunction, chronic pelvic pain, premenstrual syndrome, depression, migraine headaches, and hot flashes. And it can dramatically reduce your risk of cancer.

Could you also take a full vegetarian approach? Yes, and it's a perfectly viable way to go. I'm a vegetarian myself and can guarantee that a well-thought-out vegetarian diet can absolutely meet all your nutrition needs. The idea that meat is a necessary protein source has long been disproved. It's now universally accepted that a plant-based diet can meet our protein needs, while at the same time reduce our intake of dietary hormone-disrupting chemicals and lower our risk of acquiring food-borne diseases. (We'll be talking more about all that in a minute.) So I'm fully behind you if you decide to follow a vegetarian regime.

Before we get into our principles of eating for best hormonal balance, let's start with a brief nutritional assessment. Take a few minutes to sit down and fill out the following questionnaire. It will help you assess how your eating habits and diet are affecting your hormonal balance and quality of life. Adding up your numerical answers will give you your total score. The lower your score, the less chance you have of diet-induced hormonal imbalance. The higher your score, the more likely it is that your diet is a major source of hormonal imbalance and the more important it is to follow the Perfect Balance diet principles.

YOUR HORMONE BALANCE NUTRITION INVENTORY

4	3	2	1	0
WHAT IS YOUR WAIST MEASUREMENT (INCHES)?				
More than 40 inches	39.9–37.5 inches	37.5–35 inches	34.9–32.5 inches	Less than 32.5 inches
HOW OFTEN DO YOU EAT FOOD FROM VENDING MACHINES?				
Daily	3–6	1–5	Rarely	Never
HOW MANY SERVINGS OF FRUIT AND VEGGIES DO YOU HAVE EACH DAY?				
Less than 1	1	2–3	3–4	5 or more
WHAT ARE YOU GENERALLY DOING 1½ HOURS AFTER YOU EAT DINNER?				
Sleeping or getting ready for bed	Looking for food	Loosening my clothes	Feeling full and uncomfortable	Feeling just right
HOW OFTEN DO YOU EAT OUT?				
More than once a day	About once a day	2–5 times per week	1–2 times per week	Occasionally
FOOD LABELS IMPACT MY CHOICES OF FOODS. . .				
Never	Rarely	Sometimes	Always	Don't eat food with labels
I EAT ORGANIC FOODS. . .				
What's organic?	Rarely	Occasionally	When available	Almost exclusively
HOW OFTEN DO YOU EXPERIENCE BLOATING?				
Constantly	Every evening	Frequently	Occasionally	Never
HOW OFTEN DO YOU HAVE FOOD CRAVINGS?				
Constantly	Daily	Weekly	Monthly	Rarely

SCORE

10 OR LESS

Great! You've got good eating habits, and your diet is most likely not contributing to hormonal imbalance. Keep up the good work.

11–20

Not bad, but there's room for improvement. Follow the upcoming principles and you'll fix things fast.

21–30

Time to change your ways! Your diet and eating habits are getting in your way and could be contributing to symptoms of hormonal imbalance.

31–40

Immediate call to action! Alert! Your diet and eating habits are putting you at risk of major health problems. Start on the Perfect Balance diet today.

ASK DR. GREENE

Q: HOW MANY CALORIES DO I NEED?

A: Not as many as you think. As a woman, you need fewer calories than a man, even one who's the same size you are. Since men have more muscle, they need more calories (muscles burn calories, fat doesn't). So the more muscle you have, the more calories you burn and the fewer are stored as fat. When you have less muscle, you burn fewer calories and it's easier to gain weight. To get on the right personal dietary track, you first have to know your basal metabolic rate (BMR), that is, how many calories you actually need to be healthy. The following formula calculates your sedentary calorie needs (in other words, all the calories you need when you're totally at rest).

DETERMINE YOUR CALORIE NEEDS: HARRIS BENEDICT FORMULA

1. Multiply your weight in pounds by 4.3. Write down the number.

2. Multiply your height in inches by 4.7. Write down the number.

3. Multiply your age in years by 4.7. Write down the number.

4. Add the top two numbers (weight and height) and subtract the last one.

5. Now add 655 to that final number.

6. The final number is a good estimate of your BMR.

PRINCIPLE №1: WATCH YOUR CALORIES

One of the most important factors when it comes to food and hormones is calories—and the bottom line is that we consume too many of them. It's not that we eat too much food, necessarily, but rather that so much of the food we eat (the burgers, chips, fries, and so forth) is calorically dense. (*Caloric density* is technically the number of calories per 1 gram of food.) When food is packed tight with calories, you don't have to eat much of it to exceed your calorie needs. Whole foods, on the other hand, naturally contain more water and fiber and thus are less calorically dense. That means you can eat more of them and still have a relatively low caloric intake. A quarter cup of calorically dense raisins, for instance, is about 100 calories. You could down that handful in the blink of an eye and still be hungry. An entire cup of grapes, on the other hand, which are essentially raisins before all the water has been squeezed out, is only 60 calories. That means you could eat almost 2 *cups* of grapes for the same amount of calories. And the grapes would probably satisfy your hunger because their fiber and water content slows down the absorption of sugars, keeping you from getting hungry again as fast.

TOO MANY CALORIES PROMOTE HORMONE HAVOC

Let's take a look at exactly what happens hormonally when you consistently consume high-calorie fare. After every calorie-dense meal, your insulin level skyrockets. That encourages blood sugar absorption by your fat cells, which makes the fat cells grow. As they get larger, they begin to convert your testosterone precursors into estrone (the "bad" estrogen), and your testosterone level drops, causing you to lose muscle mass at a more rapid rate. That in turn promotes fatigue and possibly

CALORIES AND CHOLESTEROL

Consuming fewer calories improves levels of HDL "good" cholesterol, keeps blood levels of inflammatory markers low, helps stabilize blood sugar levels, and offers protection against cancer by reducing free radical formation, and more and more studies are finding it helps us live longer. In addition, the fact that it helps avoid obesity is hugely important from a hormonal standpoint. We've seen that obesity is both a symptom of and contributor to hormonal imbalance and some weight-related health problems associated with insulin, thyroid, and leptin imbalance.

A QUICK FREE RADICAL REFRESHER

One of the biggest benefits of reducing your calories in terms of brain health is combating free radicals. The more calories you consume, the more free radicals you produce. When you eat too many calories, your body's antioxidants (which fight against free radicals) simply can't do their job effectively. As a result, the free radicals cause *oxidative stress* and end up damaging your DNA and proteins. When you reduce your calories, you reduce the oxidative stress, which keeps the brain healthy, slows the aging process, and reduces your risk of cancer.

SNACK TIMES

To avoid overeating, consider snacking part of your daily meal plan rather than as a bonus. The best snacks are whole foods like veggies, nuts, seeds, and fruits. Processed foods marketed as snacks are, needless to say, the worst possible foods to eat between meals, since they are calorically dense and result in a real free radical burst with all of the ensuing consequences.

overeating, since you may misinterpret your low energy level as a need for more food. The excess estrone reduces the amount of water reabsorbed by your kidneys, which causes fluid retention and creates cellulite and higher blood pressure. Eventually, your estradiol (the "good" estrogen) level gets lower because you don't have as much testosterone that can be converted into it. Without enough estradiol, which your brain needs to improve your mood, you get depressed and might even seek out sugary comfort foods that will worsen your situation.

As you stress out over your progressively expanding waistline, your *cortisol* level rises. The chronic elevation of this stress hormone exacerbates your depression, worsens your insulin resistance, raises your blood pressure further, and decreases the effectiveness of your immune cells, making you more susceptible to infections and cancers. Now, thanks to your high-calorie, low-energy-output lifestyle, your liver produces more of the carrier proteins to which testosterone and thyroid hormone bind. That further lowers your free testosterone and thyroid levels and makes both hormones less active, which promotes fatigue, weight gain, and depression. Total hormonal chaos—just by regularly consuming too much calorically dense food.

Your brain takes a hit from all this havoc, too. As your cardiovascular status worsens, so does the blood flow to your brain. The associated high blood pressure decreases the flexibility of the blood vessels that's necessary to keep your brain nourished with oxygen-rich blood. At the same time, the insulin resistance lowers the glucose available for your brain to use as fuel—another trigger that raises your appetite. While you're experiencing chronic hunger and fatigue, your brain is deprived of the vital estradiol that improves not only brain blood flow, but also brain functioning. Since your brain is still working in this hostile environment, free radicals are produced, but you have less estradiol to act as an antioxidant. And if you're not getting other antioxidants via veggies and fruits, your brain is exposed to the free radical damage and isn't even able to make effective repairs.

PRINCIPLE № 2: GO ORGANIC WHENEVER POSSIBLE

It's estimated that each of us eats between thirteen and fifteen pounds of food additives and chemicals per year, 90 percent of which are in processed foods. Only about 1 percent of these chemicals by weight is actually used to protect us, the consumers, from harmful microorganisms. The other 99 percent of the chemicals have been added to the food to make it look prettier, lengthen its shelf life, or taste like something it's not (there are no cherries in that Cherry Coke). Flavorings aside, of the remaining food additives used in foods available in the United States, 540 are considered "safe for human consumption," 320 are listed as "reasonably safe," and 150 are ranked "questionable safety." At least 70 commonly used food additives can provoke food allergies, and 30 are considered to be harmful to consumers. And this chemical epidemic isn't limited to packaged processed foods; our produce isn't as pure as it once was, either.

WHAT IS ORGANIC?

It was only recently, in December 2000, that the term *organic* acquired a formal and official meaning. Today, to be officially categorized and labeled as organic food, a product must be grown and produced without the use of sewer-sludge fertilizers (the mudlike postsewage treatment matter that includes cleaning products, disinfectants, and other toxins that go down your drain), synthetic fertilizers, and pesticides; or treated with hormones, radiation, antibiotics, or genetically modified products.

Fortunately, organic products are becoming more popular and therefore easier to come by than ever before. Aside from health food stores and farmer's markets, most good supermarkets carry at least some organic items. There are a few variations on organic product labels to watch for:

- "100% Organic" can be used only when produced *exclusively* with organic ingredients.

- "Organic" means that at least 95 percent of the ingredients are certified organic.

- "Made with organic ingredients" is the designation used for products that contain at least 70 percent organic ingredients.

- "Natural" is not organic. When applied to food products, the term has no regulatory definition. It is essentially a marketing tool.

Hormone-disrupting pesticide residue on conventionally grown fruits and veggies can't simply be washed off once you get home. Washing, of course, reduces the amount of chemicals you're exposed to, but it doesn't get rid of them altogether. Organic produce can be a bit more expensive than conventional, so if you're on a limited budget, you may have to compromise here and there. Here's what to do: Go organic when buying the produce that's been found to hang on to pesticides the most tenaciously and relax your standards with the fruits and veggies that are least impacted by agrichemicals. Definitely go organic when buying produce noted in the following list.

THE DIRTY DOZEN: THE MOST CONTAMINATED "CONVENTIONALLY GROWN" PRODUCE THAT YOU SHOULD BE SURE TO BUY ORGANIC

- Apples
- Bell peppers
- Celery
- Cherries
- Imported grapes
- Nectarines
- Peaches
- Pears
- Potatoes
- Raspberries
- Spinach
- Strawberries

The following items have been found to be *less* impacted by agrichemicals, so this is where to compromise and go with conventional produce if you need to. But still be sure to give them a good rinsing before you eat them.

THE BETTER BUNCH: THE LEAST CONTAMINATED PRODUCE THAT YOU DON'T *HAVE* TO BUY ORGANIC

- Asparagus
- Avocados
- Bananas
- Broccoli
- Cauliflower
- Corn

- Kiwi
- Mangos
- Onions
- Papaya
- Pineapples
- Peas (sweet)

BIOMUTAGENS

I categorize pesticides and herbicides as BioMutagens—toxic chemicals that disrupt hormone activity and cause a laundry list of problems from birth defects and sterility to diseases like cancer. Take, for example, the insecticide *DDT*. This toxin was first used in 1939 and resulted in a Nobel Prize for its creator. Ultimately, though, it was banned (in 1972) after it was found to be responsible for reducing the bald eagle population and driving our national symbol to near extinction. Because DDT, like many other pesticides, is a hormone interrupter, it weakened the shells of the eagle eggs, making them so brittle that when the mother eagle sat down to nest, the shells broke and fell apart.

Even though DDT has been banned for over thirty years, it's still one of the most commonly detected toxins in our food supply (these poisons are extremely long-lived). In humans, DDT mimics a weak estrogen that can block the testosterone receptor. In fact, it's linked with abnormal male sexual development in humans. Other pesticides have recently been linked to delayed sexual maturation in school children ten to nineteen years of age who were simply living near cashew plantations that used the chemicals.

From the perspective of hormonal balance, the issues related to pesticides are hugely important. Your body's hormone-producing endocrine system is even more sensitive to toxin exposure than your respiratory, nervous, or cardiovascular systems, and their effects can manifest decades after the original exposure. Hormone-disrupting chemicals can completely upset natural hormonal balance. The antiandrogenic properties of DDT, for example, reduce the effects of testosterone and growth hormones (by binding and blocking the estrogen receptors) and increase the dominance of estrogens. *Endosulfan,* the most commonly detectable pesticide in our food, is an antiestrogen, which restricts estrogen activity and shifts the balance toward testosterone and progesterone. *Atrazine,* a popular weed killer that contaminates the drinking water of about 20 million U.S. citizens, has such broad hormonal activities that it can't be placed in any particular class of hormone disruptors. These Bio-Mutagenic environmental hormones, including pollutants like *PCBs (polychlorinated biphenyls),* often have unpredictable and delayed effects for us and are especially dangerous to our most susceptible citizens, our children.

Studies have found that children born to women exposed to these chemicals have a higher incidence of behavioral problems, some of them gender inappropriate, suggesting that the hormone-disrupting properties of the toxins affected them during brain development. Incidentally, fish, especially swordfish, salmon, tuna, and other longer-living fish once touted as the perfect "brain food," has become one of the foods most hazardous to pregnant women. (Toxins become concentrated in the fish meat and easily pass not only through the placenta, but into breast milk, as well.) As a result of this alarming finding, the U.S. Food and Drug Administration (FDA) issued an advisory in January 2001 warning pregnant women to avoid longer-lived predatory fish.

PRINCIPLE №3: HORMONE POWER CARBS—YES! HORMONE CHAOS CARBS—NO!

Regardless of what you might have heard, not all carbs are bad for you. There are good carbs and bad carbs. You want to eat the good ones and avoid the bad ones. Forty percent of your diet should consist of *Hormone Power Carbs* (aka unrefined complex carbohydrates), which are essentially a form of stored plant energy. These are the starches and whole sugars that naturally accompany fiber in whole foods like vegetables, fruits, and grains. The fiber helps slow their release into the bloodstream, which helps avoid roller coaster—like fluctuations in insulin levels that lead to hormonal imbalance. In the digestive

HORMONE POWER CARBS VS. HORMONE CHAOS CARBS

At least 75% of your daily carbohydrate calories should be Power Carbs. Only 25% or less should be Chaos Carbs.

SOURCE	POWER CARBS	CHAOS CARBS
Grains	Barley	Rice, instant
	Wheat berries	Rice, short-grain wild
	Rice, long-grain wild	Tapioca
	Wheat, whole kernels	Caramel corn
Breads	Oat-bran bread	Bread, white
	Multigrain	Bagel, white
	Whole-grain	Kaiser roll
	Pumpernickel	Baguette
Legumes	Baked beans	Sweetened baked beans
	Chickpeas	Peanut butter with hydrogenated oils
	Kidney beans	Refried beans prepared with lard
	Soybeans	
Vegetables	Artichoke	Potatoes, French-fried
	Asparagus	Potatoes, instant
	Eggplant	Parsnips
	Peppers, all	Beets
Fruit	Grapefruit	Canned fruit cocktail
	Blueberries	Peaches in heavy syrup
	Cherries	Caramel apple
	Plums	Dried banana chips
Beverages	Milk, skim	Soft drinks (nondiet)
	Milk, soy, low fat	Sports drinks
	Hot cocoa	Sweetened instant iced tea
	Juice, tomato	Whole-milk latte
Sweets and Treats	Nonfat frozen yogurt	Whole-fat ice cream
	Angel food cake	Doughnuts
	Dark chocolate	Packaged cookies
	Low-fat granola	Cheesecake

SWEET TIMES

Your brain and hormones process sweets in different ways depending on when, where, and how you eat them. You're much better off eating sweets after a meal, since you'll feel satisfied with a smaller amount, and they're actually less fattening than when you eat them on their own, since the simple sugars are better absorbed and less insulin is secreted.

ASK DR. GREENE

Q: HOW DO HORMONE POWER CARBS AND CHAOS CARBS RATE ON THE GLYCEMIC INDEX?

A: Hormone Power Carbs have a healthy low number on the *glycemic index (GI)*. The GI measures the rate in which a specific carb triggers an elevation in blood glucose levels. The lower numbers on the index reflect foods that *do not* provoke elevations. Power Carbs are foods with a GI less than 55; Chaos Carbs have a GI above 70. If you do occasionally eat foods that are high on the glycemic index (like white bread, doughnuts, and soda pop)—and we all do from time to time—eat them with a protein- and a fiber-rich food to slow their absorption.

system, Power Carbs are easily and gradually digested back into the glucose the brain uses as its primary fuel. Glucose gives you quality energy; without it you'd feel fatigue, confusion, and hunger.

Power Carbs actually create hormone balance by *lowering* insulin levels and stabilizing or reducing blood sugar levels. Reducing average blood sugars (especially for those who are obese) also dilates blood vessels and actually promotes better blood flow. This improves circulation to the heart as well as the brain.

The bad carbs are the *Hormone Chaos Carbs,* the simple processed sugars found in cookies, chips, candies, cakes, doughnuts, rich salad dressings, sodas, and other processed foods. Chaos Carbs are devoid of fiber and are absorbed so rapidly into your bloodstream that they cause a surge of blood sugar, followed by a drastic drop that throws your hormone balance way out of kilter. Insulin levels shoot up, fat hormones act up, thermoregulatory hormones are thrown off—almost every hormone group is affected in one way or another. Simple sugars also promote weight gain without providing nutrition or satisfaction and leave you hungry, craving more—which is why they're often referred to as "empty calories."

TRANS FAT AND HIGH-FRUCTOSE CORN SYRUP

One of the most common processed food ingredients is trans fat, which is hidden in most commercial candies, cookies, cakes, muffins, crackers, nondairy creamers, frostings, margarines, popcorn, and French fries. I say "hidden," because food manufacturers aren't required to list trans fat as an ingredient on their labels until 2006. As of this writing, then, a product can be labeled "low fat" when it is in fact full of trans fat.

Trans fat is a toxic, unnatural oil that has been molecularly changed through *hydrogenation.* And while it might give processed food a longer shelf life and commercial appeal (artificial but alluring freshness, taste, and appearance), it also clogs arteries, is harmful to the heart, and raises bad cholesterol levels (LDL) as it lowers the good cholesterol (HDL). Hormonally, foods with a high fat content have been shown to not only reduce brain blood flow, but also impair the ability of appetite-suppressing hormones. So fats, especially trans fats, which aren't broken down and absorbed into cells effectively, encourage overeating. They also stimulate taste receptors in your

ASK DR. GREENE

Q: IS THE ATKINS DIET HELPFUL OR HARMFUL FOR HORMONAL HEALTH?

A: Absolutely harmful. Because the Atkins diet doesn't contain enough carbs, the body's preferential fuel, it encourages your body to use your own muscle as fuel—which reduces muscle mass and causes an imbalance of insulin, leptin, and adiponectin levels, slowing your metabolism and creating cravings and fatigue. It also alters your muscle-to-fat ratio (creates more fat, less muscle), which tips your sex hormone balance so that estrone, the "bad" estrogen, dominates over estradiol and testosterone. So your libido suffers, and you can develop hot flashes or insomnia. Because the diet is so meat heavy, it encourages a further accumulation of BioMutagens. A high-animal-fat diet has been linked to a marked increase in endometriosis and a 400 percent increase in breast cancer risk! Finally, while you can lose weight on the Atkins diet, about 20–40 percent of the loss is muscle tissue loss, and that increases the susceptibility to weight gain once you go off the diet.

TIP

Before eating, make sure you're fully hydrated. Since your brain can't differentiate thirst from hunger, having a glass of water thirty or so minutes before a meal is likely to decrease your food intake.

mouth, sending additional signals to your brain that boost your appetite and encourage you to continue eating—a double whammy to your waistline.

High-fructose corn syrup is just as bad as trans fats—if not worse. It's essentially corn without any of its healthy nutrients, fiber, or water, so that all that's left is the simple sugar. This preservative and concentrated sweetener is in practically every processed food we eat and is one of the most hormonally disruptive products that we're all exposed to on a daily basis. It's in everything from soft drinks to ketchup and mayo to prepared pasta sauce. The dramatic rise in insulin you get after eating highly processed sugars causes your blood sugar to plummet to very low levels about three to five hours later, often resulting in a strong sense of fatigue—and it promotes unhealthy high triglyceride levels, which contributes to heart disease.

PRINCIPLE №4: GET PLENTY OF FIBER

A high-fiber diet has consistently been found to lower risk of obesity, intestinal ailments, heart disease, colon cancer, and diabetes (as well as improve control of blood sugar for those with diabetes) and to lower the risk of mortality in general. And it has surprising hormonal benefits. It lowers insulin levels and helps balance sex hormones; plays a critical role in helping you get rid of excess amounts of estrone, the "bad" estrogen, by sequestering it in your bowels so it can't be reabsorbed into your bloodstream; and by facilitating removal of estrone from your body, fiber can improve your libido, reduce hot flashes, and prevent bloating. You should get at least 30 grams of fiber each day.

WHAT IS FIBER?

Fiber is a complex carbohydrate found exclusively in plants—it's the ingredient that eases the absorption of healthy Power Carbs. Veggies, fruit, beans, seeds, and nuts are all packed with fiber. Whole grains in particular are wonderfully fibrous in their most natural state and provide some of the best sources of antioxidants, trace elements, and phytoestrogens. Because fiber is indigestible, and since the body doesn't produce the necessary enzymes to break it down and absorb it, it is in effect calorie-free. There are two types of fiber—insoluble, which among other things helps protect against cancer; and soluble, which greatly helps lower cholesterol and balance hormones.

Insoluble fiber regulates bowel functions, preventing food from passing through too quickly (diarrhea) or too slowly (constipation). It is an excellent colon health remedy and also helps your body to absorb all of a food's healthy nutrients without exposing your colon to unhealthy chemicals that may also be passing through. (By creating bulk, it binds and speeds toxins right out of your system.)

Soluble fiber is more actively involved in regulating hormone balance. It slows the emptying of the stomach and thus contributes to a prolonged sense of satiation following a meal. It also suppresses your appetite by slowing the absorption of sugars. Drinking orange juice, in which the fiber has been removed, for instance, raises your blood sugar much faster than eating an orange. The lack of fiber in the juice also makes it much easier to drink too much. You'd have a hard time overeating oranges with all its natural fibrous pulp, but you could gulp down a couple of glasses of orange juice in a flash. It's the ability of soluble fiber to slow the absorption of sugar that stabilizes

WHOLE-FOOD SOURCES OF FIBER	OFTEN CALLED	FIBER TYPE
Oats, beans, legume guar	Gums	Soluble
Soybeans, apples, citrus fruit, potatoes, cauliflower, cabbage, carrots, green beans	Pectin	Soluble
Psyllium	Mucilage	Soluble
Barley, wheat bran, whole grains, beets	Hemicellulose	Both
Strawberries, pears, peaches, radishes, green beans	Lignin	Insoluble
Beans, peas, corn, wheat, cabbage, broccoli, peppers, apples, carrots, beets, radishes, and other root veggies	Cellulose	Insoluble

WEIGHT CONTROL BONUS

The more fiber present in a food, the lower the food's caloric density. And since natural fiber in foods is usually accompanied by plenty of water, you feel more satisfied on fewer calories. So fiber translates to fewer calories, less risk of insulin problems, less risk of the fat-regulating hormones running amok...and ultimately improved balance.

FIBER TIPS

- Be sure to drink plenty of water with your fiber.

- Don't be discouraged if one form of fiber causes some gas or bloating. Keep experimenting until you find the perfect fit, then increase your fiber intake gradually. Flaxseeds are a good source of fiber. Grind them up in a coffee grinder and sprinkle them on salads, soups, yogurt, even desserts.

- Apples, bananas, oranges, and grapefruit are all good sources of fiber. And berries are fabulous—lots of fiber, lots of water, few calories.

insulin levels. It lowers your risk of cancer as it feeds the beneficial bacteria that live in the colon, allowing them to produce the potent cancer-fighting chemicals that take on damaging free radicals and promote healthy immune functions.

GO FOR WHOLE GRAINS

Whole grains are wild forms of grasses that have been domesticated by our ancestors over thousands of years. The advantages of whole grains vs. processed grains are so important that you should make a concerted effort to find whole-grain sources in your neighborhood and incorporate them into your diet. All good health food stores stock whole grains.

PRINCIPLE №5: EAT MORE HIGH-PERFORMANCE VEGETABLE PROTEINS, FEWER ANIMAL PROTEINS

When you substitute plant proteins for some animal proteins in your diet, you automatically reduce your intake of dietary hormone-disrupting chemicals and lower your risk of acquiring foodborne diseases. That's not to say you have to forgo meat altogether—we are, after all, taking the "flexitarian" approach here—but you should definitely eat more vegetable protein and less animal protein. There are lots of good reasons for this—but first, the basics:

WHAT ARE PROTEINS?

Proteins are the building blocks from which we're made. About 20 percent of our body is composed of small molecules connected together to make proteins. The proteins we produce naturally in our body perform important functions throughout our system, including immune system functions, nerve impulse transmission, and muscular contractions that allow us to move. (Many hormones are in fact proteins.) The proteins we take in as food are used to build and strengthen those necessary bodily proteins, and they're also recruited as an alternate fuel source.

HOW MUCH PROTEIN DO YOU NEED?

As a woman, to promote optimum hormonal balance your daily protein intake should be about 30 percent *less* than your total carbohydrate intake. To absorb protein effectively, you actually will burn carbohydrate calories. If you don't have enough carbs to burn protein, you'll lose muscle. Most plant proteins naturally have the balanced ratio—approximately 1.3 carb to 1 protein—necessary to be absorbed effectively.

All proteins are made up of amino acids. While there are about a hundred different amino acids, our body needs only twenty-one to build the different kinds of proteins it needs to function. As long as we take in an adequate number of calories, our body can produce thirteen of the twenty-one amino acids that it needs to build proteins. The other eight amino acids come from our food—these are called *essential amino acids.* They're a necessary, "essential" part of our diet, and they're readily available in both plant and animal proteins. But plant proteins are much better for you than animal proteins, both for your health in general and hormonally.

THE DISADVANTAGES OF ANIMAL PROTEINS

One of the most problematic issues with meat products is that animals store environmental toxins and industrial pollutants, such as dioxin and PCBs, in their muscles and bones. When you consume animal products, many of these BioMutagen "hormone disruptors" make their way into your system, and since some are especially long-lasting (if not indestructible), they stay with you a

BEST BETS FOR WHOLE GRAINS

GRAIN	PREPARATION GRAIN-TO-LIQUID RATIO	COOKING TIME
Amaranth	1 cup to 3 cups	25–30 minutes
Quinoa	1 cup to 2 cups	15–20 minutes
Barley	1 cup to 4 cups	30–40 minutes
Triticale	1 cup to 4 cups	1 hour
Bulgur	1 cup to 2 cups	15 minutes
Wild Rice	1 cup to 4 cups	40 minutes
Millet	1 cup to 4 cups	25–30 minutes
Brown rice	1 cup to 2½ cups	35–40 minutes
Buckwheat	1 cup to 5 cups	20 minutes
Oats	1 cup to 3 cups	30–40 minutes
White rice (enriched)	1 cup to 2 cups	20 minutes
Wheat berries	1 cup to 4 cups	1 hour
Couscous	1 cup to 1½ cups	5 minutes
Whole oats	1 cup to 2 cups	45 minutes
Rye berries	1 cup to 4 cups	1 hour

YIELD	SERVING SUGGESTIONS WAYS TO PREPARE AND ENJOY
2½ cups	Breakfast porridge, thickener for soups/stews, and mixed with other grains
3½ cups	Can be combined or substituted for rice in any soup, salad, pilaf, and the like
4 cups	Thickener for soups/stews, pilaf, hot/cold salads, or mixed with vegetables
2½ cups	Flour for baked goods, pastas, and cereals, or mixed-grain dishes and soup
2½ cups	Mix with other grains for multigrain salads or pilaf, bean dishes, or cold soup
3–3½ cups	Mix with other grains to add texture and flavor in soups/salads/pilafs
4 cups	Breakfast porridge, thickener for soups, and blends well with quinoa and bulgur
2½ cups	Can be combined or substituted for rice in any soup, salad, pilaf, and so on
3 cups	Breakfast porridge, thickener for soups/stews, salads, stuffing, and as flour
3½ cups	Flour for baked goods, granola, breakfast porridge, oat burgers
2 cups	Flour, mix with other grains to add texture and variety soups/stews, or pilaf
2½ cups	Salads, soups, breakfast porridge, stuffing, pilaf, or mixed with other grains
1¾ cups	Hot/cold salads, salsas, casseroles, or drizzled with olive oil
2½ cups	Breakfast porridge, flour for baked goods, pilaf, soup, oat burgers
2⅔ cups	Flour for baked goods, breakfast porridge, granola, and soups or stews

long time and end up accumulating in your fat cells. The effects of the exposure depend on the type of chemical you're exposed to, but they include infertility, delay of puberty, increased cancer risk, and a plethora of amorphous
symptoms, syndromes, and illnesses. Even naturally occurring toxins are
stored in animal muscle. And though many of these botanical toxic elements
are not harmful to an animal that eats it, it could have adverse effects on the
species next up on the food chain—which in some cases could be you.

Ill-conceived factory farming practices are another big problem. Aside
from the estimated 25 million pounds of antibiotics that are used in U.S. animal agriculture each year, high doses of potent growth hormones and sex hormones (estradiol, progesterone, and testosterone) are injected into livestock to
make the animals grow or produce milk faster and remain in their fat and
muscle. Though the actual health risks are not yet known, some studies have
linked the growth hormones with breast cancer as well as early onset of
menses in adolescents, and I believe this is just the tip of the iceberg.

Of course, getting too much protein from animal sources—especially red
meat—has also been found to clog arteries. America has the highest per capita
consumption of animal products in the world. And we have the highest rates
for obesity, heart disease, cancers, and many other problems associated with
chronic disease. If we didn't at least consider a correlation, we'd be doing our-
selves a disservice. More and more studies are linking high consumption of
animal products with cancers of the breast, colon, lung, and prostate. Consuming a heavy concentration (more than 20 percent of daily calories) of meat or
dairy has also been shown to increase women's risk of osteoporosis and kidney stones. (It causes the acid content of the blood to increase, which provokes
the bones to release calcium and phosphorus, buffering the acid and restoring
the pH to normal. That results in loss of bone and an increased risk of kidney
stones.)

Reducing the amount of animal foods you eat will lessen your risk of
many of these problems. Try not to have more than one serving of meat and
one serving of dairy a day at most. Cutting out marbling in beef and removing
fatty skin from chicken and other poultry is always a good idea, since the toxins tend to settle in these areas.

ORGANIC MEAT AND POULTRY

The only thing meat has to offer us is protein, calories, and iron, and you can
easily get that from cleaner plant protein sources. But if you do choose to eat
meat, organic is absolutely the way to go whenever possible.

Many consumers believe that free-range animal products are a healthy option. And they may be. "Free range" essentially means that livestock are uncaged and the animals are free to roam and eat what they will. But since there are no official guidelines, free-range animal products may or may not be injected with hormones and antibiotics. That, as well as how much of the time the animals are let out to pasture, is left to the discretion of the individual producer. So while there's a good chance

VARIABLE ANIMAL PROTEIN SOURCES

- Cod
- Halibut
- Snapper
- Wild pink salmon
- Turkey breast without skin
- Chicken breast without skin
- Pork tenderloin, trim excess fat
- Pork boneless sirloin chops, trim excess fat
- Beef sirloin (all cuts), trim excess fat
- Beef flank steak, trim excess fat
- 90–95 percent lean ground beef, drain fat

that free-range meats are healthier for you than commercial meats—since commercially raised animals are kept in cages, constantly fed questionably processed feed full-time, and regularly shot up with hormones and antibiotics—without stricter guidelines, I don't feel comfortable endorsing free-range meats.

On the other hand, I am comfortable endorsing organic meat if you wish to eat meat, since it actually does have federal guidelines that are enforced by the U.S. Department of Agriculture (USDA). To be certified organic, animal products must meet the following criteria:

- Livestock must be fed 100 percent organically grown feed or forage in pastures free of synthetic pesticides.

- Use of synthetic hormones or vaccination is prohibited.

- Use of sewage as fertilizer is prohibited.

- X-rays may not be used in production and packaging.

FARM-RAISED VS. WILD FISH

The advantages of farmed fish vs. wild-caught fish is an ongoing, hotly contested debate. While farmed fish, born and raised in confined, controlled areas, were once considered a healthy, less expensive alternative to wild fish, it's been discovered that farmed fish can be seriously unhealthy due to pollutants, questionable feed, and a high, unhealthy fat content (as opposed to the beneficial omega-3 fats found in wild fish). They're also treated with pesticides to control parasites and subjected to pen disinfectants and antibiotics. Some farmed fish are also genetically modified and once they're harvested are often shot up with dyes to render them more attractive in the marketplace. The bottom line: You're not eating healthier if you're buying farm-raised fish. Always choose fresh-caught wild fish when given the option.

In terms of meat, poultry, and fish, the term *natural* is misleading. It is essentially a marketing tool, with no relation to how the animals are raised or what they're fed. So while "natural" may sound healthier, there's no official difference between natural meat and commercially raised meat.

Vegetable proteins give you the same protein bang for your buck but have several advantages. They don't accumulate as many toxins as animal proteins, since they're short-lived and they obviously don't consume other toxins. They're packed with fibrous Hormone Power Carbs, and they contain cleansing unsaturated fats rather than clogging saturated fats. They boost your energy level, provide you with the essential amino acids, and, most important, promote hormone balance by stimulating your brain to release growth hormone (GH) that is crucial to muscle development and proper neurotransmitter functioning. Plus, they contain fewer calories than meat proteins.

SOY: ONE OF THE BEST SOURCES OF PROTEIN

Soybeans are one of your best sources of plant-based proteins and offer a major contribution to brain health. In fact, soy is now considered by many to be "the new brain food." Besides promoting good brain blood flow and containing every amino acid, including tryptophan, it's also packed with cleansing fats, B vitamins, antioxidants, and many other vital brain health nutrients. Studies have shown that both younger and older women are more alert and have better visual recall, sustained attention, and advanced planning skills when they make soy a regular part of their diet.

POPULAR SOY PRODUCTS

SOY MILK — A creamy liquid made from whole soybeans and often fortified with calcium and vitamin D and/or B$_{12}$ (10 grams protein per 8 ounces).

SOY FLOUR — Powder created by grinding roasted soybeans for addition to recipes. Defatted flours add more protein with fewer calories because they are more concentrated (12 grams protein per $^1/_4$ cup).

COOKING METHODS MAKE A DIFFERENCE

Smoking, frying, and charcoal grilling meats and fish are damaging to your hormonal health. Your best bets: baking, steaming, and poaching. These methods allow you to avoid the ultra-high temperatures and subsequent chemical reactions that form hormone-disrupting BioMutagens, as well as the cooking smoke that contains hormone disruptors and polycyclic aromatic hydrocarbons (PAH) that are well-known carcinogens. (Since BioMutagens are stored in animal fats, be sure to cut out the marbling in red meat and remove the skin from chicken and other poultry.)

SOY PROTEIN POWDER — Protein isolated and dried from defatted soy flakes to contain about 90 percent protein, an amount higher than any other soy product (23 grams protein per ounce).

SOY MEAT ALTERNATIVES — Foods processed to cook and often appear, taste, and smell like various kinds of meat and cheese, such as bologna, salami, mozzarella, and cheddar. Like any processed foods, some are healthier than others (10–12 grams protein per burger, for instance).

WHOLE GREEN SOYBEANS — When harvested at about 80 percent maturity, they are often found in Japanese foods such as edamame. They tend to be larger and sweeter than commercially grown soybeans. Can be steamed and added to a variety of recipes (11 grams protein per $^1/_2$ cup).

ASK DR. GREENE

Q: WHERE DO EGGS FALL IN THE PERFECT BALANCE DIET IN TERMS OF PROTEIN?

A: Eggs, although technically animal protein, deserve special inclusion in our high-performance protein category reserved primarily for vegetable protein. They're a high-quality protein source and like most proteins promote growth hormones, but their key importance lies in the *choline* found in egg yolks. Choline is terribly important for brain health. It's a major building block for the myelin sheath that insulates our nerves as well as for important memory-boosting neurotransmitters like acetylcholine. It is, in fact, a vital component of brain cells. Choline has become so important, the USDA has recently published guidelines suggesting that women should have at least 425 mg of choline a day. (That's found in about two eggs.) Though there are other sources of this vital chemical, especially grains, none is as potent a source as eggs.

WHOLE DRIED SOYBEANS— Beans that are matured, harvested, and dried to improve shelf life. They must be rehydrated and cooked before eating (19 grams protein per $^1/_4$ cup).

TEMPEH— Small cakes made from soybeans and mixed with another grain like rice, then fermented to produce a mild smoky or nutty flavor (about 20 grams per 4 ounces).

TOFU— A soft vegetable cheese made by treating soy milk with binding agents to produce a small cake (13 grams protein per 4 ounces).

TEXTURED SOY PROTEIN— Low-fat soy protein processed into ground beef–like texture (11 grams protein per $^1/_4$ cup).

SOY: A TOP PHYTOESTROGEN

Not only does soy provide a great quantity of protein, it also contains *phytoestrogens* (aka plant estrogens), plant-derived compounds, such as isoflavones, that mimic some of the effects of estrogen. Phytoestrogens have been shown to offer a reduction in uterine cancer and a moderate decrease in the risk of breast cancer and heart disease. They also may reduce hot flashes and night sweats, slow skin aging, and strengthen bones.

Studies further indicate that a soy-based diet causes measurable reductions in estrogen, progesterone, and thyroid hormone levels. Anytime we can successfully lower hormone levels without provoking symptoms, we believe

TEN HIGH-PERFORMANCE PLANT PROTEIN SOURCES

FOOD	PROTEIN CONTENT (GRAMS)	CALORIES PER SERVING
Soybeans	21	240
Black beans	18	225
Kidney beans	16	230
Chickpeas	18	270
Green peas	16	230
Lentils	16	215
Barley	16	700
Rice	5	230
Potato	5	220
Lima beans	16	25

that the body is responding with greater sensitivity to its own hormonal messages, therefore achieving a greater state of hormone balance. So phytoestrogens are more hormone modulators than hormone replacements—they enhance your response to the hormones you produce, rather than serve as stand-ins. Too much soy can actually act as competitive inhibitors and interfere with your normal hormone functioning. It would be nearly impossible for you to consume too much soy by eating whole soy foods, but high-dose soy supplements could cause an imbalance, so be cautious there. Some studies found that soy supplements available in many health food stores can achieve blood levels of phytoestrogens three thousand times higher than those reached after eating soy-based foods.

BEST TIME FOR PROTEIN

Eating proteins in the morning keeps your brain more alert during the day. So eat higher-protein breakfasts and prenoon snacks, then gradually introduce carbohydrates into subsequent meals later in the day.

PERFECT BALANCING FOODS VS. HORMONAL IMBALANCE TRIGGER FOODS

As you can see, knowing what to eat is as important as knowing what *not* to eat.

Hormone-balancing foods are abundant, but with the vast variety of food choices we're offered today, it's not always easy to decide which are the best at achieving hormone balance. Here are some of my favorite perfect balancing foods:

OATMEAL—Loaded with soluble and insoluble fiber, this power carb will stabilize your insulin level while you gradually absorb the brain-boosting sugars. Since this food is rich in fiber, it leaves your stomach slowly, so your ghrelin levels remain suppressed, helping to shut off your appetite.

EGGS—These performance proteins promote the release of growth hormone and keep you awake and alert throughout the morning. Choline is one of the macronutrients in eggs that gives your brain a much needed building block for one of your memory neurotransmitters, acetylcholine.

NONFAT ORGANIC MILK—One cup gives you 9 grams of protein to keep you alert *without* the added BioMutagens and synthetic growth hormones that your body can't process normally. It also provides 30 percent of your daily calcium to strengthen your bones and help you burn fats.

SOYBEANS—Loaded with cancer-fighting phytoestrogens, these protein powerhouses are the "thinking woman's" best friend.

ORGANIC CHILI—A great insulin-stabilizing meal that includes beans for fiber and protein such as texturized vegetable protein or 90–95 percent organic lean ground beef. This meal suppresses your ghrelin level, which keeps you feeling satiated longer.

WHOLE-WHEAT PASTA—These Power Carbs keep insulin levels low but still supply the flavor and substance of pastas made from processed Chaos Carbs. It is digested, then released slowly as glucose when you need fuel for your muscles and brain.

POMEGRANATE—This exotic fruit actually contains a small amount of estradiol that will be absorbed slowly owing to the carbohydrates and proteins in the fruit. So instead of creating an imbalance, it will actually boost your own estrogen production and improve the way you feel. In addition, this fruit is a powerful antioxidant.

GREEN TEA—Hot or iced, this drink fights free radicals with its anti-inflammatory and antioxidant properties, especially if you add a little mint for additional flavoring. If that's not enough, green tea also contains compounds thought to prevent certain cancers.

RED WINE—A glass or two before dinner will raise your testosterone level. This can give you that last bit of energy to get you through the rest of the day while boosting your libido. Wine is also rich in antioxidants to protect your brain against free radicals.

DARK CHOCOLATE—Contains many antioxidants that protect your brain. It also has several brain-boosting chemicals, including phenylethylamine (PEA), currently thought to be a primary neurotransmitter associated with passionate love. In addition, chocolate triggers the brain's reward center for those who enjoy it.

Hormonal imbalance trigger foods shift your hormones out of balance and create chaos. Here are common trigger foods to avoid:

POPULAR BREAKFAST CEREALS—With most of the fiber, vitamins, and nutrients removed, the nutritional value is worsened by added high-fructose corn syrup. Eating these first thing in the morning, while your cortisol level is peaking, causes your insulin level to shoot way up—promoting fat production and a brief energy burst, followed by hunger and fatigue.

DOUGHNUTS—These high-fat pastries trigger a similar rise and fall of insulin. Doughnuts also have unhealthy trans fats. This lethal high-fat/Chaos Carb combo blunts your brain's response to leptin and other appetite-suppressing hormones—and high-fat sweets worsen the insult by stimulating your taste buds for a longer period of time. The result: You stay hungry longer.

FRUIT JUICE—Without the fiber of the whole fruit to slow the absorption of the fruit's sugar, juice not only raises your insulin level, it gives you additional calories without satisfying your appetite. Even worse, many of today's popular fruit drinks have added high-fructose corn syrup!

HOT DOGS OR COLD CUTS—These high-fat processed proteins are laden with hormone-disrupting preservatives as well as synthetic hormones. Many of them even contain known BioMutagens like nitrosamines. They deliver their final blow with their saturated fats, which provoke many inflammatory pains (like menstrual cramps and joint aches); and their salt content promotes bloating as an extra insult through their effect on the hormone aldosterone.

REGULAR WHOLE MILK—Unless it's organic, when you drink milk you are getting a nice dose of synthetic bovine growth hormone. There is some evidence it can interfere with your normal growth hormone and may be contributing to the increase in early onset of puberty that we're seeing in girls today.

APPLESAUCE—Unless you cook it up yourself, it's probably made from apples laden with hormone-disrupting pesticides that are ground up and mixed with additional sugar in the form of corn syrup. Your blood sugar remains high just long enough for all your fat cells to absorb this Chaos Carb and convert it to even more fat.

POTATO CHIPS—Salt, low fiber, starch, and plenty of trans fat are in this highly processed snack. The salt can promote the release of antidiuretic hormone, enhancing fluid retention while promoting insulin release. Your fat cells interpret this signal by filling its tank—storing up even more calories—while your brain feels as though it's "running on empty."

FRIED CHICKEN OR HAMBURGER—The fat content of these popular high-protein foods reduces the sensitivity of your brain to leptin. That's more likely to get you to "supersize" in order to feel full. The clogging fats of these meals will also reduce brain blood flow by narrowing your blood vessels.

FRENCH FRIES—High in saturated fat and calories, these rapidly absorbed Chaos Carbs will produce plenty of free radicals to attack your brain as well as your blood vessels, especially if you're using ketchup with its high-fructose corn syrup. French fries will cause an insulin spike and blunt your leptin levels, while prolonging hunger with their lingering taste.

SOFT DRINKS—One can of soda contains the equivalent of about ten spoonfuls of sugar, causing a rapid rise in insulin that will suppress your growth hormone levels. Their potential free radical damage is also high.

(The most common phytoestrogens, and the ones often sold in soy supplements, are *genistein* and *daidzein,* the two most beneficial isoflavones.)

Since soy is a complete protein and provides all your essential amino acids, you could technically eat it as your sole source of protein; about a half cup per day would fully satisfy your protein needs. But since most of us crave a bit more variety, I suggest you eat a variety of plant-based proteins. The FDA and most nutritionists and health researchers recommend consuming at least one serving of soy per day (25 grams) to reap all its health benefits. (To earn the imprimatur of the FDA, a soy food must contain at least $6^1/_2$ grams of soy protein—so if not otherwise listed on the label, it could take up to four servings of a particular soy food to fulfill this recommendation.)

PRINCIPLE №6: EAT PLENTY OF CALCIUM- AND MAGNESIUM-RICH FOODS

The body needs several dietary minerals to function properly, but when the focus is on hormone balance, calcium and magnesium deserve specific mention.

Calcium is the most abundant mineral in your body. While 99 percent of it is in your teeth and in your bones, where it provides the strength and hardness needed to maintain good posture and prevent bone fractures, the other 1 percent circulates in your body fluids and plays a critical role in promoting nerve signaling, muscle contraction, and hormone release. Calcium is also involved in maintaining healthy cell membranes, enhancing the function of various enzymes, and ensuring that your blood is able to clot when it's supposed to. It's unlikely that your calcium levels will ever get low enough to pose serious health risks, but low levels can promote some subtle hormone imbalances.

When calcium levels fall significantly, your body releases *calcitriol,* a hormone that first shuts off the mechanism that allows you to burn fats for energy (as fuel), then activates the enzymes that promote fat production. This double whammy is the major reason chronically low calcium levels can contribute to excess weight gain. Now the good news: Calcium can also help you lose weight and maintain a healthy weight once you reach it.

HOW MUCH CALCIUM AND MAGNESIUM DO YOU NEED?

For optimum hormonal balance and health, try to get 1,200 mg per day of dietary calcium and 200 mg per day of dietary magnesium.

BEST CALCIUM SOURCES

DAIRY	VEGETABLES (1-CUP SERVING)	FRUITS (1-CUP SERVING)
Nonfat milk, 1 cup (300 mg)	Chinese cabbage (400 mg)	Blueberries (33 mg)
Yogurt, plain, nonfat, 1 cup (490 mg)	Broccoli tops (349 mg)	Strawberries (68 mg)
Yogurt, 2% fat, fruited, 1 cup (370 mg)	Collards, cooked (414 mg)	Raspberries (82 mg)
Swiss cheese, reduced fat, 1 oz. (350 mg)	Cauliflower (163 mg)	Cantaloupe (64 mg)
Muenster cheese, natural, 1 oz. (200 mg)	Spinach, fresh (156 mg)	Blackberries (43 mg)
GRAINS	OTHER	BEANS AND NUTS
Whole-wheat bread, calcium fortified, 1 slice (190 mg)	Soy milk, fortified, 1 cup (150–500 mg)	Almonds, raw, 2 oz. (150 mg)
Cornbread, 1 slice (110 mg)	Soy yogurt, fortified, ¾ cup (250 mg)	Black beans, cooked, 1 cup (120 mg)
Spaghetti, calcium fortified, ⅔ cup (300 mg)	Orange juice, calcium fortified, 1 cup (300 mg)	Sesame seeds, 2 tbsp. (160 mg)
Flake breakfast cereal, fortified, 1 cup (345 mg)	Tofu, calcium fortified, 4 oz. (200–330 mg)	Northern beans, cooked, 1 cup (160 mg)
English muffin, 1 each (100 mg)		Soybeans, 1 cup (175 mg)

One study found that when you consume calcium along with any kind of fat, it reduces the number of fat calories absorbed into the system. Investigators theorize that by establishing adequate calcium intake during your early twenties and maintaining it in later years, you may be able to reduce weight gain excess by about one pound per year. Although this might not sound like

BEST MAGNESIUM SOURCES

SEAFOOD	VEGETABLES	FRUITS (1-CUP SERVING)
Crab, cooked, 4 oz. (58 mg)	Broccoli, cooked, 2 large stalks (120 mg)	Avocado, Florida, ½ (103 mg)
Prawns, cooked, 4 oz. (49 mg)	Potato, baked with skin, 1 medium (55 mg)	Banana, 1 medium (34 mg)
Salmon, cooked, 4 oz. (40 mg)	Spinach, cooked, ½ cup (66 mg)	Raisins, golden, ½ cup (28 mg)
Oysters, cooked, 4 oz. (42 mg)	Sweet potato, ½ cup (61 mg)	Kiwi, 1 medium (23 mg)
	Artichoke, 1 medium (47 mg)	
	Acorn squash, cooked, ½ cup (43 mg)	
GRAINS	BEANS, NUTS, AND SEED	OTHER
Wheat germ, toasted, 1 oz. (90 mg)	Peanuts, roasted, 2 oz. (65 mg)	Milk, nonfat, 1 cup (40 mg)
Cereal, shredded wheat, 2 biscuits (80 mg)	Pumpkin seeds, 1 oz. (152 mg)	Yogurt, low fat, 1 cup (37 mg)
Cereal, bran flakes, ½ cup (60 mg)	Soybeans, cooked, ½ cup (74 mg)	Tofu, raw, regular, ½ cup (127 mg)
Whole-wheat bread, 1 slice (24 mg)	Small white beans, cooked, ½ cup (61 mg)	
	Black beans, cooked, ½ cup (60 mg)	

much, it could translate to over twenty-five pounds between the ages of twenty and fifty.

Magnesium is another important mineral in terms of maintaining hormonal balance. One of its critical functions is to keep your neurons healthy and stable. When neurons become overly active, they trigger excess release of stress hormones like epinephrine and *CRH (corticotropin-releasing hormone),* which can lead to depression and compromise your immune system. So if your magnesium level is low, your body may not be able to respond to colds, the flu, or even chronic infections like herpes as well as it could if you had adequate levels in your diet.

Low magnesium levels can also contribute to problems related to blood pressure and heart rate—and insulin resistance. Studies have shown that higher magnesium consumption translates into a nearly 40 percent risk reduction in diabetes. A diet rich in whole grains, nuts, green leafy vegetables, and bananas has been shown to provide all the magnesium you need in your diet.

SUPPORTING PLAYERS

Those six principles are the most important components of the Perfect Balance diet, but other key dietary factors are also important.

FATS

Fat fulfills some of our most important structural biological needs. It helps repair body tissues, stimulates the immune system to function properly, helps us absorb important vitamins, and makes up and helps support a good part of our cellular membranes. It is, in fact, essential to our health and well-being. But just as with proteins, moderation is the name of the game, and some fats are better than others. Too much of the wrong fat (saturated fats and trans fat) can clog arteries that are essential for maintaining the blood flow to your brain and can cause serious problems, like heart disease.

Unsaturated cleansing fats (omega-3 and omega-6), on the other hand, can reduce inflammatory chemicals in your bloodstream, so they can help ease menstrual cramps and pain. Adding a spoonful of fibrous omega-3-packed, ground flaxseed to your breakfast cereal and eating cold-water fish, especially during the last two weeks of your menstrual cycle, will reduce menstrual cramping.

The bottom line on fats:

- Less than 30 percent of your total calories should be from fat—lower is better.

- In general, if a fat is solid at room temperature, it is a "clogging fat" that can interfere with effective blood flow. Fats that are liquid at room temperature are "cleansing fats" that can help clean out blood vessels.

- The healthiest cooking oils are olive oil and canola oil.

WATER

All systems in our body depend on water. It plays an indispensable role in digestion and in the absorption, transportation, and use of nutrients. Without water, we'd be unable to regulate our body temperature or get rid of the toxins and waste products our body produces. Your regulatory hormones influence your brain and kidneys so that your body maintains the necessary amount of water. That explains how hormonal imbalance can cause bloating, high blood pressure, or dehydration and shock. As a woman, you have to be even more vigilant about taking in adequate amounts of water, particularly if you're older, which automatically makes you susceptible to dehydration. Since the onset of thirst lags behind the body's need for water, by the time you begin to feel thirsty you've already lost 0.8–2 percent of your body weight in water, and a 2 percent drop in water is equivalent to about a 20 percent drop in energy level. So you need to stay hydrated.

Another important factor: It takes water to flush out the excess salt in your diet—and the average American diet is packed with salt. While we need about 500 mg of salt a day, most of us consume about eight times that, nearly 4,000 mg a day. Too much salt can promote the release of antidiuretic hormone, which enhances fluid retention and promotes insulin release, which in turn signals your fat cells to store more calories. Water helps flush out that excess salt. If you don't take in enough water each day, you'll tend to retain salt and feel

IF YOU FEEL HUNGRY, YOU MIGHT JUST BE THIRSTY

Hormone brain studies have shown us that the earliest sensation for thirst is actually perceived by us as hunger. So at the first sign of hunger or fatigue, try drinking a glass of water first, then wait a half hour. There's a good chance your hunger will pass and you'll feel refreshed.

KNOW YOUR FATS

FAT TYPE	FOOD SOURCE
Saturated fats	Butter, ice cream, whole milk, fatty meats, and to a lesser extent coconut and palm oils
Monounsaturated fats	Olives, olive oil, canola oil, peanut oil
Polyunsaturated fats	Soybean oil, safflower oil, sunflower oil, corn oil
Trans fatty acids	Margarine, shortening, baked goods, deep-fried foods, common snack foods, fast food, crackers, and processed food
Hydrogenated oils	Margarine, shortening, baked goods, deep-fried foods, common snack foods, fast food, crackers, and processed food
Partially hydrogenated oils	Baked goods, deep-fried foods, common snack foods, fast food, crackers, and processed food
Omega-3 fatty acid	Flaxseed (ground, oil), rapeseed oil, pumpkin seeds, soybean oil, walnut and walnut oil, fatty fish (sardines, salmon, mackerel, herring, halibut)
Omega-6 fatty acid	Sunflower oil, corn oil, sesame oil, pumpkin oil, soybean oil, walnut oil, wheat-germ oil, mackerel

bloated or look puffy, or both. An average 130-pound woman should drink eight 8-ounce glasses of water per day. Add a glass or two more if you're on the heavy side, a glass or two less if you're lighter. And to diminish bloating caused by a rise in progesterone levels (during the second half of your menstrual cycle), double your fluid intake for a few days when you feel bloated.

A final word: For every gram of carbohydrate your body stores as glyco-

HEALTH RISK	HEALTH BENEFIT
Cause of high LDL levels	None
High caloric value	Helps to reduce blood cholesterol levels, extra-virgin olive oil can decrease blood pressure, helps reduce risk of rheumatoid arthritis
High caloric value	Helps to reduce blood cholesterol levels
Raises LDL levels ("bad" cholesterol), lowers HDL levels ("good" cholesterol), increases risk of cancer and heart disease	None
Raises LDL levels ("bad" cholesterol), lowers HDL levels ("good" cholesterol), increases risk of cancer and heart disease	None
Raises LDL levels ("bad" cholesterol), lowers HDL levels ("good" cholesterol), increases risk of cancer and heart disease	None
Excessive bleeding with high doses	Reduces risk for heart attack, stroke, heart disease, blood clots, and cancer; lowers LDL cholesterol and triglyceride ("bad" cholesterol) levels; lowers blood pressure
With high doses, excessive bleeding when cut	Lowers inflammatory markers, thins blood, acts as a precursor for central nervous system health

gen, it stores 3–5 grams of water. That little fact adds up to one of the major reasons people initially lose weight on ultra-low-carb diets—no carbs, less water retention. It's not weight they're losing, it's water. And that water is rapidly replenished when they go off the diet and return to their normal eating habits. Essentially, it's "false" weight loss. On a positive note, drinking cold water *can* help you lose *real* weight. Warming water to body temperature requires some energy—not a lot, but some. If you drink eight glasses of cold water throughout the day, you burn off about 67 extra calories per day as your body heats up that water. And remember to begin each day with a large glass of water. Sleep is very dehydrating.

ANTIOXIDANTS

Eat plenty of foods containing antioxidants. Plants produce antioxidants—their natural stay-fresh system. One of the simplest guidelines when it comes to choosing fruits and vegetables is their color. The brighter the color, the higher the antioxidant content.

BEST ANTIOXIDANT SOURCES

FRUITS	VEGETABLES	NUTS	LEGUMES
Blueberries	Kale	Walnuts	Red kidney beans
Raisins	Spinach	Pecans	Black beans
Prunes	Brussels sprouts	Hazelnuts	Pinto beans
Blackberries	Alfalfa sprouts	Almonds	
Strawberries	Broccoli flowers		
Raspberries	Beets		
Plums	Red bell pepper		
Oranges	Onion		
Red grapes	Corn		
Cherries	Eggplant		
Cranberries	Artichokes		
	Russet potatoes		
	Sweet potatoes		
	Yams		

ANTIOXIDANT TIPS

- Eat at least five servings of antioxidant foods a day.

- If you're going to take antioxidant supplements, take them with your largest meal of the day.

- Many herbs have super antioxidant powers: cloves, cinnamon, oregano, sweet marjoram (aka Italian oregano), dill, winter savory, coriander (cilantro), garden thyme, rosemary, peppermint, and lemon verbena.

- Green and white teas are rich in antioxidants.

- Dark chocolate is the most powerful antioxidant food. One bar (100 grams) neutralizes free radicals as effectively as two days' worth of fruits and vegetables.

- Dark and aged red wines, high in antioxidants, are being investigated as a potent source of *acutissimin A,* a cancer-fighting chemical. So one or two glasses of red wine a day provides myriad health benefits, including reduction in heart disease, stroke, Alzheimer's disease, and cancers. (It's best to have an extra glass of water for each glass of wine that you drink to avoid extra fluid loss, since alcohol is a mild diuretic.)

- Hot cocoa is a potent antioxidant. It has more antioxidant polyphenols and cancer-fighting flavonoids than either tea or alcohol.

A QUICK WORD ON VITAMINS, FUNCTIONAL FOODS, AND SUPPLEMENTS

If you stick to a well-rounded diet rich in whole foods, you really shouldn't need many supplements. If you do choose to take them, don't exceed the recommended amount. Some vitamins can actually provoke serious risks when taken in excess. As for herbal supplements, no herbs are considered an "essential nutrient." So though some may have benefits in certain situations, which we'll talk about in later chapters, there is no evidence that consuming any particular herb on a daily basis would be a boon to your overall health. My advice: Because supplements can contribute to medical problems—especially for people with existing health problems—it's always a good idea to discuss them (as well as over-the-counter medications) with your health care provider. Consider risks as well as benefits and decide for yourself if you need to correct imbalance artificially or if you can trace back the dietary cause and correct the problem at its source.

TWO-WEEK PERFECT BALANCE MEAL PLAN

This fourteen-day diet plan is designed for the generally healthy woman, so if you have food allergies or bowel difficulties, be cautious. It's high in insoluble and soluble fiber, high in omega-3 and omega-6 fatty acids, and low in calories and saturated and trans fat. The 1,600 calories per day are balanced among the Power Carbs, performance proteins, and cleansing fats. The variable animal protein sources in the following list will guide your selections when it comes to meat sources. Each substitution is for a 3-ounce serving size of cooked meats.

Whether you follow the flexitarian plan or go all-out veggie, this will put you on the road to hormonal balance—and feeling better on a day-to-day basis. As with any change, new eating habits take some getting used to. So give yourself time to ease into these hormone balance principles and don't expect to be perfect. Think 80/20—follow the hormone balance principles at least 80 percent of the time and allow yourself to splurge 20 percent of the time. It will help keep you from feeling deprived. (You might try sticking to the guidelines during the week and easing up on restrictions during week-ends.) Even at 80 percent you'll feel better, look better, and most certainly lose weight. Once you start to feel the differences in your body—trust me, there will be no going back to the old ways. To quote one of my favorite patients, "Good health is addictive."

THE MENU

DAY	BREAKFAST	LUNCH
DAY 1—MONDAY	2 4-inch buckwheat pancakes 1 tsp. trans-free margarine 1 cup strawberries 1 cup nonfat milk	Southwest bean salad: ⅓ cup black beans, 1 packed cup mixed greens garnished with jicama, corn, and pimento 2 tbsp. low-fat dressing 1 oz. baked tortilla chips ¼ cup fresh salsa 8 oz. calorie-free beverage such as green tea or mineral water with lemon
DAY 2—TUESDAY	½ cup oat bran breakfast cereal ¾ cup blueberries ½ cup nonfat milk 8 oz. calorie-free beverage	½ whole-wheat pita ¼ cup hummus with tomato, lettuce, and red onion 1 cup barley-mushroom soup 1 cup nonfat milk
DAY 3—WEDNESDAY	2-egg scramble 1 oz. part-skim mozzarella cheese 1 slice whole-wheat toast 1 tsp. trans-free margarine 1 cup nonfat milk	1 small baked potato ½ cup vegetarian bean chili 1 tbsp. low-fat sour cream 8 oz. calorie-free beverage

DINNER	SNACK
3 x 3–inch square eggplant lasagna	1 celery stalk filled
½ cup marinated vegetable salad	with 1 tbsp. peanut butter
1 cup minestrone soup	2 tbsp. raisins
8 oz. calorie-free beverage	1 cup nonfat milk

3 oz. teriyaki tofu (calcium enriched)
1 cup mixed stir-fried vegetables:
   carrots, broccoli, bean sprouts,
   snow peas, and red pepper
2 tbsp. sesame seeds
½ cup brown rice
2 pineapple rings
8 oz. calorie-free beverage

3 cups air-popped popcorn
1 medium apple
8 oz. calorie-free beverage

3 oz. grilled shrimp
2 corn tortillas
½ cup sautéed peppers and onions
1 cup tropical fruit salad
8 oz. calorie-free beverage

1 cup low-fat yogurt
½ cup raspberries
10 almonds
8 oz. calorie-free beverage

DAY	BREAKFAST	LUNCH
DAY 4—THURSDAY	1 cup low-fat cottage cheese 1 medium pear 1 oz. walnuts 8 oz. calorie-free beverage	1 grilled soy protein burger with lettuce tomato, pickle, and red onion 1 whole-wheat bun 1 tbsp. low-fat mayonnaise 2 tsp. mustard ½ cup low-sugar baked beans 8 oz. calorie-free beverage
DAY 5—FRIDAY	1 mixed berry smoothie: ½ cup low-fat plain yogurt, 2 tbsp. 100% cranberry juice, ½ cup frozen mixed berries 8 oz. calorie-free beverage	1 whole-wheat tortilla ⅓ cup refried beans 1 oz. jack cheese 2 tbsp. pico de gallo 1 tbsp. low-fat sour cream ½ cup grilled zucchini 8 oz. calorie-free beverage
DAY 6—SATURDAY	2-egg omelet: ⅓ cup black beans, ½ cup pico de gallo, and 1 oz. shredded jack cheese 1 cup cantaloupe 8 oz. calorie-free beverage	1 slice whole-wheat bread 2 oz. sliced turkey breast with lettuce, tomato, and red onion 1 oz. Swiss cheese 1 cup hearty barley-and- vegetable soup 8 oz. calorie-free beverage
DAY 7—SUNDAY	1 cup cooked old- fashioned oatmeal 2 tbsp. raisins 2 tbsp. dried cranberries 1 cup nonfat milk	½ medium tomato stuffed with ½ cup lentil salad 1 medium apple 1 cup nonfat milk

DINNER	SNACK

DINNER

1 quinoa-stuffed pepper
¾ cup steamed cauliflower
1 tsp. trans-free margarine
1 cup three-melon salad
1 cup nonfat milk

3 oz. grilled salmon steak
6 asparagus spears sautéed in garlic
    and 1 tsp. olive oil
½ cup wild rice
1 cup garden salad
1 cup nonfat milk

½ cup roasted vegetables:
    cherry tomatoes, red and green
    bell peppers, and button mushrooms
¾ cup whole-wheat pasta
1 packed cup romaine
2 tbsp. low-fat Caesar dressing
2 tbsp. shredded Parmesan cheese
1 cup nonfat milk

3 oz. grilled chicken breast
½ medium sweet potato
1 tsp. trans-free margarine
1 packed cup baby spinach greens
2 tbsp. fat-free vinaigrette dressing
1 oz. crumbled blue cheese
8 oz. calorie-free beverage

SNACK

1 slice pumpernickel bread
2 tbsp. low-fat cream cheese
7 carrot sticks
8 oz. calorie-free beverage

4 oz. dried fruit
¼ cup low-salt pumpkin seeds
8 oz. calorie-free beverage

1 Mueslix bar
1 medium orange
8 oz. calorie-free beverage

1 cup low-fat yogurt
¼ cup low-fat granola
8 oz. calorie-free beverage

DAY	BREAKFAST	LUNCH
DAY 8— MONDAY	1 low-fat bran muffin 1 cup nonfat milk 1 medium peach	Chef salad: 1 cup packed mixed greens and 2 oz. grilled turkey breast topped with tomato, cucumber, mushrooms, grated carrot, and egg 2 tbsp. low-fat dressing 1 cup nonfat milk
DAY 9—TUESDAY	2 slices multigrain French toast ¾ cup mixed berries topping ¼ tsp. cinnamon Artificial sweetener to taste 1 cup nonfat milk	1 cup spicy Texas vegetarian chili 1 tbsp. low-fat sour cream 3 x 3–inch slice cornbread ¾ cup low-fat apple coleslaw 8 oz. calorie-free beverage
DAY 10—WEDNESDAY	1½ cups mixed fruit: grapefruit, berries, and banana ¼ cup low-fat granola 1 cup nonfat milk	¾ cup grilled vegetables: red and green bell pepper, cherry tomatoes, and onion 1 whole-wheat tortilla 1 oz. skim mozzarella cheese ¾ cup Aztec bean salad 8 oz. calorie-free beverage
DAY 11—THURSDAY	1 biscuit shredded wheat cereal ¼ small cantaloupe ½ cup nonfat milk 8 oz. calorie-free beverage	1 cup five-bean soup ½ cup cottage cheese 1 nectarine 8 oz. calorie-free beverage

DINNER	SNACK
3 oz. baked red snapper	2 oz. low-salt mixed nuts
½ cup sautéed summer squash	1 cup fresh pineapple
1 tsp. trans-free margarine	8 oz. calorie-free beverage
1 tbsp. shredded Parmesan cheese	
1 cup chickpea salad mixed with avocado, yellow pepper, banana peppers, red onions, and cider vinegar	
8 oz. calorie-free beverage	
1 large portobello mushroom	1 cup mixed raw vegetables
½ small zucchini	2 tbsp. low-fat dill dip
½ tomato	8 oz. calorie-free beverage
2 tbsp. fresh basil	
1 tsp. olive oil	
¾ cup whole-wheat pasta	
1 cup tart-apple-and-pecan salad	
2 tbsp. fat-free vinaigrette dressing	
1 cup nonfat milk	
3 oz. lemon chicken breast	2 graham cracker wafers
¾ cup sesame-sautéed broccoli	1 tbsp. natural peanut butter
2 tsp. toasted sesame seeds	8 oz. calorie-free beverage
1 tsp. sesame oil	
1 cup Chinese salad	
1 cup nonfat milk	
2 small slices low-fat homemade garden vegetable pizza on whole-wheat crust	1 cup low-fat yogurt
1 cup Greek arugula salad	4 Brazil nuts
2 tbsp. low-fat dressing	8 oz. calorie-free beverage
8 oz. calorie-free beverage	

DAY	BREAKFAST	LUNCH
DAY 12—FRIDAY	¼ cup 10-grain cereal 1 oz. slivered almonds 2 tbsp. golden raisins Dash of cinnamon 1 cup nonfat milk	3 x 3–inch focaccia 2 oz. grilled chicken breast 2 slices tomato 4 endive lettuce leaves 1 tbsp. raspberry mustard 1 orange 8 oz. calorie-free beverage
DAY 13—SATURDAY	1 mixed berry smoothie: ½ cup low-fat strawberry yogurt, 2 tbsp. 100% orange juice, ½ medium banana 8 oz. calorie-free beverage	1 whole-wheat pita melt topped with 1 tsp. olive oil ½ cup spinach leaves ½ medium sliced tomato 2 oz. melted feta cheese 1 small orange 1 cup nonfat milk
DAY 14—SUNDAY	2-egg omelet: 1 oz. low-fat Swiss cheese, ⅓ cup spinach, ¼ cup mushrooms, ¼ cup tomato 1 medium fig 1 cup nonfat milk	1 lentil burger 1 multigrain roll brushed with 1 tbsp. low-fat Italian dressing ½ grilled red pepper 2 plums 8 oz. calorie-free beverage

DINNER	SNACK
3 oz. pan-roasted sea bass 1 medium baked artichoke ¾ cup barley-mushroom pilaf 1 cup nonfat milk	1 serving high-fiber cracker 2 tbsp. low-fat cream cheese 8 oz. calorie-free beverage
3 oz. rosemary-baked chicken ½ cup roasted baby red potatoes ¾ cup Brussels sprouts 1 cup nonfat milk	2 oz. low-fat Swiss cheese 1 medium apple 8 oz. calorie-free beverage

Broccoli and tofu stiry-fry with
   almonds: 3 oz. calcium-enriched
   seasoned tofu, ¾ cup broccoli,
   2 tbsp. slivered almonds
¾ cup multigrain pasta
1 baked spring roll
8 oz. calorie-free beverage
	1 cup barley pudding (made with
	   nonfat milk and 2 tbsp. raisins)
	8 oz. calorie-free beverage

CHAPTER FIVE

BALANCING HORMONES WITH EXERCISE

Exercise is vital in terms of hormone balance and brain health. The exercise-brain-hormone connection is not something commonly discussed, but it's hugely important. Since our bodies were meant to move, *all* the systems in our body function best when we're active—and that includes our hormones and our brain. Exercise actually feeds the brain by creating hormonal changes that promote brain blood flow. That keeps you more alert and stimulates areas of your brain that would otherwise remain dormant. When you don't exercise, your hormones shift into a "power saving" mode that you experience as fatigue. Exercise not only makes you feel more energetic, it actually stimulates the brain's reward centers—the same ones that are boosted by things like chocolate, cocaine, and sex.

Exercise also helps balance the "energy equation." Unfortunately, over the last three or four decades, as our calorie consumption has *increased,* our activity level has *decreased,* creating a serious energy and hormonal imbalance that's at the root of many of our most common diseases. The upcoming Perfect Balance guidelines are designed so that your incoming energy (calories) is in sync with your outgoing energy and hormonal imbalances are equalized.

EXERCISE LOWERS STRESS HORMONES AND RELEASES "FEEL GOOD" NEUROTRANSMITTERS

Since short-term stress is a necessary adaptation for responding to threats, it keeps your performance at peak levels. But when stress is ongoing, it becomes toxic and is a major health risk. Exercise is your best weapon against that kind of chronic stress. Here's how it works: When the stress is short-term, you perceive a situation to be threatening, and your brain sends a signal through a special network of nerves in the sympathetic nervous system. The hypothalamus processes it and sends out a stress alert signal—primarily to the adrenal glands. The adrenals then release the stress hormones (and other chemical messengers) that ready your brain, muscles, and the rest of your body for action. Cortisol, the primary stress hormone, increases your heart rate, blood pressure, and blood sugar levels. Digestion shuts down temporarily; blood flow is diverted away from the skin to support your heart and muscles; and your immune system prepares to respond in case you're injured or your muscles need to be repaired from the physical exertion. Once the threat passes, all emergency stress systems are called off and things get back to normal, in what's known as the *relaxation response.*

When you're *chronically* stressed, however, this relaxation response doesn't occur—unless we give it a gentle prodding. That's exactly what exercise does. It helps initiate the relaxation response through a complex interaction of hormones (thyroid, cortisol, and sex hormones) and neurotransmitters (dopamine, serotonin, and endorphins). The release of the feel-good endorphins serotonin and dopamine causes a heightened sense of well-being and euphoria, and this in effect functions as a natural antidepressant. Exercise also helps you sleep better by stabilizing cortisol levels that have been disrupted by daily stressors. Further, it helps you heal and lowers your risk of infection by increasing blood flow and boosting your immune system. The lactic acid produced by your muscles during vigorous exercise stimulates the release of *growth hormone (GH)* by your pituitary. Once released, GH not only promotes health in your muscles and bones, it also helps control blood sugar and stimulates your body's natural repair capabilities to identify and fix any injuries.

EXERCISE AND THE SEX HORMONES

As an adult, the structural integrity of your muscles and bones is maintained by estrogen and testosterone. Estrogen primarily strengthens your bones. Testosterone builds up your muscles. As we've discussed, starting around your mid-twenties, you begin to produce less and less of these hormones—especially testosterone. There's also a simultaneous natural decline in the density of your bones, collagen levels, and muscle mass. The good news: Exercise can help slow this natural age-related decline of estrogen and testosterone and thus slow down or even prevent muscles and bones from breaking down (a process known as *catabolism*). This makes exercise a brilliant preventive measure against osteoporosis, weakness, weight gain, and even collagen loss.

EXERCISE NORMALIZES INSULIN LEVELS

It's always better for your insulin level to be as low as possible—and exercise helps keep it that way. Lowering insulin levels initiates a domino effect of beneficial hormonal changes. First, your *triglyceride* levels—those unhealthy fats in the bloodstream—drop along with the insulin. As insulin levels normalize, your triglycerides decline further and are used more efficiently as fuel. With repeated exercise, as you tap into your fat fuel reserves, you'll lose those extra pounds around your midsection, which further reduces insulin levels. It also induces muscles to open up their glucose channels, which allows sugar in the blood to enter the muscles more easily. That lowers the need for insulin and corrects—partially or completely—insulin resistance.

EXERCISE BOOSTS TESTOSTERONE PRODUCTION

Exercise promotes the release of testosterone from your ovaries and offsets its natural decline. Studies show that after exercise, your testosterone level increases by 13–18 percent (depending on the duration and intensity of your fitness session). The elevation in testosterone promotes muscle growth, which then initiates a cascade of beneficial effects. You're able to lose weight more easily by increasing your fat-burning potential (bigger muscles burn more fat), your libido picks up, you feel more confident, and your mood improves.

Exercise-induced testosterone also improves your stamina by promoting the storage of glycogen—the first fuel source your muscles use when you start exercising. If you feel fatigued when you begin to exercise, it's generally because you don't have enough glycogen stored in your muscles. That improves with time as increased testosterone levels enhance your muscle health and stamina. In effect, the more you exercise, the more glycogen you store and the more stamina you have. Several studies have found that when women are fit and exercise regularly, their testosterone level actually begins to rise *in anticipation* of exercise.

EXERCISE OPTIMIZES ESTROGEN LEVELS

Exercise boosts estrogen's efficiency in two major ways. First, when you exercise regularly, your liver produces less of the carrier protein to which estrogen typically attaches. That makes it easier for estradiol to enter your brain, muscles, and other cells, where it can promote its beneficial effects. Second, regular exercise encourages fat loss. With less fat, your body produces less estrone (the "bad" estrogen), which of course can block beneficial estradiol from reaching its target cells.

Steady estrogen levels also improve the efficiency of your kidneys, which helps you maintain lean body mass by ensuring there's adequate water content in your muscles. This prevents cramping and fatigue and increases agility and strength. Estrogen also helps stimulate your neurons to fire more rapidly and efficiently, which is important when it comes to exercise, since agility is defined by the speed and accuracy of your movements. Finally, estrogen promotes blood flow, which provides your muscles with the good, steady supply of oxygen and glucose necessary for optimal muscle functioning.

EXERCISE IMPROVES BRAIN FUNCTIONING

Regular exercise increases the connections among brain neurons, which improves cognitive function, memory storage, and recall and actually makes your heart more efficient at pumping oxygen-rich blood to your brain. In fact, exercise can increase your cardiac output—the amount of blood your heart can release each time it beats—by as much as 200–400 percent. And your brain's ability to accept the oxygen is commensurate. With regular exercise, oxygen release from your red blood cells increases by about 300 percent, bathing your brain in the glucose and oxygen that allows it to thrive.

The following three-step process, when combined with the Perfect Balance diet, will get you well on your way to health, wellness, and hormonal balance.

THREE EASY FITNESS STEPS TO HORMONAL BALANCE

STEP №1: MASTER THE EXERCISE-HORMONE CONNECTION

Coordinating your exercise with your hormones puts you in charge—you get to decide which exercise combination is most beneficial to your hormones on any given day. Because chemical changes are closely interwoven with exercise, you can bring on associated hormonal effects when they can best be used to your advantage. Exercising in the evening, for instance, delays melatonin production, which can help you adjust to jet lag, accommodate changes in work shifts, or move smoothly into daylight savings time. Exercising in the morning, on the other hand, boosts testosterone, which promotes self-confidence and stamina throughout the day and gives you a brief spike in cortisol to heighten alertness—perfect if you're heading to a morning board meeting. When I'm dealing with serious deadlines, I actually do short intervals of exercise throughout the day to keep those hormones boosted and my energy level high. Here are some other ways to time your exercise to suit your life—and your hormones:

- TO ENHANCE YOUR SEX LIFE: Physical activity in the early evening boosts blood flow to your brain and your pelvis, raises your testosterone level (which is usually highest in the morning), and reduces common early evening fatigue. That trifecta increases your sex drive and arousal response and enhances sexual activity. Some studies suggest it can even improve orgasm.

- TO STAY AWAKE LATER THAN USUAL: Exercise around your normal bedtime. It will generate hormonal changes that shift your internal clock and keep you awake for several more hours.

- FOR MORE STAMINA: If you're a person who feels more sluggish than energized in the mornings, exercise as early in the day as possible. It will optimize your cortisol and testosterone levels. And within a short period of time, it will improve your stamina.

ASK DR. GREENE

Q: I OFTEN FEEL AS THOUGH MY CRITICAL THINKING SKILLS IMPROVE AFTER A WORKOUT. WHY IS THAT?

A: Exercise is frequently the key that unlocks creative solutions. While the area of your brain responsible for triggering muscle movement is fairly small and contained, the areas involved in initiating and controlling movement are located throughout your brain. So during exercise you use areas of your brain that may not otherwise be active when you're sitting still, and that promotes creative thinking. One recent study showed that listening to music while exercising activates more regions of your brain and further improves memory. By activating more regions of your brain, you often find answers to problems that have long eluded you. It's no secret that top executives work out regularly and ardently.

• TO COUNTER INSOMNIA: Don't do a serious workout late in the day. Try a nice relaxing yoga session in the evening. It will lower your stress hormone level and enhance sleep quality.

• TO LOSE WEIGHT: Exercise early in the day. Some caffeine, coffee or tea, before exercising can help accelerate your weight loss by boosting your fatty acid levels. Your muscles then use these fatty acids preferentially as fuel during your early morning exercise.

• TO WORK YOUR MENSTRUAL CYCLE TO YOUR ADVANTAGE: If you have significant PMS and feel more sluggish or irritable just *before* your period, be careful during strenuous exercise *just after* your period when your estradiol levels are low, since your coordination may be adversely affected and you'd be more likely to fall or develop an injury.

• TO BUILD THE MOST MUSCLE: Strength workouts can be most effective in the late afternoon—followed by low-fat, nutrient-dense meals to promote muscle and bone growth. Eating Power Carbs and proteins *after* your strength-training workouts boosts both insulin and GH levels to promote muscle growth while your body has the fuel and amino acids it needs. Occasional sweet treats can also provide an extra insulin boost. Chocolate in particular is a good choice, since it contains polyphenols, antioxidant chemicals that promote muscle healing.

- **TO REACH YOUR PEAK PERFORMANCE:** Your reaction time may be compromised when estrogen levels are low. The delay is usually so slight, most of us would never notice. But if you're a swimmer or sprinter reacting to a starting gun, or if you need to counter a 110 mph tennis serve, that fraction of a second could count. You can track your menstrual cycle and plan ahead to ensure that you perform when estrogen levels are high. Also, if you're competing in an early morning sporting event, wake up several hours earlier than usual to adjust your biological clock, and turn on bright lights to turn off sleep-promoting melatonin and help wake up your body.

STEP № 2: BALANCE ENERGY INPUT WITH ENERGY OUTPUT

Balancing the energy you take in as food calories with the energy you expend is known as *energy balance*. When you take in more energy/calories than you put out, you gain weight. When you burn more energy than you take in, you lose weight. It's as simple as that.

You'll remember from the last chapter that the term *basal metabolic rate (BMR)* is used to describe the number of calories you need while at rest. It's the number of calories you need simply to maintain your body temperature, get rid of waste, breathe, pump your blood, and think, and it varies to a degree in relation to your size, muscle (lean body mass), and hormonal status.

ACTIVE METABOLIC RATE

While your basal metabolic rate refers to your needs while resting, your *active metabolic rate (AMR)* takes your physical activity into consideration and reflects your total energy needs. Your AMR is the sum of your BMR, your activity level (this is your wild card), and the calories you use to digest your meals (which varies depending on what you eat):

ACTIVE METABOLIC RATE =
BMR + PHYSICAL ACTIVITY + CALORIES USED FOR DIGESTION

This formula tells you how many calories you should limit yourself to in order to achieve a state of energy balance. Add your basal metabolic rate (see page 66 for formula) to your exercise-related calories (see chart). That will give you your daily calorie needs—your AMR.

ACTIVITY	CALORIES/ 15 MINUTES	CALORIES/ 30 MINUTES
Aerobics (high impact)	165	320
Aerobics (low impact)	135	270
Circuit training (with weights)	185	320
Cycling (12 mph)	100	200
Elliptical trainer	235	548
Kayaking	75	150
Rowing machine	150	350
Running (10-minute-mile pace)	180	360
Sex (average pace)	24	49
Stair climber	155	310
Swimming (freestyle)	130	250
Walking (flat, 17-minute-mile pace)	65	130
Water aerobics	70	140
Weeding a garden	90	160
Weight training	130	270
Yoga	70	120

But there's a bonus: When you eat a low-fat, high-fiber, nutrient rich diet you burn about 10 percent of the calories you consume just digesting your food. With the popular high-fat diets, on the other hand, the fats are so easily absorbed that the metabolic boost is minimal—you burn very few calories in the digestive process. Think of it as gastronomic aerobics. If a 140-pound, five-foot-five-inch woman follows the Perfect Balance diet and goes for a forty-five-minute walk and does fifteen minutes of yoga each day, her AMR increases to almost 2,100 calories per day. That means she could eat 850 calories more a day and not gain weight. The chart above gives you a

CALORIES/ 45 MINUTES	CALORIES/ 60 MINUTES
500	660
400	540
455	580
300	410
690	905
225	300
475	650
540	730
75	97
460	618
380	510
200	275
210	280
230	320
385	510
185	240

good idea of the potential each type of exercise has in terms of burning off calories.

STEP №3: DIVERSIFY EXERCISES

By varying your exercise regimen, you affect different hormones and create the greatest overall health benefits. Short-duration exercises that require maximum exertion, like weight training, for instance, raise your testosterone, growth hormone, and norepinephrine levels. Intense, prolonged aerobic exercise boosts insulin sensitivity and briefly raises epinephrine and

HOW VALUABLE IS EXERCISE?

Studies have shown that just thirty minutes of aerobic exercise daily reduces the risk of various diseases by huge percentages:

BREAST CANCER:
20–30 percent risk reduction

COLON CANCER:
30–50 percent risk reduction

DIABETES (TYPE 2):
30–40 percent risk reduction

OSTEOPOROSIS (INCLUDING HIP FRACTURE REDUCTION):
50 percent risk reduction

STROKE:
30–50 percent risk reduction

PREMATURE DEATH:
30–50 percent risk reduction

HEART DISEASE:
40–50 percent risk reduction

cortisol levels. And varying your regimen promotes new brain activity and growth.

THE TOTAL FITNESS TRIAD

Total fitness incorporates endurance, strength, and flexibility. Endurance exercises stimulate the heart, which keeps blood pumping to the brain and hones brain skills; strength/weight resistance exercises promote sex hormone balance by building muscles and promoting growth hormone; and flexibility exercises minimize stiffness, aches, and pains while improving coordination. All three help balance stress hormones. Ideally, you want to commit to an hour per day for your personal fitness and aim for a 40 percent endurance, 30 percent strength, and 30 percent flexibility program; alternate endurance exercise with strength training; and try to practice a meditative exercise like yoga or tai chi *at least* three days a week. If weight loss is a personal goal for you, increase your exercise time for more energy output.

Endurance exercises are *aerobic*—activities like jogging, running, hiking, and good old-fashioned jumping jacks. Aerobic exercises lower your insulin resistance and help you lose weight, and they rely on your ability to take in oxygen and pump it efficiently to your muscles. Essentially, aerobics is all about blood flow, which is why these exercises also benefit the brain (remember, what's good for the heart is good for the brain). As your endurance improves, you promote more blood flow to your muscles and brain and improve your heart and lung health.

Try to do one of the following aerobic activities four or five times a week. Start with twenty minutes a day (break it up into two ten-minute sessions if it seems like too much); then add another five minutes each week or two until you reach at least forty minutes each session (or two twenty-minute sessions).

- WALKING/HIKING—One of the most fundamental and least-appreciated forms of aerobic exercise. You actually burn about the same number of calories walking as you do running; you just do it at a slower rate. For example, it will take 100 calories to go a mile whether you're walking or running, it will just take you more time to walk the mile than it will to run it.

- JOGGING OR RUNNING—Can be practiced at any age. Find a running partner or listen to a book on tape while you run. If it's a good one, you'll hardly notice the time go by. (Books on tape are great for long walks, too.)

- CYCLING—A terrific exercise and very practical alternative means of transportation. Many cities now have special "bike to work" incentive programs. Make sure that you have good equipment. The seat should be wide enough to support both of your sitting bones and will probably be more comfortable if the front of the saddle is tilted downward slightly.

- SWIMMING—An excellent form of aerobic exercise because it minimizes risks of injury or overheating. This is my most recommended exercise for women in the second and third trimester of pregnancy.

- SPORTS—Good aerobic sports include tennis, racquetball, squash, skiing, ice-skating, in-line skating, hockey, soccer . . . you get the idea. Any sport that keeps you moving at a good clip and makes you breathe a bit harder is aerobic.

Strength training is typically *anaerobic.* These exercises promote muscle and bone growth rather than prompting your heart to beat more efficiently, like aerobic exercises. With strength-training exercises, your muscles use their stored calories as fuel and keep weight off by promoting the production of anabolic hormones like testosterone and GH.

Your muscle strength depends on a few things: the amount of energy stored in your muscles, the number of fibers in your muscles, and the ability of your nerves to coordinate groups of muscles to work together. With regular weight-bearing exercise, muscles get stronger and store more fuel; more muscle fibers are stimulated to work together; and protein is built for future exercise sessions. Weight-bearing exercises do more than build muscle strength alone—they also build strong bones by creating a bone strain that triggers bone-building cells to absorb and deposit calcium. Ideally, you should do thirty to forty minutes of strength-training sessions three to four days per week. (If you find yourself lugging sacks of mulch around in the garden, lifting and stacking bricks, or moving furniture, that counts, too!) Choose from the following options:

- WEIGHT LIFTING—The unifying concept here is to move an object of defined weight to build muscle in a specific muscle group—the biceps, hamstrings, lower legs, upper and lower abdomen, and so on.

- ISOMETRIC EXERCISES—These work muscles against fixed objects for brief periods of time to build muscle force. They can be as simple as pushing against the wall or pushing one arm against the other. The advantage of isometrics is that they don't require equipment, and you can do them just about anywhere.

- PILATES (officially the Pilates method of body conditioning)—These exercises, which often incorporate specially designed equipment, improve your posture as they strengthen your body. Emphasizing body alignment and correct breathing, Pilates relies on the abdomen, lower back, and buttocks as a power center (called "the powerhouse"). The main goals are muscular harmony, balance, flexibility, and strength for the entire body.

- BAND TRAINING—These exercises use elastic bands of rubber with handles on the ends. You position the bands and pull in various directions to build strength in different muscles. For instance, pulling handles apart with your arms builds strength in your chest and back; placing a band around your knees and pushing your legs apart builds hip and thigh strength.

Flexibility training involves doing simple basic stretches for twenty to thirty minutes at least three times a week to help you maintain agility, coordination, and suppleness and reduce the risk of injury. Research reveals that certain flexibility exercises like tai chi and yoga not only enhance balance and flexibility, but improve hormone balance by lowering stress hormone levels. Yoga, which stretches the muscles as they gain strength, is one of the best ways to improve flexibility. At the same time that it works and stretches your body, it helps clear, center, and calm the mind—sort of like one-stop shopping for well-being.

Tai chi is a form of martial arts that combines body awareness and balance through a long series of slow, precise, and graceful movements, almost like a dance. The slow movements promote relaxation, flexibility, and coordination and emphasize breathing to quiet the mind and reduce stress. Tai chi is a gentle, safe exercise at any age and a great alternative if you find yoga difficult because of arthritis, knee problems, or other injuries. Several studies have demonstrated that regular practice reduces the incidence of falls in elderly people prone to balance disorders.

Remember: As you forge ahead with your exercise regime, have fun! Our brains are designed to appreciate novelty and surprise, so try new exercises and activities as the opportunities arise. Exercise promotes more exercise, and considering that all evidence tells us regular physical activity is healthy and essential, this is one addiction you can engage in without a trace of guilt.

CHAPTER SIX

MIND BALANCING FOR HORMONAL HEALTH

Mental and emotional health is enormously important to your overall well-being, and as we've seen, both are intricately linked to hormones. When you're anxious, tense, or worried—and most of us are to one degree or another in this multitasking, uncertain world of ours—your body is flooded with stress hormones (cortisol, prolactin, epinephrine, and others) that can dramatically affect your physical health. Mind-centering techniques such as meditation, yoga, and biofeedback (see page 191) can help reduce those stress hormones (and in turn balance your growth, metabolic, and sex hormones) and safeguard your health. As these mind-body methods improve your awareness of stress signals, they give you the ability to control stress rather than letting it control you. Much like exercise, these kinds of mind-body connections counter the effects of toxic chronic stress and help pull hormones back into a state of healthy equilibrium so that your body is better able to repair and replenish itself.

With the recent advances in modern medicine, we've been able to study objectively and examine the mind-body connection in an entirely new way. Neuroimaging has allowed scientists to track how our thoughts impact our body—both positively and negatively. By visually mapping chemical changes in the brain, we now understand much more about the brain's considerable healing power—and it's something we can use to our full advantage. The mind, it turns out, is a very powerful resource and tool.

You can clearly see the mind's extraordinary powers when you examine the placebo effect. (*Placebo* is Latin for "do no harm.") The placebo effect refers to experiencing a therapeutic benefit—having a tumor shrink, a tremor decrease, or a pain relieved, for instance—in response to a treatment that contains no known medicinal properties, usually some sort of "sugar pill." For example, studies have recorded Parkinson's disease patients responding to a placebo treatment much the same as they would to one of the FDA-approved drugs used to treat Parkinson's-induced tremors. With both the drug and the placebo, their tremors decreased, and the patients had an increase in brain activity in exactly the same region of the brain.

A HEALTHIER IMMUNE SYSTEM

One of the major health benefits of taking time out to calm and relax the mind is the boost it offers your immune system. By reducing the levels of cortisol and other stress hormones, mind balancing restores the immune system to its normal state and initiates a cascade of beneficial effects. It starts by reestablishing your natural pattern of daily hormone fluctuations, which facilitates your body's normal defense and repair mechanisms. This makes you much less susceptible to viruses, inflammatory immune system disorders, and chronic infections. Studies have found that people involved in mind-centering practices have fewer infections and faster healing times after major surgery, and cancer patients who practice have higher survival rates. On the other side of the coin, people who are unhappy or tense are three times more likely to develop colds and other respiratory infections.

Nobody knows exactly why some of us get headaches while others have stomach pains, develop depression, or suffer from high blood pressure. It's most likely a complex interaction of genetics, diet, and lifestyle, but it all comes back to the way the body responds to stress and subsequent hormone interaction. We get ulcers and other digestive problems, for instance, because stress hormones put normal stomach function "on hold," and they can remain in that state for only a limited period of time before illness sets in. Blood pressure problems are similar in this respect. When stress hormones are constantly revved up, your blood pressure is, too, and your risk of heart disease, vascular dysfunction, and stroke is two to four times higher than normal. There's also the age factor to consider. Your blood vessels become less elastic and pliable with age, which makes it more difficult for your body to adapt to sudden elevations in blood pressure, like the kind you might have in a truly stressful moment. While drugs known as *beta-blockers* can help these problems to a degree, relaxation techniques do these medications one better. They turn off the stress signal at its source, your brain. They provide the same results as the beta-blockers, they have no side effects—and they're free.

SWEEPING EFFECTS OF STRESS ON YOUR BODY

Although there's no evidence to suggest that chronic stress actually causes infertility, it can certainly exacerbate it. Constant elevated stress hormones have been shown to delay puberty, provoke irregular menstruation, promote miscarriage, worsen infertility, and cause premature ovarian failure. Studies of self-described "high stress" couples have found that they experience miscarriages at double or triple the normal rate.

Chronic stress and the inevitable emotions it fosters—anxiety, depression, hopelessness, and the like—can also decrease libido, an obvious deterrent to pregnancy. Loss of libido, in fact, is a common physiological response to stress, since the area in the brain that initiates the stress response is also responsible for signaling the ovaries to release testosterone and estrogen. These signals can't occur at the same time. It's an either-or situation, stress or normal sexual functioning. The stress response also directs blood away from the pelvis—another libido deterrent. The good news: A growing body of research shows that mind-centering techniques can switch your brain from signaling the stress response to signaling normal sex hormone production and activity. Not only do pregnancy rates rise in couples when they begin practicing stress reduction exercises, but miscarriage rates drop, as well.

IMPROVED LONGEVITY

Though we can't reverse the aging process, we can greatly slow its progress and promote long-term health by improving the hormonal milieu associated with relaxation. Calming your mind and body through the relaxation response is, in fact, one of your best tools for slowing aging and managing long-term health.

Essentially by countering chronic stress, relaxation reduces the net loss of cells that accelerates aging. As we get older, our cells get injured or die faster than we can repair or replace them. When the cell loss is in the muscles, we lose strength; when it's in the brain, we lose memory. Both are accelerated by chronic stress. Chronic stress halts the body's natural DNA-repairing system, which can potentially lead to the development of cancers. We all develop abnormal cells from time to time, but they're usually attacked by the immune system, which prevents them from dividing and becoming tumors. If chronic stress renders the immune system less effective, the abnormal cells can continue to grow, and the risk of cancer is increased. The bottom line: By warding off chronic stress, relaxation keeps our immune system functioning better, slows down cell loss, and helps us live longer.

FOUR STEPS TO BALANCING MIND, BODY, AND HORMONES

Your answers to the following questionnaire will provide tremendous insight into the role stress is currently playing in your life. After you've filled it out and totaled your answers, you'll end up with a numerical score. The lower your score, the lower your stress hormones and the closer you are to hormonal balance. The higher your score, the more stressed-out you are and the more likely it is that your stress hormones are causing or contributing to an imbalance. Healthy low stress hormone levels are our goal. If you don't meet that goal the first time you fill in this quiz, chances are you will the next time if you follow the tenets of the hormone-balancing program. Take this quiz every three weeks or so as you follow the stress relaxation guidelines and watch your score improve.

HORMONE BALANCE STRESS TEST

	ALWAYS (4)	OFTEN (3)	REGULARLY (2)	SOMETIMES (1)	NEVER (0)
Do you have indigestion?	4	3	2	1	0
Do you feel lonely?	4	3	2	1	0
Are you unusually prone to illnesses?	4	3	2	1	0
Do you feel anxious?	4	3	2	1	0

HORMONE BALANCE STRESS TEST

	ALWAYS (4)	OFTEN (3)	REGULARLY (2)	SOMETIMES (1)	NEVER (0)
Have your sleep patterns changed recently—do you sleep too much or too little?	4	3	2	1	0
Do you feel as if no one is on your side?	4	3	2	1	0
Do you worry a lot in comparison with your friends or family?	4	3	2	1	0
Do you feel shy or timid?	4	3	2	1	0
Do you avoid friendships and social situations?	4	3	2	1	0

SCORE

10 or less Great! No problems here. Keep up the good work!

11–20 Not bad, but you could feel even better if you practiced one or more of the upcoming mind-balancing techniques.

21–30 Your stress hormones are getting the better of you. You need to take time out of your schedule to relax and get back on an even keel before you become more stressed-out.

31–36 Call to action! Your stress hormones could be seriously interfering with your health and well-being. Make your mental and emotional health a priority. Promise yourself to take time out of every day for relaxation and rejuvenation.

Now that you've got a pretty good idea of where you stand, let's talk about some of the evidence-based steps that have been proven to help balance stress hormones and tap into the mind's own amazing healing powers.

STEP №1: CREATE A SAFE PLACE FOR RELAXATION

Your surroundings can be a source of stress—or a place of healing. That's why it's extremely helpful to set up a place of health and healing where you can let down your guard and relax. Here are a few easy ways you can manipulate your own space to encourage a more centered mind:

SMART LIGHTING: Lighting is a big contributor to elevating mood and energy levels, since it helps regulate the production of *melatonin,* a hormone that stabilizes mood and energy levels. When your melatonin levels are steady and regular, it helps normalize your body's production of stress hormones, sex hormones, and growth hormone (GH). Regular exposure to bright lights (at least 6,000 lux for at least two hours a day) has also been shown to be extremely effective at restoring neurotransmitter balance—especially serotonin—in the brain, which gives another positive boost to mood and energy. (This same kind of lighting has been found to be effective in treating the fatigue, anxiety, and lack of motivation caused by *seasonal affective disorder,* a condition caused primarily by a lack of sunlight and a long period of darkness.)

RELAXING COLORS: We all respond to color viscerally, whether we realize it or not. The hot colors like reds and oranges tend to stimulate, while cool colors such as lavender, blues, and greens tend to have a calming effect. So take that into consideration when designing your space. While a stimulating lively yellow in the kitchen would work well with your morning coffee, you'll want a cool, calming color in your meditation or relaxing areas.

PLEASANT SOUNDS: Soothing sounds calm the mind. Certain sound frequencies trigger the brain to relax, withdraw from the external world, and focus inward. The sound of water has been shown to have this effect. Since most of us don't live close to the ocean or a stream, a good alternative water sound source is a small tabletop fountain with recycling water. The bubbling water of a fish tank has consistently been found to lower blood pressure, and the fish bring down the blood pressure another peg, since they provide a calming visual accompaniment. Music can also influence your thought processes—it can perk you up and get you dancing around the house, or it can calm your mind. Slow, rhythmic sounds are the best for relaxing, since heartbeat and respiration tend to synchronize with the musical rhythm. There's some wonderful meditation music in most record stores now—check the "New Age" sections. Many of them consciously stick to between sixty and seventy beats per minute—just slightly less than your heartbeat.

SOOTHING SMELLS: When creating a relaxing environment, fragrance is an important ingredient. The smell receptors in your nose are in direct connection with the amygdala and hippocampus areas of your brain, which explains why odor can have such a powerful effect upon emotion and memory, respectively. Aromatherapy capitalizes on this by using essential oils to provoke certain responses. Try some of these fragrant oils recommended by the National Association for Holistic Aromatherapy:

> Eucalyptus to boost the immune system
>
> Ylang-ylang to relax and relieve muscle tension
>
> Geranium to reduce depression and promote calm

Peppermint to relieve indigestion and aches, including headaches

Lavender to relax

Lemon to promote relaxed readiness and encourage immune functions

Clary sage to encourage relaxation and relieve aches

DIMINISHED MENOPAUSAL SYMPTOMS

When it comes to menopausal symptoms, mind balancing can be a real blessing. Relaxation techniques, especially deep breathing and meditation, have been clinically shown to reduce the frequency and intensity of menopausal symptoms as well as the psychological distress they often induce. Again, the main factor is the reduction of stress hormones. Vasomotor symptoms (like hot flashes and night sweats) that disrupt mood, sleep, and quality of life tend to be more intense and last longer when a woman is under chronic stress (and stress hormones are abnormally high). The more "stressed out" she is, the more severe her menopausal symptoms are. Structured relaxation helps tremendously in countering stress and the menopausal repercussions and also helps avoid premature menopause.

Tea tree to boost immune function

Chamomile to relax (and aid sleep)

Rosemary to promote wakeful readiness while relieving tension

STEP №2: TRY DEEP BREATHING

You can fool your brain into interrupting the typical shallow breathing and tense muscles characterized by chronic stress by consciously inducing a state of calm and relaxation through breathing techniques. And by modifying your physiological responses, you can actually alter your behavior and your mood. Modifying your breathing and deliberately relaxing any of the muscles that tense up during times of stress help relaxation and have a positive influence on your heart rate, nervous system, blood pressure, and circulation.

By actively controlling your breathing for at least a few minutes several times a day, you can relieve tension and create a state of calm. And you can do it anywhere, no special equipment or clothing needed. The key is to make your breathing as slow and deep as possible and to take about twice as long to exhale as you do to inhale. These are the basics for deep relaxation breathing:

1. Exhale deeply, contracting the belly.

2. Sitting erect, inhale slowly as you expand the abdomen, completely filling your lower lungs.

3. Continue inhaling as you expand your upper chest.

4. Raise your shoulders up toward to your ears to be certain you have optimized your lung capacity.

5. Hold for a few comfortable seconds.

6. Exhale in reverse pattern, as slowly as possible, releasing your shoulders first, then relaxing your chest, and finally contracting your belly.

7. Repeat at a rate of no more than six breaths per minute. Repeat ten times.

If you want to monitor your success, take your pulse before and after three or so minutes of slow deep breathing. If your pulse is several beats slower after you've done your deep breathing than it was before, you'll know you're on the right track. Do these deep-breathing exercises at least twice daily. Late morning and late afternoons are ideal times, since it encourages cortisol levels to decline gradually throughout the day, the way they normally do when you're not stressed. Make deep breathing a habit.

STEP №3: TRY MEDITATION

Meditation has been scientifically proven to reduce stress and improve health. Via neuroimaging techniques, scientists have studied the changes that occur in the brains of various religious practitioners during their meditative practices. The similarity between their brain activation and blood flow patterns (to the mood-controlling frontal lobe) and the resultant reduction in their stress hormones clearly show that we can all benefit

HEALTH BENEFITS OF OPTIMISM

Optimists see the glass as half-full, and it stands them in good stead. Between 1962 and 1965, a group of investigators from the Mayo Clinic performed personality testing on nearly five hundred study participants. They recently followed up on them some thirty years after the original test and found not only that the "pessimists" had lower overall scores in terms of their health, but that over the three decades, the "optimists" had about a 50 percent higher survival rate. Other studies have had similar results. Psychologist Dr. Richard Wiseman, author of *The Luck Factor*, has shown that the way we assess various situations changes how effectively we accomplish our goals. And a positive outlook wins every time.

from meditative practices—whether they are religious or nonsectarian. Meditation essentially clears the mind of extraneous thoughts and shifts the brain patterns into deep relaxation, or "restful alertness." Studies have found that after eight weeks of regular meditation (four to five days a week), the stress response shifts from the "fight or flight" mode to acceptance, reducing heart rate, blood pressure, and oxygen consumption.

STEP №4: BE SOCIAL

Isolation exacerbates the stress response. Studies have shown that the surviving member of an elderly couple lives longer when he or she is socially engaged; and teenage girls with few close friends and distant relationships with their mothers have higher levels of insulin resistance (an emerging surrogate marker for stress). Neuroimaging shows that social rejection activates some of the same regions of the brain as pain, with just as much intensity; the greater the degree of rejection or loss, the greater the increase in blood flow to these areas.

Many studies have also found that women release more of the hormone *oxytocin* from their brain following social contact. This signal triggers the relaxation response and thus relieves stress. It is in fact the same hormone that the brain releases during breast-feeding and following an orgasm. Something as simple as a hug, a pat on the back, or other reassuring gesture from a loved one can promote a surge in oxytocin. Even laughter among friends relieves stress hormones. Following laughter, blood pressure, heart rate, and stress hormone levels go down. All things considered, it's easy to see how the hormone-brain-body connection is one of the major keys to prolonged health and well-being.

PART TWO

TROUBLESHOOTING FOR HORMONAL BALANCE

CHAPTER SEVEN

YOUR VIRTUAL OFFICE VISIT

Now that you're totally in tune with the Perfect Balance diet and lifestyle plan, it's time to discuss solutions for any symptoms of your hormonal imbalance that didn't improve with the program, including problems related to sex and sexuality, mood, hot flashes, sleep, and memory. Since each of you can't visit my office, this is my way of bringing my practice to you. In this chapter, I'll take you step by step through the same kind of diagnostic process we'd go through if you'd come to see me. Once we establish the nature of your problem, we'll discuss solutions in the following troubleshooting chapters.

Good medicine is still an art in many ways—especially when it comes to diagnosis. And whether you're self-diagnosing or have the help of a physician, the art is often in asking the right questions and listening carefully to the answers.

Diagnostic tools like blood tests can often be useful, of course, but certain questions need to asked and answered *before* we can even ascertain what tests would be most helpful. Blood test results are often limited because they essentially tell doctors how you compare with other women, while what doctors really need to know is how you compare with yourself at a time when you were feeling your best. Consider, too, that hormone-related blood tests can give you only a glimpse of the big picture because they simply reflect your hormone levels at the time of the test. They can't tell you what your levels were before you entered the office or what they'll be tomorrow. And remember that hormones are always changing—levels shift from day to day and week to week and can even cycle within a given day. When you do bloodwork, it's important to have a time reference on each report noting where you are in your menstrual cycle and the time of day. (I even like to know how my patients were feeling at the time of the test.)

Saliva testing is a slightly different story. Since certain hormone levels in your saliva are more stable than those in your blood, some doctors believe that saliva tests are more effective than blood tests. I rarely recommend them, though, for a number of reasons. They're not considered accurate enough at this point to earn the approval of the FDA. It also remains to be seen if the level of a hormone in saliva is an accurate reflection of the hormone levels in the bloodstream. Saliva testing is a good concept, and I believe that one day it will be much more helpful than it is now, but it still has a ways to go. However, both blood and saliva tests can be helpful for reference and to track improvement *after* you've started therapy.

THE INITIAL EVALUATION

Before you consider bloodwork or saliva testing, complete the following questionnaire. This is the type of form my patients fill out at their first visit to my office. It will create an inventory of all your complaints, which will enable you to take the next steps toward hormonal balance.

YOUR HORMONE BALANCE INVENTORY

CHECK YOUR PERSONAL SYMPTOMS

	YES	SOMETIMES	RARELY	NO
1. Does the idea of sex generally seem uninteresting?				
2. Do you often find you have a word "right on the tip of your tongue" but can't access it? Or forget a name or number just after you hear it?				
3. Do you avoid intimacy?				
4. Do you wake up in the middle of the night?				
5. Do you feel you're looking older than your age?				
6. Are you overly concerned—to the level of preoccupation—with cancer?				
7. Do you feel cranky and irritable?				
8. Are your joints, muscles, or lower back achy?				
9. Do you feel detached from others?				
10. Do you eat a lot of prepackaged or fast foods?				
11. Do you get headaches that last more than one day?				
12. Do you wake in the middle of the night to urinate?				
13. Do you suddenly feel warmer for no apparent reason? Or throw the covers off in the middle of the night?				

	YES	SOMETIMES	RARELY	NO
14. Do you feel you're dragging through the day with little energy?				
15. Do you wake up feeling tired?				
16. Are you unhappy with the people and things in your life?				
17. Are you failing to accomplish personal goals?				
18. Do you feel weaker than you did a year ago?				
19. Do you feel your heart beating fast and hard at times?				
20. Do you experience hot flashes?				
21. Do you get dizzy or shaky?				
22. Does your family have a history of cancer?				
23. Do you have difficulty falling asleep?				
24. Is your skin dry, itchy, or scaly?				
25. Do you skip screening tests such as Pap smears or mammograms?				
26. Have you had a recent onset of dental problems?				
27. Are you experiencing vaginal dryness?				
28. Are you anxious or nervous?				
29. Do you feel pain during or after intercourse?				

	YES	SOMETIMES	RARELY	NO
30. Are you experiencing memory loss?				
31. Do you feel unappreciated?				
32. Do you have an increase in facial hair or hair loss?				
33. Do you have headaches or neck aches?				
34. Do you carry a pocket fan, or are you usually the warmest person in the room?				
35. Do you have trouble concentrating?				
36. Do you have difficulty emptying your bladder?				
37. Are you dealing with "postpartum blues"?				
38. Does achieving an orgasm seem about as unlikely as winning the superlotto?				
39. Do you experience pelvic aches and pains before your menstrual cycle?				
40. Do you urinate more frequently than other women you know?				

Your answers to the questionnaire correlate directly to the following chapters, where you'll find explanations and solutions through lifestyle strategies and specific hormone formulations to your particular symptoms. On pages 142–43 is the key to your individual solutions and where you'll find them.

SEX: If you've answered "Yes" or "Sometimes" to questions 1, 3, 27, 29, and 38, you're experiencing problems related to libido, arousal, orgasm, or vaginal atrophy.

PROBABLE CAUSES: a deficiency of estrogen and/or testosterone.

SOLUTIONS in chapter 8.

CHRONIC PELVIC PAIN: Questions 8, 12, 36, 39, and 40 are directly related to chronic pelvic pain, other chronic aches that vary with monthly cycles. Seemingly unrelated symptoms such as urinary frequency can contribute to pelvic pain disorders.

PROBABLE CAUSES: unstable or persistently low estrogen levels.

SOLUTIONS in chapter 9.

MIGRAINE HEADACHES: If you've answered "Yes" to questions 11 or 33, you may have migraine headaches. Even if your headaches are not migraines, they may become worsened by hormone imbalance.

PROBABLE CAUSES: unstable or persistently low estrogen levels.

SOLUTIONS in chapter 9.

MOOD: "Yes" or "Sometimes" to answers on questions 7, 9, 16, 19, 28, 31, and 37 indicates your symptoms are related to PMS or premenstrual dysphoric disorder, postpartum depression, or menopause-associated mood disorders.

PROBABLE CAUSES: stress, estrogen deficiency, progesterone sensitivity, and/or testosterone deficiency.

SOLUTIONS in chapter 10.

HOT FLASHES: If you've answered "Yes" to questions 13, 20, and 34, you're experiencing the thermoregulatory imbalance associated with hot flashes and night sweats.

PROBABLE CAUSES: estrogen deficiency, testosterone deficiency, progesterone excess, or elevated thyroid hormone.

SOLUTIONS in chapter 11.

SLEEP: "Yes" to questions 4, 15, and 23 are directly related to sleep disturbances.

PROBABLE CAUSES: lifestyle and diet, estrogen deficiency, progesterone excess or deficiency.

SOLUTIONS in chapter 12.

MEMORY AND COGNITION: "Yes" to questions 2, 17, 30, and 35 means you need to take measures to boost your memory and cognition.

PROBABLE CAUSES: low estrogen, low testosterone, progesterone excess, or elevated stress hormones.

SOLUTIONS in chapter 13. (Also includes ways to protect against devastating problems like Alzheimer's disease and stroke.)

BALANCE: "Yes" to questions 14, 18, 21, and 39 indicates that you could use some help with movement, coordination, dizziness, and strength.

POSSIBLE CAUSES: estrogen-progesterone imbalance, estrogen deficiency, testosterone deficiency or sensitivity.

SOLUTIONS in chapter 14.

APPEARANCE: "Yes" or "Sometimes" to questions 5, 24, 26, and 32 tells you that a hormonal imbalance can be keeping your skin and hair from looking their best.

POSSIBLE CAUSES: estrogen deficiency, testosterone excess, stress hormone elevation.

SOLUTIONS in chapter 15. (Also includes information on teeth and eyes.)

CANCER: "Yes" to questions 6, 10, 22, and 25 signifies that you need the real facts about cancer. Not surprising, since there are so many misconceptions floating about on the relationship between sex hormones and certain types of cancer.

SOLUTIONS in chapter 16.

THE CONSULTATION

The next step is determining the crux of the problem. At the beginning of a diagnosis, I always discuss a few important issues that help to establish the hormone-brain connection and provide insight into the specific hormonal imbalance. So here's what I want you to do: Consider all the problems that you answered "Yes" to in your Hormone Balance Inventory in terms of the following questions and ideas. Jot down your answers and any related thoughts. (Make sure to have them available when you talk to your doctor.)

WHAT WAS HAPPENING IN YOUR LIFE WHEN YOU FIRST NOTICED THIS PROBLEM?

Write down as much as you can remember about what was going on at that time in your life. Pay particular attention to major events like the birth of a child, starting a new medication, or changing your diet, and record any illnesses, injuries, or surgeries. Did you start forgetting things soon after a hysterectomy, for example?

HOW LONG HAVE YOU HAD YOUR SYMPTOMS?

It's definitely worth noting if the symptoms have always bothered you and are simply getting worse or if they are fairly recent in onset. Write down any past treatments, noting when you tried them and how you responded (include herbs and any other complementary treatments like acupuncture). This information will help you consciously determine how seriously your symptoms are impacting your quality of life and will also keep your doctor from recommending treatments that are similar to ones you have already tried.

DO YOU HAVE ANY ASSOCIATED SYMPTOMS?

In other words, is there anything else—however minor—that cropped up around the same time as your symptom? Symptoms often come in groups. Even if one symptom pales in comparison with another, the two may be related. In fact, sometimes the less annoying, more minor symptoms can provide the most important clues. For instance, if unexplained weight gain is your major symptom and you also notice small skin tags (pencil point–size fleshy appendages) under your arm or on the back of your neck, it would be a good indication of insulin resistance.

HAVE ANY ESPECIALLY STRESSFUL EVENTS OCCURRED IN YOUR LIFE RECENTLY, OR ARE ANY CURRENTLY GOING ON?

Stress is a serious contributor to many hormone imbalances. Sometimes even changes that are positive and exciting, like moving into a new house, can be a source of stress. Or you may have been feeling stress for so long that you've gotten used to it and don't recognize the feeling as stress. Take a look at the following stress scale and consider if any of the events apply to you. If you have experienced one or more in the last year, circle the score associated with the event.

STRESS HORMONE LIFE EXPERIENCE CORRELATION SCALE*

LIFE CHANGE	SCORE
Death of spouse or partner	10.0
Marriage dissolution	7.0
Death in immediate family	6.5
Major illness	5.5
Marriage	5.0
Termination from employment	4.5
Retirement	4.5
Major change in health of family member	4.5
Pregnancy, childbirth	4.0
Sexual difficulties	4.0
Major change in financial status	4.0
Taking out a mortgage	3.0
Son or daughter leaving home	3.0
Beginning or ceasing formal schooling	2.5
Major change in living conditions	2.5
Change in residence	2.0
Major change in amount of recreation	2.0
Major change in social activities	2.0
Major change in sleeping habits	1.5
Major change in eating habits	1.5

TOTAL: _____

*Modified from Holmes-Rahe Social Readjustment Scale

Determine your score by adding the numbers you circled and write your total in the space provided.

- If your score is less than or equal to 10, it is unlikely that stress is a factor at this time.

- If your score is between 10 and 20, try some of the relaxation techniques in chapter 6 to bring your stress under control. It should be fairly easy to do at this stage.

- A score between 20 and 30 indicates that stress is probably compromising your quality of life. The warning flag is waving.

- A score above 30 means that stressful life situations are probably compromising your health. Adjusting those situations is crucial at this point, since your stress hormones are working overtime and throwing your entire hormonal system out of whack.

UNDERSTANDING HORMONE THERAPIES

Now a quick word about prescriptive medications. Since we'll be discussing specific prescriptive hormone therapies in the next chapters, there are a few things you need to know. First, while I consider hormones more a supplement than a medication, the FDA does view them as medicine, so you'll need to see a health care provider for the treatment prescriptions I recommend. Second, there's the off-label usage issue.

Drugs can't legally be marketed without formal approval from the FDA. Every medication that's available by prescription has an "indication" assigned by the FDA that lists the ailments the medication is federally recognized to treat. That indication is designated after years of research on the drug or hormone in regard to the particular problem for which it is approved. But that doesn't mean the drug can be prescribed only for its approved use—especially if it's a hormone. Physicians (and nurse practitioners) may legally prescribe the medication for other uses if, in their judgment, the medication is safe and effective. This is referred to as an "off-label usage." And that's not only acceptable, but sometimes preferable.

Prometrium, a BioIdentical progesterone capsule, for instance, is officially approved for menopausal women using estrogen "to prevent endometrial hyperplasia" (hyperplasia refers to the overgrowth of cells). But I often prescribe it for pregnant women in certain situations to help prevent

ASK DR. GREENE

Q: DOES TAKING HORMONES HAVE ASSOCIATED RISKS?

A: Some hormone therapies may involve some degree of risk for some women. But the risks associated with any of the hormones I recommend for specific symptoms in the upcoming chapters are very low—especially BioIdentical hormones. They're so chemically identical to your own hormones that using them is essentially like adding back a little of your own naturally produced hormone. BioIdentical hormones are, in effect, no more harmful to your health than your own hormones.

miscarriage. Because the formulation is identical to progesterone, and proges-terone deficiency has been shown to be a major cause of miscarriage, I feel it would be indefensible for me *not* to offer Prometrium to a pregnant woman with vaginal bleeding. But I am always careful to inform my patients that this application would be considered an off-label usage. (Incidentally, large studies are currently under way that may soon enable Prometrium to be approved ["labeled"] for this use.)

You'll find that many of the regimens I recommend in the following chap-ters involve off-label use of different hormones or medications. All my recom-mendations are fully evidence based—that is, they are all well supported by scientific research involving the hormone-brain connection. And they allow you access to treatments and potential benefits based on established clinical expertise. (Because not all doctors are aware of the latest research supporting these off-label usages, I've provided a comprehensive reference list in appen-dix 5 that can be shared with your doctor so that he or she can review the find-ings regarding any of my recommendations. You can also find up-to-date information supporting my Perfect Balance solutions on my website, www.SpecialtyCare4Women.com.)

A quick word about all the alleged "dangers" of estrogen replacement: In 2003, the FDA took the unprecedented action of putting a black box warning on all hormone therapies that contain estrogen.

A step like this is typically taken when a substance has been proven to cause harm. But most of the risks listed, including the risk of breast cancer, do not have any statistical significance, so in my opinion, the label is inaccu-rate. (In the introduction, I explained how misleading I felt the results of the WHI study were in regard to the reported increase in breast cancer risk for women taking a combination estrogen/progestin; and how the estrogen-only phase of the study found that estrogen *did not* cause an increase in heart disease or breast cancer risk.) Still, the FDA decreed that this statement had to appear on all estrogen products, including those that are BioIdentical. There are *no* data to support that all estrogens and progestins should be treated the same, and there's no compelling information that suggests BioIdentical hormones are harmful when used appropriately. Despite this, as of this writing there is no discussion by the FDA to remove the label. This warning is as follows:

ESTROGENS INCREASE THE RISK OF ENDOMETRIAL CANCER

Close clinical surveillance of all women taking estrogens is important. Adequate diagnostic measures, including endometrial sampling when indicated, should be undertaken to rule out malignancy in all cases of undiagnosed persistent or recurring abnormal vaginal bleeding. There is no evidence that the use of "natural" estrogens results in a different endometrial risk profile than synthetic estrogens of equivalent estrogen dose.

CARDIOVASCULAR AND OTHER RISKS

Estrogens with or without progestins should not be used for the prevention of cardiovascular disease.

The Women's Health Initiative (WHI) reported increased risks of myocardial infarction, stroke, invasive breast cancer, pulmonary emboli, and deep vein thrombosis in postmenopausal women during 5 years of treatment with conjugated equine estrogens (0.625 mg) combined with medroxyprogesterone acetate (2.5 mg) relative to placebo (see CLINICAL PHARMACOLOGY, Clinical Studies). Other doses of conjugated estrogens and medroxyprogesterone acetate, and other combinations of estrogens and progestins were not studied in the WHI and, in the absence of comparable data, these risks should be assumed to be similar. Because of these risks, estrogens with or without progestins should be prescribed at the lowest effective doses and for the shortest duration consistent with treatment goals and risks for the individual woman.

That's a real shame, since estradiol is the primary hormone linked to the most profound benefits of brain protection and is the most potent in terms of alleviating the typical symptoms of hormonal imbalance. Also, I want to point out that there's no intimidating black box warning on men's testosterone replacement, despite the fact that prostate cancer is the leading cause of death and illness in men in the United States and Europe. In fact, by comparison, men have a far greater risk of developing prostate cancer than women do of breast cancer. Yet men seeking to improve their quality of life (sex life, mood, energy level, and even memory) filled nearly 2 million prescriptions for testosterone in 2002 in the United States alone. I have no problem with men taking testosterone, and I don't believe it causes prostate cancer any more than I believe that estrogens cause breast cancer, but this does highlight one of the inequalities in public policy making for men and women. It's another reason you want to be in the driver's seat when it comes to your health care.

THE PERFECT BALANCE HORMONE BIOSYSTEM

When it comes to hormone therapies, not all estrogens and estrogenlike products are the same, nor are all forms of testosterone or progestin. I developed the Perfect Balance BioSystem to help you understand the differences and why one hormone therapy will be more effective in correcting your particular hormonal imbalance than another. Once you understand your treatment options, you'll be better able to choose the most appropriate strategy and to guide your doctor when your doses need adjusting. The BioSystem is categorized according to how your brain recognizes various therapies and how well they can relieve symptoms. You'll find a full, easy-reference chart of my favorite products in each category in appendix 1. The BioSystem also tags toxins (BioMutagens) that contribute to hormonal imbalance and lists the most common BioMutagens, with tips on how to avoid them.

I hope that my BioSystem will also clarify some of the terms being used—in the medical community and in the population at large. The word *bioidentical,* for instance, means different things to different people and even to different health care providers. Up to now it's had no universal meaning, and there have been no terms to describe the other kinds of hormone therapies we'll be discussing here. Hopefully this will help clear things up. While some doctors may already prescribe their version of bioidentical and other hormones, they generally don't take the brain-hormone connection into account or consider how hormones interact with one another when they write their prescriptions. That's why you often end up using a hormone combination that fails to help you achieve hormone equilibrium and feel your best. The BioSystem clearly defines the parameters of hormone therapy options and allows you to help your doctor help you.

BIOIDENTICAL HORMONES

BioIdentical hormones are designed to correct a deficiency—to supplement a key sex hormone that your body is not producing in sufficient quantities. BioIdentical hormones are so identical to the hormones that your own ovaries produce that your brain can't tell the difference between them and the real thing, and it responds to them exactly the same. BioIdentical hormones are, in fact, so identical to your own natural hormones that, like herbs and other

KEY POINTS OF BIOIDENTICAL HORMONES

- Safest therapy—as safe as your own hormones.

- Easiest to balance. Dosage can be easily tweaked.

- Integrates organically with your system and has the ancillary characteristics of your own hormones. Your body can convert one BioIdentical to another just as it can your own hormones.

- You'll know intuitively if you have to increase or decrease your dosage, since any symptoms will be similar to your previous experiences with natural hormonal imbalances.

- Most effective at reducing symptoms.

- No side effects when dosage is correct.

products produced by nature, they can't be patented. Because your body knows precisely how to use them and we can accurately predict their effects on your brain—and thus how you'll respond to them—BioIdentical estrogen, testosterone, and progesterone are my first-choice prescription options when they're appropriate.

Because BioIdentical hormones have the same chemical structure as your own hormones, they can bind to the enzymes that normally convert one of your natural hormones to another. That means that even if your dosage isn't perfectly suited to your needs, your body can convert one BioIdentical hormone to another and thus correct any subtle imbalance. Your body is also able to get rid of some excess BioIdentical hormones, as well, while non-BioIdentical hormones can accumulate and actually create new symptoms as a result. So BioIdentical hormones produce the fewest side effects and are safest for long-term use.

BioIdentical hormones are typically made from phytoestrogens extracted from yams that have been put through various chemical changes in the lab. The enzymes necessary to make the changes are active only at very high temperatures (around 200 degrees Fahrenheit), which is one of the many reasons you can't produce BioIdentical hormones yourself just by eating yams. (Cooking yams doesn't yield BioIdentical hormones, either, since other enzymes are also needed, and only 2 percent of each yam can be turned into the viable BioIdentical hormone.)

Because digestion changes the composition of BioIdentical estrogen and testosterone, they are not as effective when taken orally. Transdermal or transvaginal applications are currently the best prescription methods. They can be applied via patches, creams, gels, or vaginal ring and reach the bloodstream via skin absorption. BioIdentical progesterone, on the other hand, is such a large molecule that it's difficult to absorb through the skin and is best taken in pill form or by means of a vaginal cream, which is absorbed by the mucosal membrane. The patches (which are applied daily, biweekly, or weekly depending on the formula) and rings (which remain in the vagina for up to three months) are produced commercially and, with a prescription from your health provider, can be purchased in any pharmacy. Some creams and gels are also prepackaged or can be tailor-made by compounding pharmacies in whatever strength your doctor orders for you. (Your doctor should be able to recommend a good compounding pharmacy. If not, see appendix 2 for some suggestions.)

Because BioIdentical estrogen, testosterone, and progesterone are each absorbed by your body at a different rate, they're not manufactured in combination preparations. So if you need to supplement both estrogen and testosterone, for instance, you'd need two individual prescriptions. While single preparations might be slightly less convenient, it allows doctors to adjust the dosage of each hormone more precisely for better individual symptom management based on your personal needs—surely worth the trade-off for many women. Because figuring out your ideal dosage and deciding on the best application takes a little more experience and requires a bit more time, BioIdentical hormones are not prescribed nearly as often as the standard one-size-fits-all treatments. Hopefully that will change soon.

While you might hear the term *bioidentical* applied to other sex hormones, such as estrone, estriol, DHEA, androstenedione, pregnenolone, or

KEY POINTS OF BIOSIMILAR ESTROGEN

- Practical—available in pills and in combination formulas.

- The only estrogen useful for birth control.

- Inexpensive.

- Produces minimal side effects.

- Tried and true—been tested and used for over fifty years.

ASK DR. GREENE

Q: ARE "NATURAL" HORMONE PRODUCTS BIOIDENTICAL?

A: Hormone supplements marketed as "natural," such as soy or yam creams or capsules commonly sold in health food stores, may be extracted from plants, but most of them are far from BioIdentical since they're not recognized by your brain, and they're not necessarily safer than "non-natural" products. "Natural" is really more of a marketing strategy than a valid way of judging or rating hormones. To some people natural might mean a product is plant derived, to others that no processing was involved in its creation. That's the reason I don't use the term *natural* or *synthetic* and why I devised this BioSystem to provide crystal-clear definitions of treatment options.

allopregnenolone, they're not viable choices for hormone supplementation or symptom relief, and they're actually more likely to cause or worsen imbalances than correct them. The only BioIdentical hormones you should consider are estradiol, testosterone, and progesterone.

BIOSIMILAR HORMONES

These are estrogens that are very similar, but not identical, to the hormones your own body makes. (Currently, there are no BioSimilar forms of progesterone or testosterone.) They're fairly predictable in terms of how they make you feel, since your brain reacts to them in much the same way it does to BioIdentical hormones, but the dosing is not as easily adjustable. Because they're patented formulations and available only in the dosage amounts the manufacturers choose to produce (usually two to four options), you may end up getting more or less than you need. So you can't do the same kind of subtle tweaking of quantities the way you can with BioIdentical hormones. And because your body is not able to covert BioSimilar hormones to other hormones, you may end up with a little too much or too little, which can affect the way you feel.

But BioSimilar hormones do have some advantages in terms of convenience. They have been chemically modified so that digestive enzymes don't affect them. That means BioSimilar estrogen can be taken in pill, capsule, or injection form (as well as vaginally or transdermally). And unlike BioIdentical estrogen, BioSimilar estrogen can be combined with another product for con-

YOUR VIRTUAL OFFICE VISIT

venient use, such as BioSimilar estrogen/BioLimited progestin preparations. This is why most birth control pills (which always contain estrogen and progesterone) are usually a combination of BioSimilar estrogen and BioLimited progestin. (The majority of the BioSimilar products on the market are made from plant extracts—yams, soy, and others.)

BIOLIMITED HORMONES

BioLimited Hormones are synthesized and formulated to replace one of your own hormones that might be causing you symptoms of imbalance with another one that will not. Because they have *limited* activity in the brain, they provide some functions of naturally produced hormones but not others and are thus able to alleviate symptoms. BioLimited hormones are used to treat particular conditions or prevent disease like endometriosis or breast cancer. Because they're designed to target receptors in certain parts of your body, their effects are "limited" in some parts of the body and active in others. BioLimited progesterone (progestins), for instance, is active in the uterus yet minimally active in the brain. That *limited* nature often serves as an advantage by safely preventing vaginal bleeding or pregnancy without creating any of progesterone's occasional unpleasant side effects like depression or fatigue.

BioLimited progestin gives modern birth control pills the ability to reduce symptoms that can occur naturally with your cycle, such as cramping, bloating, and moodiness, rather than intensifying them the way the older pills often did. The most commonly prescribed BioLimited preparations combine a BioSimilar estrogen with a BioLimited progesterone (like the popular birth control pills Yasmin and Ortho Tri-Cyclen). Because BioLimited hormones are not chemically identical to your own hormones, they're a bit

KEY POINTS OF BIOLIMITED HORMONES

- Target specific biological functions to treat specific problems.

- Reduce hormone activity in your brain and thus provoke or prevent certain symptoms.

- Readily available at any pharmacy.

- Likely to be covered by your insurance (not always true with BioIdentical hormones).

unpredictable—you may feel great on a specific birth control pill, while your friend feels awful on it. Every woman's reaction is a bit different.

BioLimited estrogens are commonly known as *SERMs—selective estrogen receptor modulators.* These hormones are active in the bones like estrogen, but they block estrogen activity in the breast. I have serious concerns about the safety of long-term use of SERMs because they also block estrogen's beneficial effects on your brain; this means they often intensify rather than relieve symptoms like hot flashes, night sweats, and forgetfulness. Still, they clearly have some benefit in treating certain cancers. The most frequently prescribed BioLimited estrogens are tamoxifen (Nolvadex), Evista, and Danazol. (The BioLimited form of testosterone, methyltestosterone, found in preparations such as Estratest, cannot be converted to estradiol and can cause skin problems, which is why I rarely prescribe it.)

BIOANTAGONISTS

BioAntagonists are hormone interrupters. They are a new category of medications that, like BioLimited hormones, have been designed to treat certain hormone-sensitive diseases, such as cancer or endometriosis, by blocking particular hormones that your body produces naturally. But in this case, they prevent *all* the activities of a particular hormone by curtailing, or *antagonizing,* its activities. BioAntagonists, in effect, neutralize the targeted hormone, creating a hormonal milieu in which that hormone is absent altogether.

Unfortunately, many hormone antagonists interrupt the hormone receptors in the brain, as well, which can create severe side effects such as mood changes, hot flashes, and memory problems. I view those side effects as a warning from your brain that it doesn't like what's going on hormonally and highly recommend that these products be used only when their benefits clearly outweigh their risks. For instance, BioAntagonists can protect your ovaries from the effects of chemotherapy in the treatment of advanced breast can-

KEY POINTS OF BIOANTAGONIST HORMONES

- Can temporarily shut off all hormone production, which helps treat conditions like endometriosis.

- Used as an adjunct therapy for certain cancer treatments.

- Should be used for only a short period of time.

YOUR VIRTUAL OFFICE VISIT

cer, which is clearly desirable if you want to have children in the future. The new antiestrogen breast cancer treatments Arimidex and Femara, now commonly prescribed to reduce the growth of any breast cancer cells that may have escaped surgery, are estrogen BioAntagonists. The "abortion pill" (RU-486) is a progesterone BioAntagonist. The bottom line: While a BioAntagonist is warranted in some situations, you should have a thorough discussion with your doctor regarding all the pros and cons before taking one for symptom management.

> ### KEY POINTS OF BIOUNKNOWNS
>
> - Results are unpredictable.
> - Tremendous variability in quality from one manufacturer to another.
> - May *decrease* the effectiveness of BioIdentical hormones.
> - May be useful for short-term symptom management.

BIOUNKNOWNS

BioUnknowns are various herbs and supplements that contain substances produced by plants (phytoestrogens) that have some hormonal activity, but the exact nature of the activity is *unknown*. Although these phytoestrogens can provide some relief from symptoms of hormone imbalance, results are inconsistent and unpredictable, and the quantities needed to achieve results have not been scientifically established. Since BioUnknowns are very different from human hormones, reactions vary from person to person depending on how their brain reacts to the particular chemicals. This category includes popular phytoestrogens like soy and flaxseed and herbs such as black cohosh, evening primrose, and red clover. Though most of the data suggest that these kinds of BioUnknowns are safe and many have clear benefits when consumed in their natural, whole-food form, we're still learning how they influence our health when extracted and concentrated. For now I feel they're safest when consumed as a food, tea, or tonic—the way they've been used in traditional Chinese medicine for thousands of years—rather than in pill form. As studies continue, we may find that they're even safer than more standard therapies, but they could also prove to be problematic. So I advise caution when using them in concentrated creams, pills, and extracts.

MOST PERVASIVE BIOMUTAGENS

BIOMUTAGEN	HEALTH RISKS
2,4 Dichlorophenoxyacetic acid (2,4 D) (Herbicide)	Fertility problems Birth defects
Polybromides (PBDEs) (Flame retardants)	Contamination of breast milk Nerve toxicity Learning deficit Possible cancer
DDT and DDE (Insecticides)	Cancer Fertility problems
Dieldrin (Insecticide)	Linked to breast cancer
Permethrin (Insecticide)	Linked to breast cancer Nerve toxin Thyroid failure
Dioxin (Pollutant)	Endometriosis Fertility problems
Phthalates (Plasticizer)	Fertility problems Birth defects Premature puberty
Perchlorate (Pollutant)	Thyroid failure Mental retardation
Polycyclic aromatic hydrocarbons (PAH) (Pollutant)	Linked to breast cancer and lung cancer Birth defects
Parabens (Preservative)	Linked to breast cancer
Nitrosamines (Contaminant)	Highly carcinogenic

HOW YOU GET EXPOSED	HOW TO LOWER YOUR BIOACCUMULATION
By skin contact, inhalation, or eating contaminated food	Avoid use on your lawn Buy organic food
By treated clothing, furniture, and electronics	Support legislation to ban use—currently under consideration in Washington, D.C., and California
By eating meat, fish, dairy products, leafy and root vegetables, and certain fruits By using cosmetics containing lanolin	Eat organic foods Reduce meat and fish consumption Avoid cosmetics with lanolin
By eating contaminated meat, fish, dairy, and root vegetables, especially squash	Eat organic foods Reduce consumption of dietary fat
By using insect sprays and foggers, lice shampoos, tick and flea sprays	Read labels of products used at home, and eliminate products with this ingredient
By eating meat, fish, poultry, and dairy products from exposed animals	Reduce consumption of animal products
By using cosmetics and plasticized nail polishes Through vinyl products	Avoid personal care products with DBP and DEHP Avoid use of vinyl or anything with the "new car" smell Avoid microwave cooking of food in plastic containers
Through contaminated drinking water By eating dairy products from exposed areas	Install water purification units in your home Eat organic dairy
By burning organic matter like wood, gasoline, tobacco, oil, or coal	Avoid smoke and other pollutants Reduce consumption of charcoal-broiled meat, fish, or smoked foods
From cosmetics and personal care products From processed foods	Avoid cosmetics that contain parabens, especially deodorants
By eating cured meats From contaminated cosmetics Can be present in beer, tobacco, and some dairy	Ascorbic acid (vitamin C) may neutralize.

BIOMUTAGENS

These are the hormone-disrupting toxins and chemicals, such as DDT, PCBs, dioxins, and parabens found in our food, water, air, household products, and sometimes even hygiene products and cosmetics that can gravely disrupt normal hormone functioning. Because they're foreign to our physiology and we often can't excrete them, they accumulate in our bodies over our lifetime and are a likely source of many cancers. There's also gathering evidence that many BioMutagens are a major source of cancers, birth defects, and problems related to infertility and miscarriage. U.S. chemical companies manufacture over seventy-five thousand chemicals for commercial use, and the federal government registers about two thousand new ones each year (about 80 percent of them go through the application process and are approved in as little as three weeks). Most are "presumed safe" until proven otherwise. The following table shows you the most common harmful BioMutagens that you should do your best to avoid.

Now you've got a heads-up on the terms we'll be using as we discuss your solutions in the following chapters. According to standards set up by the World Health Organization, women in the United States, on average, experience up to twenty-five years of compromised quality of life because of current health care practices. Let's turn that around.

CHAPTER EIGHT

OPTIMIZING YOUR SEXUALITY

Few aspects of human behavior produce such levels of joy or misery as our sexuality, yet until the advent of neuroimaging, this key component of our lives had been considered one of science's "unexplained mysteries." Understanding the science behind the elusive and intricate pattern of hormones that weave through our brain to influence our sexuality can empower our sex life. It is very rewarding to have my patients tell me that by helping them correct their hormone imbalances, I've helped them rekindle the embers of their passion. So the idea that science and sex are adversarial is another old-fashioned concept that should be filed away under "past history"—right along with the idea that sexual dysfunction is some kind of amorphous psychological disturbance. Far from it. Neither a great relationship nor a superlative sexual technique can overcome sexual disorders caused by hormonal imbalance. However, most sexual dysfunctions are treatable.

FEMALE SEXUAL DYSFUNCTION

The National Health and Social Life Survey, considered one of the most sweeping studies on the U.S. population, found that about 43 percent of

ASK DR. GREENE

Q: I'M OFTEN UNINTERESTED IN SEX. DOES THAT MEAN I HAVE SEXUAL DYSFUNCTION?

A: Your sex life is a problem only if you decide it is. Sexual dysfunction is defined by you, nobody else. If you're satisfied with your relationships and your sexual responsiveness, desire, and experiences, regardless of how they compare with those of others, then you do not have sexual dysfunction. When I'm consulting with my patients, I never discuss sexual behavior in terms of "normal" or "abnormal" because I don't want to mislead them into thinking that sexual responsiveness is a black or white issue. We each define our own sense of "normal." If your sexual responsiveness and desire are no longer satisfying to you, it's possible that a change in your hormones may have triggered an imbalance that created the problem. If it did, I can help you correct it.

women between eighteen and fifty-nine years of age have experienced sexual dysfunction at one time or another—and the percentage increased exponentially with age. This survey also found that only one woman in ten had actually sought treatment. That's a shame, because treatment is readily available and can be very successful.

Female sexual dysfunction is classified into four categories—libido (desire), arousal, orgasmic, and painful sex. Each category has specific treatment recommendations. It's common to have problems in more than one category, and as you'll see, treatments often overlap so that one solution can actually help with more than one problem.

If you discuss any of these sexual dysfunctions with your doctor, let him (or her) know if the problem is a recent development or if it's always been present. Diagnosis isn't always easy, so defining your problem accurately gives you a much better chance at solving it successfully. Surveys show that about 75 percent of women are reluctant to discuss sexual dysfunctions with their health care providers either because they feel that nothing can be done about it or because they fear their doctor won't be comfortable discussing it. If you fit into either group, this chapter is especially important for you.

LOW LIBIDO

Libido is our sex drive, our desire, and the craving for sexual gratification that's often referred to as lust. And it's highly instinctual. Virtually all men and 98 percent of women experience strong sexual yearning at some time in their lives. Modern neuroscience has shown us unequivocally that intimate relationships and the drives that shape them are hardwired into our biology.

Before we go any further, take a minute to gauge the current state of your libido. Answer these questions based upon the way you've felt during the last month (or during your last sexual relationship if you're not currently in one). Keep in mind that you should complete all the questionnaires in this chapter, since it is often possible (although it may not be obvious) for more than one problem to exist simultaneously.

	NEVER	RARELY	SOMETIMES	FREQUENTLY	DAILY
1. I have daytime sexual fantasies	1	2	3	4	5
2. I want to have sex	1	2	3	4	5
3. My sexual desire is high	1	2	3	4	5
4. I feel a strong physical attraction to my partner	1	2	3	4	5
5. My partner and I are in sync	1	2	3	4	5
6. I get aroused thinking about sex	1	2	3	4	5
7. I am satisfied with my sex drive	1	2	3	4	5
8. I am fulfilled by my sex life	1	2	3	4	5

TOTAL SCORE _____

If your numbers are 25 or above, you've got a typical libido. If you've scored low on questions 7 and 8, consider seeking treatment to improve your quality of life. (Answering "Yes" to the following questions regarding your score will help further clarify your situation.)

Does this score seem lower than
it might have been five years ago?   YES   NO

Do you wish your score were higher?   YES   NO

Does your disinterest in sex cause relationship conflicts?   YES   NO

ANATOMY OF LIBIDO

While many factors such as poor health, profound stress, complicated lifestyles, and unsatisfactory relationships can lower your libido, the ones that I focus on here are the hormonal factors.

While testosterone and estrogen (estradiol) are both necessary components of a healthy, spontaneous sex drive, testosterone is king. A healthy libido is dependent on the presence of adequate amounts of free testosterone. A minimal amount of testosterone is necessary to generate spontaneous sexual desire. My theory is that this minimum "threshold level," which is just enough to generate desire, probably represents the minimal number of testosterone receptors in the hypothalamus able to trigger enough nerves to generate sexual thoughts. So your individual threshold has to do with the sensitivity of your nerves. Having more than this adequate amount of testosterone isn't necessarily better. Beyond your individual threshold level, additional testosterone doesn't further increase libido. So if you're already in your "normal zone"—and that's different for each woman—raising your testosterone level won't further boost your desire.

Estradiol (which you'll remember can be made from testos-

ASK DR. GREENE

Q: HOW DO I KNOW IF MY TESTOSTERONE LEVELS ARE LOW?

A: One of the best indicators of testosterone level is your skin. If it's too oily, your testosterone levels are probably high—you might also have acne or oily hair. If your skin is too dry, your testosterone level is most likely low. Also, keep in mind that testosterone levels vary during your menstrual cycle, peaking around the time of ovulation.

terone) is the other important hormone for your sex drive. It's as if these two hormones program the desire center in your brain and promote the production of the neurotransmitter dopamine, which, when combined with the right amount of serotonin, is the key mediator of sexual desire and reward. With these hormones and neurotransmitters properly balanced, you're more likely to be in the mood for love. So you need testosterone, estradiol, dopamine, and serotonin; they're all essential, and if any are lacking, you can experience low libido.

As always, there's a hormone-brain connection. There are testosterone receptors located in the regions of your brain that are most active during sexual fantasy. Estradiol plays an important role in these regions, too, and provides additional support by increasing the ability of these nerves to fire, which makes it possible for key regions of your brain to respond to sexual stimulation. It's as if testosterone sets the fuse and estrogen ignites the spark.

RULE OUT OTHER POSSIBLE HORMONE CAUSES FOR LOW LIBIDO

Many medications can diminish libido. Various birth control pills and oral hormone therapy, for instance, can do it by lowering the free testosterone level. The estrogen in the pills increases the sex hormone–binding globulin, which binds testosterone (to carrier proteins), effectively rendering it inactive. Less testosterone—less sex drive. Others drugs such as antidepressants, blood pressure medications, and antiseizure treatments reduce libido through their ability to interfere with the transmission of sexual thoughts. So make sure to ask about any possible sexual-functioning side effects whenever a doctor prescribes a medication, and if you think you're experiencing sexual dysfunction, discuss any medications you're currently taking with the health professional who prescribed them.

Numerous physiological influences such as anorexia, extreme weight loss, premature ovarian failure, and surgical removal of the ovaries will also lower testosterone levels to the degree that they can decrease libido. Correcting the underlying problem may return testosterone levels to normal, but treatment might still be necessary.

PERFECT BALANCE SOLUTIONS FOR LOW LIBIDO

It's not surprising considering the complex nature of human sexual motivation that there aren't many well-designed clinical studies on low libido. I've

Mabel, a shy, dignified sixty-eight-year-old woman, had a hysterectomy and like many women had chosen to have her ovaries removed, as well. The surgery went well, but she hadn't been prepared for the profound drop in sex drive that followed her recuperation. After two years of unsuccessful adjustments to her hormonal therapy, her doctor finally told her that she and her husband should just learn to snuggle. That's when Mabel decided to seek another opinion. After forty-three years of a sexually active, mutually satisfying marriage, neither she nor her husband was ready to give it up—surgery or no surgery.

A previous doctor put Mabel on Estratest, a combination tablet of testosterone and estrogen. Mabel reported that her skin became oily and her pubic hair thickened, but she still felt no vaginal sensation during sex. She may have done well on Estratest if she'd still had her ovaries. But in their absence, all she had were side effects of synthetic testosterone. I switched her over to a BioIdentical testosterone gel and a BioIdentical estrogen patch worn for one week at a time (Climara, 0.075 mg per day).

Within three months she was having vivid dreams, her energy had improved, and she was having spontaneous erotic thoughts again. But she still had diminished sensation in her pelvis. I suggested we switch her to a BioIdentical vaginal testosterone cream (at the same dosage) that while a bit messier would assure better absorption and would help speed the recovery of her pelvic nerves. When she returned with her husband three months later, both had big smiles. She said she was feeling better than before her surgery and had been tempted to cancel her appointment, but she wanted to come back to thank me and my office staff for helping her feel "whole again."

had great success with the following solutions when I've prescribed them to my patients.

DIET

- Because our Perfect Balance diet plan encourages total hormonal balance, it will help fight low libido day or night. Be careful to keep your dinners on the light side. By eating a veggie-and-protein-based, calorically light dinner, you're far less likely to crave the "postmeal nap" often associated with high-fat, calorically dense food. There's no greater obstacle to sexual activity than having trouble staying awake.

- Studies have shown that drinking small amounts of alcohol increases sexual thoughts and sexual activity: a glass or two of wine with dinner boosts free testosterone levels—and your libido.

- Avocado may help improve libido. Because it's rich in vitamin B$_6$, it helps lower high levels of prolactin, a stress hormone that can shut down the "sexual centers" of your brain when it's chronically elevated.

- Have an after-dinner coffee. A study published in the *Archives of Internal Medicine* found that a cup or two of coffee with dinner increases sexual activity. There's some question whether that happens because of a boost in libido or simply by promoting wakefulness, but the result speaks for itself.

EXERCISE AND MIND-BODY BEST BETS

- An evening constitutional—a walk after dinner—lowers your insulin level and boosts your free testosterone level, which is naturally highest in the morning and lowest at night. The same is true of any mild evening exercise. If your evening does end with sexual activity, you're much less likely to have problems sleeping. The hormones that your body releases in response to sexual arousal, especially if followed by orgasm, promote your body's relaxation response and enhance your ability to sleep.

- Since your mind rules when it comes to sex and your libido is very reactive to sexual innuendo, sharing the evening hours with a romantic (or sexy) movie increases sex drive. An even better way to promote sexual thoughts is to read a novel with descriptive love scenes. This can be part of foreplay if you read aloud to your partner.

- New and different experiences are something that stimulates the brain in a similar way to being newly in love. So to renew excitement in an established relationship, consider games of shared sexual fantasy to bring some steam and unpredictability back to your relationship.

COMPLEMENTARY MEDICINE

- The best studied of the herbal products is Avlimil, a proprietary combination of herbs. This composite was found to significantly improve sexual desire, arousal, orgasm, and overall sexual satisfaction, although it's unclear whether or not it will help menopausal women or those with low estrogen or testosterone levels. Recommended dose is one tablet daily, and optimal benefit sets in after about ten to twelve weeks of use. No prescription is required. (Source: 1-800-AVLIMIL [285-4645], or www.avlimil.com.)

- Ginseng is an herb that's been recommended as an aphrodisiac since its debut in China about five thousand years ago—so it's got history on its side. It may promote blood flow and therefore boost arousal, but how it might impact libido is a mystery. Since no evidence-based dose recommendations are available, follow package directions. And remember, it's always better to start with low doses and work your way up gradually. Talk to your doctor before starting ginseng to make sure you don't have a condition that would make it unsafe to use.

BEST HORMONE TREATMENTS

Low libido is one of the conditions that I feel often warrants a blood test—this one for testosterone. The result is then used not to determine the course of treatment, necessarily, but as a reference for comparison once you've started on treatment, to make sure the BioIdentical supplement is being absorbed. It's worth repeating this test a few months after your libido has been restored to document your normal zone. Make sure to tell your health care provider that you want to have your free testosterone level measured. If your free testosterone level is in the lower third of the normal range, I'd suggest supplementation with BioIdentical testosterone.

As I write this, several BioIdentical testosterone preparations for women are in final development by pharmaceutical companies, including a patch and a gel that should be readily available through any pharmacy in the near future. In clinical studies, a testosterone patch dramatically improved sexual functioning in women whose ovaries had been removed. And because these products are BioIdentical, there are no significant side effects (unless you're taking too much or too little and your dosage has to be adjusted by your doctor).

Until these kinds of products complete the FDA approval process and are readily available, I recommend BioIdentical testosterone compounded into a gel by an experienced pharmacy. (Your doctor can write you a prescription and suggest an appropriate pharmacy.) You simply rub the gel into your thigh once each day. I recommend starting with 1.0 mg. Apply the gel in late afternoon or early evening to create peak blood levels by midevening. After twelve weeks, if you're not experiencing significant benefit, consider increasing the dose by 0.5–1.5 mg and continue for another twelve weeks. Most women notice a considerable improvement by this time. If not, have another test for free testosterone level about four hours after an application of the gel to determine how well you're absorbing it. If your levels haven't increased much, talk to your doctor about going to a higher dose, like 5 mg. It's also important that the testosterone and estrogen be balanced appropriately. That's rarely a problem

ASK DR. GREENE

Q: WILL HAVING A HYSTERECTOMY LOWER MY SEX DRIVE?

A: Only if your ovaries are removed. When your ovaries are gone, the resultant loss of estrogen and testosterone can profoundly reduce your energy level, strength, mood, and libido. Having the ovaries removed at the time of hysterectomy should be done only when absolutely necessary, not as a routine part of pelvic surgery.

if you're still cycling, but if you're in menopause, your health care provider should help you determine the best balancing dose based upon how you feel or the oiliness of your skin.

AROUSAL DISORDER

Arousal (or excitement) is much more biologically driven than libido. Rather than being dependent upon a specific chemical cocktail of testosterone, estradiol, and neurotransmitters, arousal responses are more of a reflex reaction. This isn't to say hormonal balance isn't an important factor. The regions involved in arousal (the vagina, clitoris, and vulva) absolutely must have adequate levels of testosterone and estrogen in order to achieve optimal sexual responsiveness.

Arousal disorder is essentially a virtual disconnect between your mind and your pelvis. You're interested in sex and your mind is active, but your body doesn't respond anatomically to your partner's stimulation. It is in a way a female form of erection disorder. Without these anatomical changes—all of which are highly influenced by sex hormones—lovemaking can feel blunted, uncomfortable, or just impossible.

DETERMINE YOUR SEXUAL RESPONSIVENESS

Take a few moments to rate the statements below. Circle the number that best describes how you felt during the last month.

If your score is on the high side—say, above 18 (out of the total 30)—and if you find your lack of sexual responsiveness troubling, you have arousal disorder. The lower your score, the fewer symptoms you have and the less likely it is that you have arousal disorder. About 20 percent of women between the ages of eighteen and fifty-nine experience problems with sexual arousal. The number jumps to 40 percent for women going through their menopausal transition without hormone therapy.

SEXUAL RESPONSIVENESS EVALUATION

	ALWAYS	OFTEN	SOMETIMES	RARELY	NEVER
1. I get aroused easily	1	2	3	4	5
2. I flush when thinking about sex	1	2	3	4	5
3. I experience good vaginal lubrication	1	2	3	4	5
4. I enjoy sex	1	2	3	4	5
5. I experience a pleasurable sensation in my vagina during sex	1	2	3	4	5
6. I'm comfortable with my body	1	2	3	4	5

TOTAL _____

THE ANATOMY OF AROUSAL

Arousal doesn't happen just during intercourse. You can become aroused reading a sexy book, watching a racy movie, or just thinking about sex. But whatever the cause, the effect is the same. The first sign of arousal is an increase in heart rate. As your excitement builds, your breath quickens, your breasts swell slightly, your nipples become firm, and various muscles throughout your body contract and release as if ready for some sort of action. Your face and chest might flush and redden. As your interest builds, there's a marked increase in blood flow to your pelvic region that creates many changes. Your clitoris swells and becomes more prominent, increasing in sensitivity as well; lubricating secretions begin to well up at your vaginal opening; and your vagina actually lengthens and widens at its deepest regions. As this process continues, a pleasurable sensation builds and blood flow increases to your pelvis, causing your most sensitive vaginal areas to swell. At this level of arousal, heart rate, respiratory rate, and flushing have peaked, and various muscles around the vagina contract more frequently and at random. On average, it takes about eight to ten minutes to get to this level of excitement. (For some women it could take thirty minutes or longer.) This all sets the stage for an orgasm.

One study provided some fascinating insight into what happens hormonally to coordinate all these changes. It found that during the phase of progressive excitation, there is an increase in levels of epinephrine, norepinephrine, testosterone, and prolactin. As these hormone levels peak, so does the amount of pleasure. In other words, these hormonal changes probably induce the pleasurable sensation of arousal, including the building sense of tension. Except for testosterone, each of these hormones is a stress hormone, and their rapid rise represents a normal, healthy stress response—a sensation of mounting tension that seeks resolution. Orgasm is that resolution.

Your vagina, vulva, clitoris, and pubic region are vulnerable to hormonal changes. So when your level of sex hormones is very low, as it is during menopause or breast-feeding, or if it stops altogether, as it does if you've had your ovaries removed, your anatomy slowly begins to go through changes. Your vulva loses much of the collagen and adipose tissue that normally protects your pubic bone from trauma during intercourse. Your clitoris loses its protective covering (often called the clitoral hood). The vaginal surface becomes thinner and loses its elasticity, making it easier for the vagina to become irritated. Even your vaginal pH—the amount of acidity in your vagina—begins to change, making you more susceptible to vaginal infections. This is known as *genital atrophy,* and after the fourth year in menopause, nearly 60 percent of women experience it. Though it isn't troubling for all women, about 20 percent experience pain associated with irritation of the vaginal opening during intercourse. The lower a woman's estradiol level, the

Jean came to see me as a vibrant seventy-six-year-old woman—a widow of two years. She had been seeing a gentleman and felt that their relationship might become sexual but was embarrassed by how her body had changed. She was greatly troubled by the loss of pubic hair and the flattening of her *mons pubis* (the prominent swelling over the pubic bone). I told her that was common after a prolonged lack of sex hormones, but that it was reversible, and if it bothered her enough, she should consider hormone therapy. We discussed starting a very slow and gradual resumption of Bioldentical hormone therapy that would improve her sexual satisfaction if she did decide to let her relationship progress in that direction.

We started her on the Climara 0.025 mg patch. After two weeks, she increased to the 0.03 mg dose and gradually upped the dosage until she was on 0.05 mg by twelve weeks. She said she had felt the "heat and moisture" return (so much so, in fact, she had thought that she'd had a yeast infection). At her twelve-week visit, she was beaming. She and her new "friend" had booked a cruise together, and they had agreed to wait until that time to "consummate" their relationship. To speed up her response, I started Jean on Bioldentical testosterone vaginal cream. At her follow-up visit, I learned that her pubic hair had returned, she had experienced an orgasm, and she had a wonderful sense of renewed confidence. We switched her testosterone to the Bioldentical gel so that she wouldn't have to continue with the vaginal applications. A few weeks later, I got a colorful postcard from the Caribbean and a note that she was "cruisin' in style."

more likely she is to experience these changes. As estradiol levels continue to decline, the pelvic blood vessels don't dilate as well. Without a rich vascular supply, the vagina can become dry, and with that dryness comes even more irritation and more thinning of the tissue.

RULE OUT OTHER POSSIBLE CAUSES

If you have problems with sexual arousal, it's important to make certain that medications you're using aren't the source of your dysfunction. For example, beta-blockers used to treat high blood pressure can interfere with the stress response of sexual arousal. And mood-stabilizing drugs like Paxil, so effective at reducing anxiety, can also diminish the tension of sexual stimulation—

which reduces sexual response. Heart disease and diabetes also cause arousal disorder. Additionally, if you've had any pelvic surgery—particularly a vaginal hysterectomy, traumatic childbirth, or bladder "lift"—make sure to have an examination by an OB/GYN trained to evaluate nerve damage, because this is another cause of arousal disorder. Once these problems have been ruled out, the following solutions should prove highly successful in correcting arousal problems.

PERFECT BALANCE SOLUTIONS FOR SEXUAL AROUSAL DISORDER

DIET

- Eating chili peppers and other spicy foods has often been advised to improve blood flow to the skin. Anecdotal reports indicate that by increasing the blood flow just below the surface of the skin, these foods enhance sexual arousal, as well. The food should be spicy enough to induce sweating. Try it about an hour or so before anticipated sexual activity.

- Walnuts are not only a heart-healthy food, they also contain manganese, a mineral that aids the production of dopamine, one of the neurotransmitters that promote sexual arousal. You'd have to eat walnuts on a fairly regular basis to yield benefits, but since they're rich in the healthy omega-3 fatty acids, you can't go wrong. About 30–40 grams per day—a small handful—should do the trick.

EXERCISE AND MIND-BODY BEST BETS

- In general, anything that improves blood flow to the pelvis will be beneficial, so aerobic exercise is great. Yoga is also beneficial to sexual functioning because the enhanced flexibility frees you to explore a variety of novel sexual positions.

- Achieving a state of relaxation is important. One of the ironies here is that sexual activity helps lower stress hormones, but elevated stress hormone levels can be an obstacle to a healthy sexual response. Meditation or deep-breathing exercises in the early evening can promote the relaxation phase necessary to facilitate sexual arousal.

COMPLEMENTARY MEDICINE

- Ginseng has been shown to heighten arousal as well as improve libido by increasing nitric oxide production in vascular areas of the vagina and vulva. Since arousal drugs like Viagra, Levitra, and Cialis also promote nitric oxide production, there may indeed be some validity to the claim, even though it hasn't been confirmed. Start with very low doses and stay on the alert for any adverse reactions.

- Dream Cream by Sensaquest is a topical cream believed to increase vaginal sensitivity. It contains L-arginine, an amino acid that stimulates blood flow. The manufacturer (a urologist and researcher) recommends applying it five to ten minutes before sexual intercourse. (You can find it at www.dreamcream.com, or by calling 1-877-283-7326.) Research on this product has been limited.

BEST HORMONE TREATMENTS

The best hormonal treatment for arousal disorder is BioIdentical estrogen therapy. I recommend using this therapy vaginally in addition to any other estrogen therapy your health care provider feels is necessary (whether you're postpartum, menopausal, or have low estrogen levels for any other reason). BioIdentical estrogens work through the same means as Viagra, by dilating the blood vessels and thereby restoring natural sexual arousal.

If you're using an estrogen product or are currently being treated for breast cancer, Estring (vaginal ring) will provide a safe low dose of BioIdentical estrogen. The ring is simply inserted and left in place for three months at a time. Most women are aware of its presence only for the first few hours after insertion. It's easy to remove at the end of the three months, at which time you can put in another ring to replace it (or if you're taking another estrogen product, the dose could be adjusted so that the Estring may no longer be necessary). For vaginal delivery of a dose of BioIdentical estrogen that's high enough to use as the sole estrogen treatment, Femring is the best bet. (Femring comes in a daily dose of 0.05 mg or 0.1 mg, is thicker than the Estring, and is also used for a three-month time period prior to changing.) Finally, there is Vagifem, a BioIdentical estrogen tablet that is inserted into the vagina with an applicator every other day. All three options are generally well tolerated.

ORGASMIC DISORDER

The female orgasm is probably the least understood aspect of female sexuality. While the male orgasm clearly promotes reproduction by facilitating the ejaculation of sperm, the female orgasm has no such obvious function. My personal theory is that its main purpose is to relieve the mounting tension of sexual excitement and to promote bonding through the release of key hormones (oxytocin, prolactin, and phenylethylamine [see page 174–75]). Is orgasm essential in terms of female sexual pleasure? That really boils down to whether or not you're frustrated by your own sexual response. If you're sexually satisfied without achieving an orgasm, then you don't have a problem. If you are unsatisfied, I can help you do something about it.

Take a moment to rate the statements below in relation to your sexual experiences within the last thirty days (or the last time you had sex). Circle the answers that most accurately reflect your experience.

The higher your total score, the less frequently you easily achieve orgasm. If you view this as a problem, the upcoming solutions will help.

	NEVER	RARELY	SOMETIMES	OFTEN	ALWAYS
1. I worry about reaching an orgasm	1	2	3	4	5
2. I work hard to try to reach an orgasm	1	2	3	4	5
3. I'm frustrated after sex	1	2	3	4	5
4. Orgasm is not pleasurable for me	1	2	3	4	5
5. My clitoris feels numb during sex	1	2	3	4	5
6. Clitoral stimulation is uncomfortable	1	2	3	4	5
7. I'm distressed about sex in general	1	2	3	4	5

TOTAL _____

Q: IS FEMALE EJACULATION A MYTH?

A: That's a question I've often been asked by *Sex in the City* fans. The answer: It's not a myth. Though we don't know why it occurs, about 10 percent of women actually do sometimes ejaculate a small amount of fluid that has a composition much like that of the male prostate fluid.

THE ANATOMY OF AN ORGASM

A female orgasm can best be described as a euphoric sensation that lasts between four and fifteen seconds and begins with a series of muscle contractions involving the outer third of the vagina. At the same time as the contractions occur, the inner aspects of the vagina widen, the uterus begins to contract, and the skin flushes even further than in the arousal state, while heart rate, respiratory rate, and muscle contractions hit their peak. Some women say they feel as though they're "passing out," while others experience more of a sense of "letting go."

Hormonally, an orgasm occurs when your brain releases a combination of neurotransmitters from the "reward center" in the hypothalamus. In fact, an orgasm actually has more to do with this hormone-brain connection than it does with any specific sexual technique or how deeply you love your partner. If your estrogen and testosterone levels are low, your brain produces less of these potent neurotransmitters, and you're less likely to achieve an orgasm. Stress hormones play an important part, too. Orgasm is associated with a brief loss of control, and since it occurs at the peak of stimulation, it involves the excitatory stress hormones. That means that an orgasm is perceived throughout your body as a change in stress hormone levels. If your stress hormone levels are high before you even think about sex, you might not be able to achieve the buildup in tension necessary to trigger the relief of a successful orgasm, since your stress hormones simply don't have the capacity to get any higher. That's why beginning sexual stimulation from a nice, relaxed state is important. It allows your hormones to respond, build naturally, and ultimately gratify you with the sensations of orgasm.

At the time of orgasm, there is a brief pulsed release of the neurotransmitter *phenylethylamine (PEA)*. PEA is an amphetaminelike chemical produced by the brain, dubbed by many scientists as the "love potion" for its link to love, sex, and euphoria. It's also been implicated in the "runner's high" associated with exercise. Following the brief ecstasy of an orgasm, testosterone levels (which have been increasing and peak at the moment of orgasm) return to their normal levels, as do the stress hormones. In contrast, levels of oxytocin (the hormone associated with bonding love relationships) rise during orgasm and remain elevated for hours after. There's also evidence that the amount of oxytocin released may correlate with the subjective intensity of an orgasm. And oxytocin plays a role in helping your body recover from the stress (albeit pleasurable stress) of sexual arousal. Finally, the hormone prolactin remains elevated for the longest period of time post-orgasm. Since elevated prolactin levels have been associated with a reduced libido, some neuroscientists suggest that prolactin may flip the "off" switch that signals an end to sexual activity.

The involvement of your pelvic anatomy in achieving an orgasm is less clear-cut than the hormone-brain connection. Anatomically, the clitoris is the most common "trigger" for initiating orgasm, but because of the rich overlap in pelvic nerves, some women can climax from stimulation to areas in the vagina (the elusive G-spot, for example) or stimulation to the perineum (the space between the vaginal opening and the anus) or to the anus itself. Some women can even achieve an orgasm without any contact at all—this is typically induced by repeated contractions of the pelvic muscles (such as Kegel exercises, for instance). There's also some debate about whether or not there is more than one type of orgasm. For our purposes, it's probably best to say that the variations of "normal" are numerous.

RULE OUT OTHER POSSIBLE HORMONE CAUSES

If your brain doesn't have adequate amounts of the neurotransmitters necessary to create the euphoric feeling of an orgasm, or if their release is blocked, you won't climax. The most common medications that can inhibit orgasm are antidepressants. Depending on which neurotransmitter they target and how accurately they do it, these medications can either decrease or increase your ability to achieve an orgasm. Paxil, for example, represses the recycling of several types of serotonin and some other neurotransmitters, which can inhibit orgasm. In contrast, Wellbutrin is designed to increase dopamine action and therefore can boost your libido and your ability to achieve an orgasm. So make sure to discuss any possible orgasm-related side effects of your medications with your prescribing physician or nurse practitioner. Untreated depression or other conditions associated with chronic stress can also inhibit orgasm.

Maria came to my office to discuss how she was doing on her BioIdentical estrogen replacement. She had delivered a baby nine months earlier and was still breast-feeding. I had helped Maria and her husband, Dale, conceive through ovulation induction and artificial insemination, then helped her through some generalized symptoms of low estrogen: vaginal dryness, hot flashes, and mild depression after her pregnancy. She was doing well on the regime, and just as we were ending the appointment, she said shyly that there was "one more thing" she wanted to talk about. I sat back down. She told me that she had never really had an orgasm and wanted to know if there was something we could do to help.

I had her watch an instructional video on a product called the Eros-CTD Therapy (Eros—Clitoral Therapeutic Device, or CTD), an FDA-approved device designed to increase vaginal blood flow and improve clitoral sensitivity by applying a gentle and adjustable suction to the clitoris. I suggested she use the device three to five times per week—repeating applications a few times during each episode with one-minute breaks in between. I encouraged her to have her husband help, since it would improve his knowledge of her anatomy. In fact, I recommended they include that in their foreplay. She agreed to give it a try. I also cautioned her against the use of a vibrator at this point, since regular use can decrease sensitivity and create dependence. I told her we could discuss that again in the future.

I am pleased to say that when she returned for follow-up, she reported that she had had an orgasm on six occasions. She still had not had an orgasm during intercourse, however, so we discussed anatomy and using variations of sexual positions to direct her husband toward her more sensitive areas. Both she and her husband were very enthusiastic and open to suggestions. I remain optimistic that their sex life will continue to improve even further.

PERFECT BALANCE SOLUTIONS FOR ORGASMIC DISORDER

DIET

The most frequent dietary problem contributing to sexual dysfunction is overeating, so following the Perfect Balance dietary recommendations will help. Here are some ways you can specifically improve your chances of achieving an orgasm:

- Chocolate is a potent source of PEA—one of the primary mediators of sexual orgasm as well as food cravings. This euphoria-inducing chemical is one of many ingredients in chocolate that can enhance your sexual experience. Having a small amount of chocolate, preferably dark, rich chocolate, before sex can improve sexual functioning and heighten the pleasure of orgasm. Look for products with the highest cocoa content.

- Ascorbic acid (vitamin C) improves the release of the neurotransmitters associated with orgasm and enhances blood flow, as well. Vitamin C can also reduce baseline prolactin levels and boost oxytocin release, which can heighten the pleasure of orgasm and may also strengthen love bonding. At high levels (more than 1,000 mg per day), it has been shown to improve sexual satisfaction. (Raw fruits and vegetables are your best sources, with the highest levels in citrus like oranges and grapefruit. Melons and kiwi are also very high in vitamin C.)

- One or two glasses of wine before sex will boost your testosterone level, reduce your inhibitions, and promote blood flow, which will enable you to orgasm more easily.

EXERCISE AND MIND-BODY BEST BETS

- Kegel exercises have been shown to markedly improve the frequency and intensity of orgasm. Performing these sexual-enhancing exercises (which also improve urinary continence) involves isolating and exercising your pubococcygeus (PC) muscle, the muscle that contracts naturally during orgasm and is also used to stop urine flow. If you strengthen the muscle, you'll orgasm more easily. To identify this muscle, go to the restroom and while sitting on the commode allow your urine flow to start. Then stop it midstream. You've just "flexed your PC." Flex and relax this muscle about thirty times. After a brief rest, repeat this for a total of two to three sets twice each day. (Some women can actually achieve an orgasm simply by doing these exercises.)

- The most important aspect of normal orgasmic function is "letting go." Many therapists and sexologists feel that an inability to let go is one of the main reasons so many women find it difficult to achieve orgasm during intercourse. The hormonal changes that follow an orgasm and the bonding

ASK DR. GREENE

Q: **HOW CAN I TELL IF MY INABILITY TO ORGASM IS A HORMONAL IMBALANCE OR JUST SHYNESS AND EMOTIONAL DISCOMFORT?**

A: Masturbation and achieving a masturbatory orgasm can be an important step toward breaking down barriers. If you're not comfortable enough with your own anatomy to explore the way different sensations feel, then unresolved tension could be a significant obstacle to sexual satisfaction. It's also possible that there was a traumatic event in your past that's manifesting itself as a posttraumatic stress response. If you're not able to achieve an orgasm through masturbation, I recommend you make an appointment with a psychologist or sex therapist to determine if you have unresolved issues related to trust that warrant additional therapy.

feelings they promote with your partner support the theory that trust is very helpful to achieving an orgasm. Reassuring yourself that it's okay to relax and enjoy your own sexual pleasure during intercourse will help to put your body at ease.

COMPLEMENTARY MEDICINE

- Various creams can be applied to the clitoris and vagina to increase sensitivity and improve your opportunity to orgasm. They work primarily by promoting blood flow. This heightens responsiveness and facilitates greater exposure of the sensitive nerves stimulated by sexual contact. Products like Alura lotion, Dream Cream, and Kama Sutra Love Oils are good bets.

- The Eros-CTD has been well studied in women with orgasmic dysfunction, resulting in its approval by the FDA (and giving it the unique classification as a proven medical device for treating female sexual dysfunction). This device increases vaginal and clitoral blood flow by creating a gentle, adjustable suction. Results are fairly impressive. You can get more information by going online to www.urometrics.com.

BEST HORMONE TREATMENTS

No one really knows the minimal level of sex hormones needed to be able to achieve orgasm. Although we do know that adequate levels of estrogen and testosterone are essential, orgasm is highly individualized, and required hormone levels just can't be measured accurately. Consider the following hormone treatments if the other recommendations aren't effective:

- To correct an insufficient estrogen level, I recommend BioIdentical estrogen administered through either a patch, a gel, or a vaginal ring. (Each of these methods avoids the unnecessary reduction of your free testosterone level.) The dosage should be adjusted until you are satisfied with your vaginal arousal response. If you are in a dose range high enough to provoke breast tenderness and are still experiencing inadequate arousal, talk to your health care provider about adding a medication like Viagra, Cialis, or Levitra.

- BioIdentical testosterone has also demonstrated an ability to statistically improve the frequency and intensity of orgasm in women. One study demonstrated that the most consistently beneficial dose with a minimal risk of side effects was 300 mcg per day, through a patch applied to the skin. FDA approval is pending. Another great alternative is a BioIdentical testosterone gel. I recommend starting on a daily dose of 2 mg and increasing the dose gradually by 1 mg every ten to twelve weeks, up to a maximum of 5 mg. Keep in mind that different compounded doses may have different potencies, so it's up to your health care provider to adjust your dose.

PAINFUL INTERCOURSE DUE TO VAGINAL ATROPHY

Vaginal atrophy refers to thinning of the vaginal tissue. When estrogen levels are low, the vagina becomes fragile and brittle. As a result, even with the best lubricant, many women will get abrasions or "friction burns" during intercourse. As the tissue gets thinner, it also tends to contract, so the diameter of the vagina becomes narrower, which can make intercourse even more painful. In addition, the skin that protects the clitoris retracts, leaving it exposed to irritation from clothing. And the fat pad of the mons and vulva thins, leaving the pelvic bones and nerves without their normal biological protection. It typically takes one to three years of estrogen loss for all these changes to occur, though some women begin to experience symptoms during perimenopause, when estrogen levels start to decline.

The same low estrogen levels occur during the postpartum period—especially during breast-feeding, since that prolongs the period of low estrogen. So it's possible to have a fairly significant case of vaginal atrophy even if you're a perfectly healthy young woman. The brief hormonal fluctuations of a typical menstrual cycle can result in pain and discomfort for some women. When estrogen levels dip, vaginal lubrication decreases, as well, which leaves even the healthiest vaginal tissue more susceptible to irritation and pain from friction. When progesterone levels rise (as they do during the third week of a typical cycle), the sensation of irritation tends to become more of a "burning"-type pain throughout the pelvis. The brain is sensitive to imbalances in estrogen and progesterone.

Deep vaginal penetration during ovulation can sometimes trigger pain. After ovulation, when estrogen levels drop and pain fibers become much more sensitive, the brain is supersensitized to anything uncomfortable. This type of pain is often positional—it typically gets worse whenever the ovary that ovulated is "bumped" during deep penetration. Once estrogen levels rise and healing occurs from the site of ovulation, the pain is usually relieved within a few hours.

RULE OUT OTHER POSSIBLE CAUSES OF PAIN DURING SEX

Certain infections, such as yeast *(Monilia)* or bacterial vaginosis, can create a chronic burning sensation. Viral infections like herpes simplex virus can resurface after years of being dormant. And even an imbalance of certain normal bacteria present in the vagina can serve as a source of chronic infections. If there is any possibility of infection, your health care provider should take cultures (which can also detect the presence of any bacteria) as part of your exam.

PERFECT BALANCE SOLUTIONS FOR VAGINAL ATROPHY

DIET

- Yogurt with "active cultures"—essentially active acidophilus bacteria—can promote your immune system's ability to fight off chronic vaginal (and intestinal) infections. Acidophilus is a friendly bacteria that normally lives in your colon and vagina, where it helps prevent yeast infections. Consuming acidophilus in yogurt or probiotic fermented milk drinks, or taking it in capsules or liquid supplement form, can restore your body's natural defenses.

EXERCISE AND MIND-BODY BEST BETS

- The best exercise is participating in regular sexual activity. Even with low estrogen levels, frequent sexual activity promotes thickening of the vaginal tissue as well as a reduction in vaginal pH—two key components to reducing pain with intercourse—and helps by preventing your vagina from narrowing. Start slow and build slowly to a time and tolerance you are comfortable with.

- Slow deep breathing during sex can help since it keeps you from tightening your pelvic muscles—a normal reflex when experiencing vaginal pain. Slow breathing effectively interrupts the pain-promoting reflex.

- Recent studies show that watching sexy movies increases vaginal blood flow, which improves your natural lubrication and may help reduce discomfort.

COMPLEMENTARY MEDICINE

- Some studies suggest that guaifenesin, a common ingredient in nonprescription cough medicines, thins vaginal mucus and helps with lubrication. The recommended dose is 200–400 mg at least two hours before bed. Drink plenty of water to get the full effect.

BEST HORMONE TREATMENTS

BioIdentical estrogen is one of the best ways to treat pain related to vaginal atrophy. The vaginal ring, which is inserted like a tampon and is replaced by a fresh ring every three months, delivers estrogen directly to the vagina. Femring is tolerated well by most women. Estring provides such a low dose that it's safe even if you're undergoing treatment for breast cancer. BioIdentical estrogens delivered by patch, gel, or cream are equally effective. Continue with your regimen as long as you remain sexually active, or restart if you decide to resume sexual activity, because without estrogen you will eventually develop symptoms of vaginal atrophy. If your estrogen levels have been low for a long time, it can take up to twelve weeks for optimal relief. These solutions are safe even if you are breast-feeding.

For quicker response, I often start many of my patients on both vaginal estrogen for a local effect and a pill for an overall effect. In addition to the rings, there are BioIdentical vaginal creams (Estrace) and a vaginal tablet (Vagifem), as well as the BioSimilar conjugated estrogen (Premarin). Any of these will do, and your health care provider can help you by adjusting the dose. Typically, after three or four months most women are able to stop the vaginal estrogen but continue the pill to maintain the improvements established by using both.

CHAPTER NINE

CHRONIC PELVIC PAIN AND MIGRAINE HEADACHES

No matter what part of your body hurts, the brain alerts you of the pain. It's how your brain interprets a pain signal that determines what part of your body will hurt and how intensely it will bother you. When the pain is the result of a burn, cut, wound, or infection, you generally know what to do about it, but when it's caused by something less straightforward, like a change in hormone levels, you can be confused as to how it should be alleviated. If the pain continues for six months or longer, it can become an illness, even if the injury that caused it has long since healed. So chronic pain, whether it's due to an old back injury, arthritis, or fibromyalgia, is essentially a disorder of your brain's sensory alarm system. It's like a faulty fire alarm that keeps alerting you to a fire that has long since been extinguished.

Acute pain is essentially useful short-term pain, an alert from the brain to take immediate action to prevent a harmful situation from getting worse. Chronic pain, on the other hand, is long-term and serves no useful purpose. These are the essential differences between acute and chronic pain:

CHRONIC PAIN	ACUTE PAIN
Vague or remote trigger	Recent, obvious trigger
No apparent biological function	Serves a protective function
Depression and irritability common	Anxiety is common
Unpredictable duration	Lasts hours to days
May not have obvious association	Associated injury or illness

An estimated 86 million Americans live with chronic pain syndrome. Though both men and women develop chronic pain, women experience it far more often, more severely, and for a longer period of time. I firmly believe the reason for that is the relationship between pain, hormones, and the brain. Women have a greater sensitivity to pain in all parts of the body because of their naturally higher levels of stress hormones and greater fluctuation in endorphins (usually due to shifts in sex hormone levels). In contrast, men have a greater *relief* of pain due to their naturally higher and more stable estrogen levels. (Remember, it's for only a few days each month that women have higher estrogen levels than men.)

THE MECHANICS OF CHRONIC PAIN

The pain signal begins its journey to your brain along two parallel groups of nerves that are located in the skin and other organs. The nerves in the first group have a slick myelin insulation coating, which makes for rapid transmission of pain. They present the first sharp pain response—the "ouch!" The nerves in the other group are unmyelinated, so the second pain response they deliver is a slower, more persistent ache. It's this slower second pain signal that's gone awry in chronic pain syndromes—and it's much more dependent on hormones. As your estrogen levels decline (as they do during the last few days before your menstrual cycle and for several days after bleeding starts), serotonin levels fall. When serotonin levels are low, any internal pain, whether it's from your pelvis, joints, or even sore muscles, becomes amplified.

Once either the fast myelinated pain signals or the slower second unmyelinated ones reach your spinal cord, they travel to your brain via the pain highway in the spinal cord known as the *dorsal horn*. (One way to treat pain is to stop the pain signal by causing a pileup along this dorsal horn pathway, which is essentially what happens with an epidural anesthetic during childbirth: It puts up a barrier that causes a temporary traffic jam of pain signals along the dorsal horn.) Once the pain signal enters the base of the brain, it splits off in several different directions. One part of the signal travels to the amygdala, where it initiates your emotional response to pain. Another goes to your cerebral cortex, where it's processed consciously and decisions are made on how to respond to it. And another part of the signal heads toward the anterior cingulated region of your brain, where it is influenced by your mood. The mood-related component is most sensitive to your sex hormones, which is why estrogen plays an important role in pain management.

ESTROGEN DULLS PAIN BEFORE IT ENTERS YOUR BRAIN

Estrogen boosts production of the neurotransmitters norepinephrine and serotonin, which help blunt incoming pain signals. Like water putting out a fire, these neurotransmitters can douse the pain before it even enters your brain. So when your estrogen levels are high, you have less need for pain medications. But when estrogen levels are low, norepinephrine and serotonin are depleted and unable to send a signal from the brain down your spinal cord to block the pain at its source.

Estrogen also promotes sensitivity to endorphins, your body's natural painkillers, as well as to pharmaceutical painkillers. Again, that pain protection is lost when estrogen levels dip down. Your tolerance for pain is usually lowest when estrogen levels are lowest, just

ASK DR. GREENE

Q: I SUFFER FROM RHEUMATOID ARTHRITIS— CAN HORMONES HELP ME?

A: Hormone balance is a vital aspect of managing rheumatoid arthritis (which is caused by your immune cells abnormally attacking your joints) as well as other autoimmune disorders such as lupus and multiple sclerosis. Estradiol helps reduce pain, stabilize inflammation, and prevent some of the erosion in your bones that can deform your joints. Progesterone and testosterone are both involved in regulating your immune system and thus can potentially reduce flare-ups. Several studies, in fact, have found that using birth control pills during the reproductive years may actually help prevent rheumatoid arthritis from developing later in life. And more recent data suggest that the "bad" estrogen, estrone, may actually worsen your problem. So maintaining a healthy weight and sticking to a diet low in animal fats can also help reduce flare-ups.

before your period and during the first few days of menstrual bleeding—and during menopause. As you age and estrogen levels fall naturally, your tolerance for pain diminishes and your risk of chronic pain increases. The estrogen-associated drop in serotonin also increases your risk of depression, which further amplifies incoming pain signals. That's why minor bumps, bruises, or injuries that wouldn't have bothered you much in your youth can put you out of commission for a few hours later in life. The pain sources haven't changed, but your brain's interpretation of them has, thanks to the scarcity of estrogen.

MIGRAINE HEADACHES

An estimated 18 percent of all women in the United States experience one or more migraine headaches per year; that's about three times higher than the

HEADACHE ASSESSMENT QUIZ

ANSWER THE FOLLOWING QUESTIONS BASED ON THE TYPE OF HEADACHE THAT INTERFERES WITH YOUR DAILY ACTIVITIES. CIRCLE ONE ANSWER PER QUESTION.

WHEN YOU HAVE HEADACHES, HOW OFTEN DO YOU . . .

1. Have moderate to severe pain?	Never	Rarely	Usually	Always
2. Have pulsating, pounding, or throbbing pain?	Never	Rarely	Usually	Always
3. Have worse pain on one side of your head?	Never	Rarely	Usually	Always
4. Have worse pain when you move or bend over?	Never	Rarely	Usually	Always
5. Have nausea?	Never	Rarely	Usually	Always
6. Have sensitivity to or are bothered by sound?	Never	Rarely	Usually	Always
7. Have sensitivity to or are bothered by light?	Never	Rarely	Usually	Always
8. Need to limit or avoid daily activities?	Never	Rarely	Usually	Always
9. Want to lie down in a quiet, dark room?	Never	Rarely	Usually	Always
10. See visual disturbances, spots, or light flashes?	Never	Rarely	Usually	Always

Source: The National Headache Society

If you answered "Usually" or "Always" to three or more questions, your headaches could be migraines.

number of men. I've no doubt that sex hormones play a role in those numbers. Since men have more stable estradiol levels, they aren't subject to the falling estradiol levels that trigger migraines for women. Migraines, relatively rare in the childhood and teenage years, begin to occur more frequently when women are in their twenties. The highest rate of incidence occurs as women hit their late thirties and early forties. By age fifty, nearly 41 percent of women have experienced a migraine headache.

Migraine headaches are the result of a series of abnormal reactions of the nerves and blood vessels that are normally involved in healthy brain functioning. These reactions are usually in response to a triggering event—one of the most common being a change in sex hormone levels. A migraine begins with pain fibers of the nerves that are overly sensitive to the neurotransmitters serotonin and norepinephrine. When nerves are overly sensitive, they're more likely to cause dilation of blood vessels in the brain. That causes the throbbing pain characteristic of a headache. Some women even experience an aura, where they see flashing lights for a two-to-six-minute period before the onset of the migraine. Neuroimaging studies reveal that during an aura, a wave of reduced blood flow moves across the surface of the brain. Since a reduction in blood flow (called *oligemia*) is usually a sign of decreased neural activity, this suggests to me that the blood flow changes associated with migraines are a form of vascular instability, similar to hot flashes.

While the brain itself doesn't feel pain, it's covered by a sheet of tissue called the *dura mater* (Latin for "tough mother"), which contains sensory nerves and does feel pain. When this dura mater becomes overly sensitized, the slightest motion results in profound discomfort. That's the source of heightened pain with movement during a migraine headache. Sound and light make it worse, too, by triggering your "startle reflex" and making you jumpy. That sudden movement shakes your brain in a way that you'd hardly notice normally, but during a migraine it can be excruciating because of the heightened nerve sensitivity in the dura mater. Add all that to the pain generated by dilating blood vessels, and you've got an unrelenting pounding headache that makes you want to crawl into bed in a dark, silent room and not move a muscle.

The estrogen connection has another important influence on migraines through its impact on sleep. Serotonin is responsible for deep sleep, and norepinephrine is responsible for the dream phase of sleep (the deepest phase of sleep). Since the levels of both these neurotransmitters go down when

ASK DR. GREENE

Q: ARE THE FREQUENCY AND SEVERITY OF MY MIGRAINES DRIVEN BY MY MENSTRUAL CYCLE?

A: Yes. While migraines had long been thought to correlate with high estrogen levels, it's actually a sudden drop in estrogen levels that's the most common migraine trigger. (That's the reason I often give my migraine patients estrogen before their menstrual cycle—it provides a backup supply for their falling estrogen and prevents the migraine.) Upon reaching menopause, when estrogen levels are naturally lower but *stable*—no more dramatic fluctuations—most women (about 70 percent) have far fewer migraine headaches (though they are more susceptible to chronic aches and pains in general). But an *abrupt* reduction in estrogen, brought on by a hysterectomy or postpartum hormonal shifts, will likely increase the severity and frequency of headaches.

estrogen levels drop, the result is a disruption in sleep, which in turn causes a shift in the sleep hormone melatonin. Remember, anything that shifts your normal hormone patterns can set off a migraine. So whenever you change your sleep habits, you're more susceptible to migraines. That's why sleep disruption, either deliberate or unintentional, is a common trigger for migraine headaches. In fact, it's such a potent headache stimulator that the sleep centers of your brain are also referred to as the "migraine generators." In contrast, you may have noticed that when you've got a migraine, a long sleep will often relieve the headache. During sleep, your brain regenerates many of your neurotransmitters. If your serotonin and norepinephrine levels are depleted because of low estrogen levels, your body tries to compensate by using an unscheduled prolonged period of sleep to make more.

Migraines have a profound effect on quality of life. (An estimated half of all employed women lose at least six work days a year to migraines; that's nearly 38 million sick days each year!) Migraine headaches are so common and so debilitating that the World Health Organization lists them among the most disabling chronic disorders of developed nations. Like almost all headaches, migraines are diagnosed and treated based upon their symptom pattern. And since there are several kinds of migraines, the more accurately you're able to describe your symptoms, the more definitive your diagnosis will be. These are the typical symptoms:

- Localized pain on one side—usually a "throbbing" sensation.

- Pain worsened by movement, lights, and noise.

- Nausea.

- Vomiting—sometimes providing pain relief.

- Headache that typically lasts between four and seventy-two hours.

- Visual change, known as an aura—experienced by 20 percent of women with migraines.

PERFECT BALANCE SOLUTIONS FOR MIGRAINES

DIET

- Begin a food diary documenting what you're eating and whether or not you develop a headache after eating it. Try to identify patterns. Skipping meals is a common invitation for a migraine, since it alters metabolic hormones like insulin and growth hormones. Overeating can be just as bad.

- Magnesium can significantly reduce migraines but can cause intestinal problems when taken in supplement form. You can easily increase your magnesium levels without these side effects by consuming more nuts, whole grains, and occasional seafood.

- Soy can trigger migraines. If you enjoy soy, opt for whole soybeans. They have significant fiber content, which slows the absorption of phytoestrogens that can act as migraine triggers. Gradually incorporate other soy products like tofu, soy butter, or soy milk, but try to avoid highly processed soy supplements.

- Many foods and beverages are known to trigger migraines. These are the most common ones:

  Alcohol (especially wine)

  Processed meats such as hot dogs, deli meats, smoked meats, and jerky

  Food with monosodium glutamate (MSG)

  Chocolate

Aged cheeses

High-fat foods like French fries, bacon, and fried chicken

Yogurt and other dairy products

Wheat

If you suffer from frequent migraines, start out by eliminating all of these. After you've gone three months without a headache, start adding back those

CASE IN POINT

Tammy, age twenty-eight, became my patient about three years ago when her sister had urged her to see me for a second opinion before going through with a scheduled hysterectomy. Another doctor had urged her to consider surgery. He felt her headaches were hormone-related since the incidents so clearly followed the pattern of her menstrual cycles; birth control pills only made them worse; and Tammy had been headache-free while pregnant with her only child. Although Tammy and her husband had originally planned to have three children, the day-to-day struggle with her headaches was making it impossible for her to work or care properly for the one child she already had. After reviewing her history, I felt she had a classic case of "menstrual migraine." Although she was confident that the hysterectomy was her best option, I felt it was unnecessary. I asked her to delay her surgery so that we could have a full month to try another option, and she agreed.

For the first week she began the BioAntagonist nasal spray Synarel to temporarily shut down her ovaries, thereby creating the same low estrogen, testosterone, and progesterone levels that she would experience unnaturally after her surgery (only in this case it was reversible). At the same time, she began to use a Climara Bioldentical estrogen patch, 0.1 mg per day—a level much lower than that which her ovaries were currently producing. I also gave her a prescription for pain medication. The second week we added Topamax (25 mg per day), one of several antiseizure medications that have demonstrated a dramatic ability to prevent migraine headaches. By the third week, Tammy was back to work and was already pleased with her improvement. She agreed to another two weeks of the combination BioAntagonist (Synarel) suppression and stable Bioldentical (Climara) to add back estrogen. I also increased her Topamax to 50 mg daily. And she was off all prescription pain medications! At week four, Tammy canceled her hysterectomy.

Tammy continued the Synarel/Climara combination for three more months. At that time, we switched her to the BioSimilar hormone combination Ortho Evra, and she continued the Topamax 100 mg daily as a migraine prevention. She and her husband are now ready to have another child. I couldn't have asked for a better resolution.

compatible with the Perfect Balance meal plan, one food every three days, to see if they trigger a headache.

EXERCISE AND MIND-BODY BEST BETS

- Aerobic exercise restores your body's natural stress response and normalizes your brain's response to pain by generating the endorphins associated with the "runner's high." But migraine sufferers do not tolerate abrupt changes in physical activity. So create a schedule that *gradually* introduces aerobics into your exercise program.

- Once you've developed your routine, maintain it. Missed workouts can trigger headaches.

- Journaling can help, since migraine headaches can be prevented by establishing and monitoring routines. Any time you stray from your routine and have a headache, write down any unusual foods you've eaten, any change in your sleep or meal schedules, and any unusual stress you may have had that day. Include sexual activity, since this can be a trigger, although more commonly for men.

- Massage is one of the most effective ways to relieve pain. Various massage techniques can interrupt some pain signals (both chronic and referred) by relaxing specific regions where nerves interact with one another—sometimes called *trigger points.*

- *Biofeedback,* another excellent therapy for managing migraine headaches, refers to any technique that provides you with information about your physiological response, whether it's by monitoring pulse, skin temperature, or brain activity. When it comes to migraines, biofeedback can help retrain the brain to interrupt the pain response after it has been set in motion. Since your heart rate is always elevated when you're in pain, and you can learn through biofeedback techniques to reduce your heart rate while you're having a migraine, you can in effect reduce the pain of the migraine. To explore this technique without spending a lot of money, get a heart rate monitor at your local fitness center (these are so popular now that you can even find one that looks like a stylish wristwatch). Try creating your own biofeedback program by wearing the monitor during daily activity and see what aspects of your daily routine tend to increase your heart rate. When you do note an increase in your heart rate, sit in a quiet place and perform slow deep-breathing exercises. Note how your heart rate goes down. The more often you practice this technique, the better you will get.

COMPLEMENTARY MEDICINE

- Try acupuncture. Typical protocol for migraines is a minimum of ten weekly twenty-minute (at least) sessions. Ask your doctor or nurse practitioner for a referral, since the success of this technique depends upon the skill of the provider.

- Riboflavin (vitamin B_2), a 400 mg daily dose, can help with migraines. One study found it reduced migraine frequency by 50 percent! Relief is not immediate, however, so make a commitment to continue for at least three months before determining if you respond to this nutritional supplement.

- Feverfew *(Tenacetum parthenium)* is the only herb that has been tested appropriately and shown to be effective for migraine relief. Start with a dose lower than what is suggested on the package label and work your way up gradually. Whenever you add any supplements to your daily regimen, do it slowly. Never introduce more than one new supplement at a time. Note your start day in your journal to document whether or not your headaches increase, decrease, or stay the same.

BEST HORMONE TREATMENTS

Since pain management is most difficult when estrogen levels are falling, the key to successful hormone therapy for pain relief is to maintain steady levels of estrogen and free testosterone (which is able to help blunt pain because it can be converted into estradiol). Avoid rapidly absorbed products, which include those swallowed in pill form. Absorption through your skin or vagina provides a much more gradual and stable rise in estrogen levels.

- If your ovaries are still producing hormones, and especially if your menstrual cycles are irregular, I recommend going with a BioSimilar hormone contraceptive. Best bets are those with more stable release patterns, like the Ortho Evra patch or the Nuvaring vaginal delivery system. An additional advantage is that these will not suppress your testosterone levels like a birth control pill (since they're not absorbed through the stomach, they don't affect the production of SHBG).

• If you're trying to become pregnant, use a BioIdentical 0.1 mg estradiol patch beginning around menstrual day twenty-five. Continue until at least the seventh day after your menstrual cycle begins.

• For menopausal women, I recommend continuous uninterrupted use of a BioIdentical estradiol patch or comparable estradiol gel. The dose should be adjusted to minimize symptoms of too much estrogen (breast tenderness or bloating, for instance) or too little (hot flashes and sleep disturbance). If you have your uterus, I would suggest BioIdentical vaginal progesterone, such as Crinone 8 percent vaginal cream, for ten days every third month.

CHRONIC PELVIC PAIN

More than 30 percent of all women have experienced chronic pelvic pain (pain lasting at least three months) at one time in their lives. The primary sources of pain (aside from vaginal atrophy, which we discussed in the previous chapter) are usually interstitial cystitis, endometriosis, and vulvodynia or vaginismus. All of these disorders are worse when estrogen levels fall. And if you experience one of these problems, you have an 80 percent chance of experiencing another. Sexual intercourse, not surprisingly, has an impact on the pain related to all of them. For many women, the pain is bearable or even nonexistent until it is heightened or triggered by sexual activity. Other women have pain that is persistent and chronic, making sex the last thing on their minds. Let's take a look at each of the problems, with an eye toward solutions.

INTERSTITIAL CYSTITIS

Interstitial cystitis (IC), the chronic inflammation of the wall of the bladder, is one of the most commonly misdiagnosed causes of pelvic pain in women. Because the most common symptoms—frequent, urgent, or painful urination—can clear up after a week or so and then suddenly reappear three months later, IC is often mistaken for a recurrent urinary tract infection. The symptoms occur because the bladder lining isn't able to protect the bladder wall from getting irritated by urine. Anything that weakens this protective layer—like a bladder infection, sexual intercourse, or a drop in estrogen level—causes the condition to flare up. Sexual intercourse can easily aggravate the situation because the bladder is just above the anterior vaginal wall, which makes it vulnerable to the typical impact of sexual activity. Also, progesterone tends to cause a thickening of vaginal secretions, making intercourse even more painful. If you experience painful sex and the pain lingers hours afterward or is worse the next morning, IC should be considered.

PERFECT BALANCE SOLUTIONS FOR INTERSTITIAL CYSTITIS

DIET AND LIFESTYLE

- Lower the amount of toxins in your body. Avoid beer, wine, alcohol, and carbonated beverages. Instead go for filtered water, decaffeinated coffee, and plenty of green tea. Minimize consumption of animal products, especially aged or salt-cured meats and cheeses. Eliminate tomatoes, vinegar, condiments, fruit juices, and other high-acid foods.

- Begin a food diary. Whenever your symptoms get worse, write down everything you've eaten within the last twelve hours. Compare the lists over time to determine if the same foods keep showing up on your worst days, then eliminate them.

- Opt for low-impact exercises, like swimming or yoga, since high-impact movements such as running can exacerbate bladder pain.

- Contact the following two excellent patient advocacy organizations—they can provide you with a tremendous amount of emotional support and access to the latest research discoveries on emerging treatments for IC: Interstitial Cystitis Association (1-800-help-ICA, or www.ichelp.org.) and Interstitial Cystitis Network (1-707-538-9442, or www.ic-network.com). And you can accurately predict if you have IC with a questionnaire developed by Dr. Lowell Parsons of the University of California at San Diego. It can be confusing to score, however, so fill it out on the website, www.orthoelmiron.com/C06.01.htm, where it will be graded for you online. You can then take it with you to your doctor or nurse practitioner for verification and treatment.

TRADITIONAL AND COMPLEMENTARY MEDICINE

- Elmiron: This oral prescription is the mainstay of treatment for IC-induced bladder pain. Elmiron prompts thickening and reinforcement of the bladder's protective lining. I recommend a dose of 200 mg first thing each morning and again just before going to sleep. Continue for at least sixteen weeks. The treatment is even safe to continue during pregnancy and breast-feeding if needed.

- Cysta-Q complex is a combination of the potent antioxidant quercetin and various herbs, including black cohosh, valerian, and passionflower. For more information, call 1-877-284-3976, or go online to www.cystaq.com.

- Prelief, made by AkPharma Inc., is a dietary supplement that when taken with high-acid foods can lower their irritability level by 50–99 percent. It has to be taken at the same time you are eating the foods. Prelief doesn't require a prescription and is available at most pharmacies and supermarkets. For more information and comprehensive lists of irritating foods, go to the AkPharma website at www.prelief.com.

BEST HORMONE TREATMENTS

The key to alleviating IC is maintaining a steady level of estrogen and testosterone. Once again, recommendations are necessarily based upon the status of your ovaries.

- If your ovaries are still producing hormones, and especially if your menstrual cycles are irregular, then I recommend going with a BioSimilar hormone contraceptive. Best bets are those with more stable release patterns, like the Ortho Evra patch or the Nuvaring vaginal delivery system. An additional advantage of either of these is that they will not suppress your testosterone level the way a birth control pill does.

- If you're trying to become pregnant, use a BioIdentical 0.1 mg estradiol patch beginning around menstrual day twenty-five. Continue until at least the seventh day after your menstrual cycle begins.

- For menopausal women, I recommend continuous uninterrupted use of a BioIdentical estradiol patch or a comparable estradiol cream or gel. The

ASK DR. GREENE

Q: CAN I GET PREGNANT IF I HAVE ENDOMETRIOSIS?

A: Yes, you can become pregnant, but endometriosis reduces your chances of becoming pregnant, possibly because of irritation of the fallopian tubes, overactive white blood cells, or scar tissue. If you can achieve a pregnancy, though, you'll typically buy yourself three to ten years of relief from endometriosis symptoms. Pregnancy is actually the most effective and most natural way to treat endometriosis.

dose should be adjusted to minimize symptoms of too much estrogen (such as breast tenderness or bloating) or too little estrogen (hot flashes and sleep disturbance). If you have your uterus, I would suggest BioIdentical vaginal progesterone (for instance, Crinone 8 percent vaginal cream) for ten days every third month.

ENDOMETRIOSIS

Endometriosis is characterized by lesions that form on the outside of the uterus, made from misplaced tissue that normally lines the uterus (endometrium). Close to 50 percent of women actually have these lesions during their reproductive years, but most never have symptoms. In women who do have symptoms, the lesions cause pain whenever normal hormone fluctuations occur. Each time estrogen levels dip, the lesions can bleed, creating further irritation. Very often the lesions heal themselves and stop responding to monthly hormone fluctuations, but as the cells go through the natural healing process, scar tissue and infertility can result.

Endometrial lesions are usually deep in the pelvis, which dramatically increases the risk of deep pain during intercourse (especially around ovulation and menstruation). The associated pain can increase or decrease depending on hormonal changes or sexual positions, or may be persistent in one particular area during the early stages of the disease. This all varies from one woman to another according to the location of the lesions.

Several risk factors increase your chances of developing endometriosis: a family history of endometriosis; waiting till your thirties to have children; and, according to some studies, having naturally red hair or a very fair complexion. But the most common cause may be the strong link between endometriosis and certain BioMutagens, such as PCB, dioxin, and TCDD (a common herbicide). NASA was first to report the link in 1991. They found that monkeys exposed to certain chemicals were more than twice as likely to develop endometriosis. That launched an investigation that subsequently reported an alarming discovery: Several pollutants and pesticides present in soil and water at only trace levels were actually present in the fat and breast milk of women at significantly elevated levels. Since then, there's been even more evidence connecting BioMutagens to the risk of endometriosis.

PERFECT BALANCE SOLUTIONS FOR ENDOMETRIOSIS

DIET

- Going organic is your most important dietary strategy, since it's the best way to avoid the food-associated hormone-disrupting BioMutagens and impurities that promote endometriosis.

- Minimize your consumption of meat, and when you do eat animal products, avoid cooking methods like grilling and smoking, which increase toxicity.

- Drink water that has been filtered with activated charcoal filters; these remove a number of contaminants.

EXERCISE AND MIND-BODY BEST BETS

- Aerobic exercise restores your body's natural stress response. By lowering your stress hormone levels, you normalize your brain's response to pain. Exercise promotes the release of endorphins, which help reduce the "sensitization" of nerves associated with chronic pain.

- Hydrotherapy, heated water agitated in a Jacuzzi or a hot natural spring, promotes circulation and helps relieve the associated pains.

BEST HORMONE TREATMENTS

While hormone therapy doesn't cure endometriosis and may not prevent it, it is the mainstay of endometriosis pain relief. The key to alleviating the pain is preventing the hormonal fluctuations associated with a normal menstrual cycle and, for most women, preventing the very low estrogen levels that heighten the pain response. These are the best strategies:

- Continuous combined hormone therapy with BioSimilar hormones that suppress your own hormone production. Any combination hormone contraceptive will work, whether it's delivered by patch, pill, or vaginal ring. The goal is to suppress menstrual bleeding (medical term *amenorrhea*), so the dosage should be adjusted by your doctor to that end.

- If you're not attempting to get pregnant, Mirena, the BioLimited progesterone-releasing intrauterine system that remains in your uterus for five years, is effective for controlling endometriosis. It's very safe, and like all effective therapies for endometriosis, it typically suppresses menstrual bleeding altogether. (Several months of irregular menstrual spotting can occur in the beginning as your body adjusts to the regimen.)

- Use of BioAntagonists (sold under names like Lupron and Zoladex) to temporarily shut down your menstrual cycle is a common treatment for endometriosis. They're typically delivered by injections that have to be

CASE IN POINT

Cindy and Jeff came to see me for intrauterine insemination. Our first consultation revealed that the underlying reason for their request was the pain that Cindy felt during intercourse—a pain that was at its worst when she was at the peak of her fertility. I convinced them it was worth our time to further evaluate the source of the pain. The fact that Cindy's pain worsened around ovulation made me suspicious that endometriosis might be a factor and could also be contributing to infertility. When I learned that Cindy's pain continued and was often worse the morning after sex, I asked her to fill out a PUF (pain-urgency-frequency) questionnaire to further define symptoms related to urination. Her score suggested that interstitial cystitis was also contributing to her pain. I recommended Elmiron to relieve pain from her bladder but suggested we still check for endometriosis—the two conditions are so often associated with each other that they are often referred to as the "evil twins." I then did a laparoscopy, which confirmed that Cindy did indeed have endometriosis. I treated the condition through surgery, and afterward Cindy continued on the Elmiron. On the next PUF questionnaire, her bladder symptom score showed a marked improvement, indicating her IC was responding to treatment, as well. She also started on an organic diet to reduce her intake of BioMutagens. Five months after their initial office visit, I got a call from Cindy telling me that she was pregnant. After nearly five years of infertility, not only had they conceived, but Cindy was once again enjoying the intimacy of their relationship.

repeated once a month or once every three months, depending on the dosage selected. My biggest concern with them is that they can't be discontinued prematurely if they make you feel bad or you decide you want to get pregnant. A better option is Synarel nasal spray, a BioAntagonist that can be stopped at any time.

- A low dose of BioIdentical estrogen therapy usually makes any BioAntagonist treatment more tolerable. It can help prevent hot flashes and mood swings, while providing better pain relief and bone strength protection. Any of these BioAntagonist/BioIdentical combination regimens can be continued for six months or longer.

For more information on endometriosis, contact the Endometriosis Association at 1-414-355-2200, or visit their website at www.endometriosisassn .org/endo.html.

VULVODYNIA AND VAGINISMUS

Vulvodynia is pain of the vulva, which includes the labia, clitoris, and opening of the vagina. We're not certain what causes vulvodynia, but a variety of conditions can trigger it, including injury, irritation (from tight jeans, nylon underwear, and the like), chronic infection (yeast infections, bacterial vaginosis, herpes), and a genetic predisposition. In some cases you may be able to nip the problem in the bud if you can identify and eliminate any specific triggers that bring on symptoms. A new "female"-friendly bike seat, shaped to direct pressure away from the vulva, for example, would be a good solution to pain brought on by regular bike riding. (First get an examination to document the location of your pain and rule out the presence of visible lesions or infections.)

Vaginismus, the more variable of the two conditions, is a painful prolonged muscular contraction or spasm of the vagina due to an unintentional reflex. Even worse, the reflex can

ASK DR. GREENE

Q. HOW DOES MENOPAUSE AFFECT ENDOMETRIOSIS?

A: Over time, with the steady, nonfluctuating hormone levels of menopause, endometriosis withers away naturally. That's the reason hysterectomy with removal of the ovaries—a treatment that induces menopause (and one I strongly discourage except in the most severe cases)—is such a common treatment option.

become a habit. For example, if you repeatedly experience pain when something is inserted into your vagina, your body will eventually develop a defensive reaction that promotes muscle contractions to block any such insertion. Your body then continues to react automatically and tries to fend off any kind of insertion—even consensual sex with a beloved partner. Your muscles contract rather than relax as intercourse begins, and you feel pain. The good news is that since this is a "learned" response, therapies that target the brain can help "unlearn" the source of distress.

PERFECT BALANCE SOLUTIONS FOR VULVODYNIA AND VAGINISMUS

DIET, LIFESTYLE, AND COMPLEMENTARY MEDICINE

- Calcium citrate has been shown to be helpful in reducing formations of oxalate, the salts excreted in urine that irritate the skin. The less oxalate you have in your urine, the less irritation to your vulva. I recommend a tablet combination of calcium citrate (1,000 mg) and magnesium (500 mg) each morning and evening.

- Avoid high doses of vitamin C. Any more than 250 mg per day can promote oxalate formation and worsen vulvodynia.

- Reach out to other women with this condition through self-help groups like the National Vulvodynia Association (1-301-299-0775, or www .NVA.org). They'll help keep you up-to-date on the latest information so you can make sure your health care provider is aware of the latest therapeutic options.

- The Complete Vaginismus Kit is a two-book set and video that tells you everything you need to know to direct your own therapy. It can also educate your partner to help you overcome this intimate challenge together, in the privacy of your own home. At $150, it's less than a typical doctor's office visit and puts you back in control. For more information, call 1-888-834-1665, or visit the website at www.vaginismus.com.

- Biofeedback has been one of the most consistently useful mind-body therapies for vaginismus. It helps you retrain your mind and bring it into a state of relaxation so that you can interrupt the learned response of reflexively contracting vaginal muscles. Contact the Biofeedback Certification Institute of America at 1-303-420-2902, or visit the website at www .bcia.org/directory to find a qualified professional in your area.

• Cysta-Q complex is a treatment that overlaps with chronic pain syndromes. It's a proprietary blend of herbal supplements originally formulated for women with IC, but at least one study has shown it can provide relief for women with vulvodynia, as well. For more information, call 1-877-284-3976, or go to www.cystaq.com.

BEST HORMONE TREATMENTS

Topical estrogen therapy has been found to be helpful for many women. I recommend a trial of BioIdentical estrogen 0.5 mg per day applied directly to the vulva. It can be dispensed as a cream by most compounding pharmacies, but have your doctor specify that they should not use parabens (a BioMutant preservative) in the formula. A good alternative is Estrasorb, a new BioIdentical estrogen cream. Since this formulation was released late in 2004, some pharmacies may not yet be familiar with it. It should be continued for at least three months but may be used indefinitely; your dose may be adjusted by your health care provider as needed.

CHAPTER TEN

IMPROVING
YOUR MOODS

Moods and emotions may seem synonymous, but in fact they are very different. While emotions are short-lived and beneficial, moods are persistent and troublesome. Emotions are temporary motivations that arise in the inner portions of our brain in response to a situation, person, object, or specific thought; they're essentially what "turn us on"—or off. When we choose to make a conscious effort, our "rational self" can override an emotional response if it seems inappropriate to a given situation.

Moods, on the other hand, are seemingly uncontrollable; you may realize that you're in a "bad mood," but your rational self can't override it. While moods can be positive, those that constitute disorders are negative—they appear suddenly, for no apparent reason, and interfere with our happiness, relationships, and effectiveness. If you've ever woken up on "the wrong side of the bed," you know how easily one of these underlying moods can influence your emotions and life for hours on end; in fact, it can ruin your entire day (and much more if you suffer from depression). I believe that our moods are deeply influenced by the hormonal changes that are occurring in the body at any given time and are a direct manifestation of the hormone-brain connection. When you can master this connection, you can in effect control your moods.

Particular hormones and various combinations of hormones are associated with different moods. Low estrogen levels can contribute to depression; elevated testosterone levels can exacerbate irritability; and high estrogen levels combined with sudden drops in progesterone can worsen anxiety. We know from brain-imaging studies that the emotional centers of the brain surround the hormonal control center (the hypothalamus) almost like the shell on a walnut. This anatomical proximity makes for an inevitable mutual interaction.

Emotions and hormones need to be in sync to produce appropriate behaviors. When they're not, mood disorders occur. The emotion of fear and the resultant rises in the hormone cortisol, for instance, produce appropriate "fight or flight" behavior. Cortisol elevates an emotion like fear or surprise and returns to normal levels when the emotion subsides. When emotions don't subside—when they turn into long-term moods—cortisol levels remain continuously elevated, which reinforces the mood. To make matters worse, the chronically elevated levels of cortisol suppress sex hormone production, resulting in depression. This explains why there's a higher incidence of depression among menopausal women whose sex hormone levels have already bottomed out.

ASK DR. GREENE

Q: WHAT EXACTLY IS A MOOD DISORDER?

A: It's an overpowering, persistent mood that you have for a prolonged period of time and that is so severe, it interferes with your ability to function and prevents you from experiencing your emotions effectively. Women are two to four times more likely to have a mood disorder than men. Mood disorders are responsible for 80 percent of all suicides.

SEX HORMONES AND MOOD

The mood disorders most obviously affected by sex hormone levels are depression and anxiety. You're much more likely to experience these problems during times of hormonal change, such as after the delivery of a baby, before the menstrual cycle, or during the transition into menopause. Modern brain imaging shows that mood disorders are the result of an imbalance of neurotransmitters, often brought on by a shift in sex hormone levels.

Mood represents the sum total effect of the neurotransmitters dopamine, norepinephrine, and "feel good" serotonin. (The male brain makes about 50 percent more serotonin than yours does. That already gives men an edge when it comes to mood stability.) Your serotonin production varies in accordance with your estrogen levels, so whenever your estrogen levels fall—and that happens frequently—your serotonin levels bottom out, as well. But that's not all. Estrogen also boosts production of dopamine and norepinephrine, which generally has an excitatory or "mood lifting" effect on your brain. But if estrogen levels are *too high,* the senses become too "lifted," making you susceptible to anxiety and irritability. When you superimpose the monthly rise and fall of progesterone on this chemical roller coaster, it becomes readily apparent that hormonal balance is a key to stabilizing moods.

WEEKLY MOOD WATCH

Before we discuss solutions for the specific mood disorders most closely linked to sex hormone imbalance, take a minute to fill out the following questionnaire. It will help you get a better idea of your own mood fluctuations. I highly recommend that you retake this little quiz at least once a week for the next six weeks to get a better idea of how your own sex hormone levels may be influencing your personal perceptions of the world. It can be an illuminating experience. To create a score, list whether or not you've experienced any of the following feelings during the previous three days. Grade each symptom using the following scale.

0—I did not experience this symptom

1—This occurred, but it wasn't bothersome

2—Happened, but it didn't prevent me from getting things done

3—This really interfered with daily activities

1. Depression _____   6. Anxiety_____

2. Dizziness or fainting_____   7. Palpitations/heart pounding_____

3. Irritability/nervous tension _____   8. Mood swings_____

4. Crying spells_____   9. Confusion/forgetfulness _____

5. Insomnia or fatigue_____   10. Appetite changes or cravings _____

TOTAL _____

Total up your score for each week. Here's the bottom line:

0–10 Great! You probably don't have a mood disorder—but keep our solutions in mind for any troubled times ahead.

11–20 Your mood changes are negatively impacting your life, but there's an excellent chance our solutions will help relieve many of your symptoms.

21–30 You probably have a clinical problem. You'll find helpful suggestions here, but you should also seek professional help and treatment.

If your scores stay in the same range as you compare them from one week to the next, it means you have a chronic mood disorder as opposed to premenstrual syndrome. So the anxiety and depression sections in this chapter will probably be more helpful to you than the PMS section. If you see that your scores fluctuate from week to week, you'll likely find that they correlate with changes in your sex hormone levels. That's the telltale sign of PMS, the common mood pattern that impacts about 60–85 percent of women, to one degree or another, over the course of their lives.

PREMENSTRUAL SYNDROME AND PREMENSTRUAL DYSPHORIC DISORDER

Many women say they almost feel like two different people during the course of a month. During the two weeks following the onset of their menstrual cycle, they feel like the most efficient, personable, dynamic women in the world; but during the ten to fourteen days that follow, their emotions run the gamut from vulnerable and weepy, to edgy and angry, to indecisive and wishy-washy. To meet the official diagnostic criteria of premenstrual syndrome, you have to experience irritability, sudden mood swings, depression, or anxiety that improves or resolves shortly after your menstrual cycle begins.

In addition, you have to experience at least three or four of the following symptoms during the seven to fourteen days prior to the onset of your menstrual cycle:

- Feeling out of control

- Change in appetite or cravings

- Insomnia or difficulty awakening

- Decreased interest in normally joyful activities

- Difficulty with concentration

- Physical symptoms such as breast tenderness, bloating, constipation, or diarrhea

Symptoms are also graded based on their severity. About 5 percent of women have symptoms that are so severe, they feel emotionally or physically impaired, which translates to *premenstrual dysphoric disorder (PMDD)*. The chance of developing PMDD increases with age.

Both PMS and PMDD are the result of the dynamic relationship between changing estrogen and progesterone levels that occur during the menstrual cycle. Anything that interrupts menstrual cycling, including pregnancy, certain hormone treatments, and menopause, disrupts PMS/PMDD.

The associated moods of PMS are the result of the interrelationship between hormonal balance and the brain. It's the brain connection that causes premenstrual syndrome to vary from one woman to the next. Because every woman's brain is unique and reacts differently to hormonal dynamics, all women experience fluctuating hormones differently. While some are more susceptible to the estrogen drop that causes depression, others are more sensitive to the progesterone loss that causes anxiety. Still others develop symptoms like irritability, impulsiveness, and aggression, because they're especially sensitive to the low estrogen/low progesterone/high testosterone combination. So it's not the hormones themselves that cause PMS, but rather their unique combination and the way each woman's brain reacts to them. Even women with the most severe PMDD don't have abnormally high or low levels of progesterone or estrogen, which explains why blood tests are useless here as a diagnostic tool.

Your ovaries produce gradually increasing amounts of estrogen beginning about five days after your menstrual bleeding starts. Most women feel quite good during these first two weeks. The problems usually start around three to seven days after ovulation as progesterone levels begin to rise.

RULE OUT OTHER POSSIBLE HORMONE CAUSES

Though no other naturally occurring hormone problems can imitate PMS and PMDD, some women can experience changes that resemble PMS from almost any hormonal birth control method. No one pill, patch, or ring is more likely to cause these problems than another; it's all about individual response. Some contraceptive methods simply bring on PMS symptoms in some women and not in others. Accurate symptom charting can confirm whether or not the one you're using is causing you problems. The good news is that by keeping track of your symptoms, you'll be able to spot which products created the problems, and with information about your unique reaction, a good health care provider can suggest a better alternative. That's one of the benefits of charting your symptoms.

PMS SYMPTOM TRACKING CHART

Start at the beginning of your period and use the following rating system to monitor how you feel on a daily basis. In the "Day of Month" row, circle the days you are menstruating. At the same time each day, rate your symptom to indicate how severe each symptom was over the past twenty-four hours. When marking your symptoms, indicate as follows:

0 = none

1 = mild

2 = moderate

3 = severe

If you forgot to fill in a day, place an X in the "Day of Month" bar to signify that you did not fill in the chart for that day. Make a photocopy of this chart and continue on the new page on the first day of your next menstrual cycle. For the best results, you should track your symptoms for three or four months.

Start by assessing which symptoms are wreaking havoc upon your life. Then review the solutions that follow and choose those that will best suit your needs. For persistent or severe symptoms, share your Menstrual Symptom Calendar with your health care provider.

DAY OF MONTH	1	2	3	4	5	6	7	8	9	10	11	12	13	14	15	16	17	18	19	20	21	22	23	24	25	26	27	28	29	30	31
Irritability																															
Loss of concentration																															
Constipation or diarrhea																															
Anxiety																															
Breast tenderness																															
Sadness																															
Sudden mood swings																															
Loss of interest in enjoyable activities																															
Feeling out of control																															
Sleep disturbances																															
Depression																															
Bloating																															
Food cravings/ change in appetite																															
Fatigue																															
Other																															

COMMON TREATMENT ERRORS

Though mood-stabilizing agents like Prozac, Zoloft, and Paxil are legitimate treatment options, they shouldn't be the first line of therapy, since in some cases they can create other side effects, such as cravings, insomnia, or sexual dysfunction. Ultraaggressive moves like a hysterectomy with removal of the ovaries should be the very last line of therapy, considered only in the most extreme cases of PMS or PMDD. I strongly caution against any irreversible changes like that. I feel the best idea for women with severe symptoms who are thinking of taking that drastic step is first to go through "artificial menopause" with a reversible BioAntagonist. That mimics the hormonal status they'll experience after a hysterectomy. If they feel better on that regime (and some women do), then it *may* make sense to proceed with surgery.

PERFECT BALANCE SOLUTIONS FOR PMS AND PMDD

Try the following lifestyle changes first—not just during PMS bouts, but throughout the month. They may bring complete relief, or at least reduce your symptoms to a more tolerable level. If symptoms still linger, try the hormone therapy route.

CASE IN POINT

One of my patients, Dayle, a twenty-one-year-old woman in the air force, had severe PMDD, which had been documented on her chart by a military physician. When she later decided to train to be a fighter pilot, she was told by her commanding officer that she could do it only if she had a hysterectomy—with the removal of both ovaries. Since she was so young and hadn't had any children, I urged her to reconsider her decision and suggested that she see a fertility counselor I work with to make sure she fully understood the permanence of the decision she was making. With my encouragement, she agreed to a trial of a BioAntagonist to temporarily induce menopause and eliminate PMDD symptoms. Initially her menopausal symptoms were horrible, but we gradually got them under control by giving her a Bioidentical combination of estradiol (a patch) and testosterone (gel compounded by a local pharmacy). In spite of feeling better for several months, she decided to proceed with the hysterectomy, and I performed her surgery. She went on to complete the pilot training that was so important to her. I believe she would have done well with continued medical therapy, but bureaucratic career obstacles—especially in the military—are not easy to overcome. Fortunately, most women never need to go to such extremes.

DIET

- Start by increasing fiber intake to 25–30 grams per day (soluble and insoluble combined). If you get two to four servings of fruits and three to five servings of vegetables a day, you'd be well on your way toward meeting your soluble fiber needs. Bran cereals are a great way to obtain insoluble fiber ($^1/_3$ cup contains 5–8 grams on average). Lentils and beans contain an average of 6–8 grams per $^1/_2$ cup serving. Incorporate both insoluble and soluble fiber into your daily diet. Taking these steps is an effective way to reduce bloating and stabilize gastrointestinal complaints such as constipation and diarrhea.

- Increase intake of Hormone Power Carbs, but reduce fat-calorie intake to avoid weight gain. Power Carbs are helpful in boosting serotonin production in the brain, which in turn helps reduce moodiness.

- Satisfy your cravings—but do it carefully. Studies show that by savoring rich foods, like letting chocolate melt slowly on your tongue and enjoying each aspect (taste, aroma, texture), you get an optimal boost in serotonin and dopamine release in your brain, which can relieve many mood-related complaints.

- Cut back or eliminate alcohol consumption during low mood periods. Alcohol can worsen depression.

EXERCISE AND MIND-BODY BEST BETS

- Don't skip the aerobic portion of your exercise. It increases serotonin production, resets cortisol, and boosts testosterone production. The result is an overall improvement in mood.

- Avoid athletics that require more balance and coordination during your symptomatic periods. Women with PMS or PMDD are at higher risk of injury due to decreased agility when progesterone levels begin to rise.

- Practice tai chi, yoga, or other similar relaxation techniques. They will reduce stress hormones like cortisol, which results in some stabilization of estrogen, testosterone, insulin, and growth hormone. Late in the day is best, because it helps establish the relaxation response and ease the transition to a restorative night of sleep, which will also help stabilize the other hormones and reset them for the next day.

- Visualization and relaxation tapes can help when relaxation is difficult to manage on your own (which can be often if you're depressed or anxious). Calming music in the car, as background atmosphere around the house, or on the job (if possible) can work wonders.

- Aromatherapy—oils, candles, herbal tea: Since smell sensations are more acute when estrogen levels are high, use calming fragrances like vanilla, lavender, or orangewood. Odors are one of the most direct paths to the "emotion" centers of the brain, and pleasant scents can calm the emotions.

COMPLEMENTARY MEDICINE

- Calcium has been shown to reduce physical symptoms of PMS by as much as 50 percent. Taking supplements may make muscles, nerves, and blood vessels less irritable. Take 750 mg of calcium carbonate (such as Tums EX) twice a day with meals for best absorption.

- Supplement calcium with magnesium. There's less supportive data regarding its ability to relieve PMS symptoms, but magnesium is a smart companion to calcium in any case because calcium alone inhibits the absorption of magnesium. Take magnesium supplements—200 mg of magnesium oxide with your morning meal.

- Take vitamin B_6 supplements. Try the B complex, 25–100 mg per day. This supplement contains a range of B vitamins, including thiamin (B_1), riboflavin (B_2), niacin (B_3), pantothenic acid (B_5), pyroxidine (B_6), and cobalamin (B_{12}), as well as biotin and folic acid. The vitamin B complex can be found in most multivitamin-mineral supplements.

- Primrose oil, 500 mg per day, can reduce breast tenderness. It contains GLA (gamma linolenic acid), which can correct deficiencies or abnormalities in essential fatty acid metabolism. Since there are few specific suggestions and fewer proven cures for breast tenderness, this is definitely worth trying.

• Consider supplementing with chasteberry (aka monk's pepper). Though we don't know how this herb acts directly, many women find it gives them relief from bloating and breast tenderness. Dosage recommendations vary by preparation; as always with BioUnknowns, start with the lowest recommended dose. (Don't use if you are trying to get pregnant.)

BEST HORMONE TREATMENTS

If you're not trying to get pregnant, your most effective regimen is one that stabilizes your hormonal fluctuation with a BioSimilar estrogen and BioLimited progestin. The BioSimilar estrogen promotes serotonin production and improves your mood, while the BioLimited progestin helps prevent exacerbation of progesterone's typical effects, like irritability and fatigue, because its BioLimited formulation is not recognized by the brain. The right balance can be most easily achieved by combining them in hormonal contraceptives. I've found that the following birth control pills are effective in eliminating symptoms of PMS and PMDD. (This is a good example of the off-label usage we talked about.)

> **FIRST CHOICE:** Yasmin oral contraceptive pill. This birth control pill has been shown to reduce mood problems, cravings, and bloating in women with PMDD. It is generally well tolerated and is not associated with weight gain.

> **GOOD ALTERNATIVES:** Ortho Tri-Cyclen, Ortho Tri-Cyclen Lo, and Estrostep.

If you're actively trying to get pregnant, try applying a BioIdentical estrogen patch when you first feel symptoms. Since it delivers a continuous low dose of estradiol, it supplements the estrogen that your body is already producing and stabilizes the unsteady estrogen-progesterone balance associated with PMS symptoms. Most important, it reduces the monthly plunge in serotonin production that normally occurs about one week before menstrual bleeding.

DEPRESSION

On the most basic level, depression is hyperactivity of the frontal lobe of the brain. The earmarks of depression include persistent feelings of emptiness or hopelessness, lost interest in formerly enjoyable activities, feeling all sorts of new aches and pains, trouble concentrating or remaining focused, and trouble

ASK DR. GREENE

Q: HOW CAN I TELL IF I HAVE DEPRESSION OR IF I'M JUST FEELING DOWN?

A: The major factors that differentiate depression from a mild case of the blues are the duration and severity of symptoms. To qualify as true depression, your feelings have to persist on a daily basis for two weeks and interfere with your relationships, activities, or work.

eating or sleeping. Because these symptoms can be subtle, it's easy to overlook them.

Though we don't know exactly why some of us are more susceptible to depression than others, it's becoming clear that there's a genetic influence and that low levels of the neurotransmitters serotonin or norepinephrine are almost certainly involved. Although most depressed people feel very tired and lethargic, neuroimaging studies show that their brains tend to be overactive. So even though they move slowly and with great effort, their brain is constantly in a hyper-alert activity state. It is simply unable to rest and recover in preparation for future stress.

Stressful events trigger the majority of first and second bouts of depression. After a second episode, you increase your chances of suffering another episode of depression *without* any kind of triggering event—it's almost as if the limbic portion of your brain (the area that generates emotions and moods) "learns" how to be depressed and doesn't need a stressor anymore. Through brain imaging, we've actually seen a direct correlation between chronic activation of the stress hormone–producing regions of the brain and depression. And we've discovered that the brain activity in these regions encourage the production of corticotropin-releasing factor, which sets off the domino effect leading to the stress response. CRF has been implicated in anxiety, nervousness, and depression, as well as in growth suppression and shrinkage in parts of the brain (which raises the risks of dementia and memory problems).

SEX HORMONES AND DEPRESSION

While stress hormones may be involved in initiating depression, sex hormones play a role in the duration and severity of the depression. Because both estrogen and testosterone promote new nerve growth and boost production of norepinephrine and serotonin, they actually help alleviate depression.

Progesterone, on the other hand, because of its highly sedative effects, can exacerbate the fatigue you feel with depression. In fact, if your hormone balance is seriously progesterone heavy, it can actually cause or worsen clinical depression. Each woman's response to her own progesterone is extremely variable and unpredictable. It can cause sleepiness, memory problems, clumsiness, and irritability for some and cause no problems whatsoever for others. The brain areas activated by progesterone are rich in GABA receptors (primarily the cortex and thalamus). That, in effect, makes progesterone a hormonal downer because it activates the same region of the brain as sleep-promoting sedatives.

When GABA activity remains elevated, the brain develops a tolerance for it. (This is true whether they're taken in pill form—as sleeping pills, for instance—or are produced naturally by the adrenal glands through the conversion of progesterone.) When a tolerance develops, their sedative (and intoxicating) effects are reduced, which leads to symptoms of withdrawal when activity is not elevated. The same thing happens when elevated levels of progesterone fall, which is why progesterone can cause depressive symptoms as levels rise and then again as they fall. All these constant fluctuations, needless to say, can make things mighty uncomfortable in terms of mood. Many women have no adverse reactions to normal amounts of progesterone but develop symptoms during periods of high progesterone production, such as the third trimester of pregnancy. Others easily tolerate the high levels but have severe reactions to progesterone withdrawal after they deliver their child—the likely trigger of postpartum depression.

These kinds of hormone-brain complexities have no doubt contributed to the difficulty in teasing out the complex relationship between sex hormones and mood disorders. We've still got a lot to learn before we can fully appreciate why and how normal hormone shifts can create such variable problems from one woman to the next. That's why I don't advocate using hormones alone to treat moderate or severe depression. But they can improve your response to treatment and in some situations may be valuable in preventing a recurrence.

In general, your risk of depression is highest whenever your hormone levels are either falling or changing dramatically—at adolescence, postpartum, perimenopause, and menopause. The following table gives you a good idea of the typical changes in brain chemistry associated with depression and how estrogen, because of its unique ability to reverse abnormal neurotransmitter changes, affects them. (This holds true for either natural estrogen or supplementation.)

CHANGES IN NEUROTRANSMITTER PRODUC-TION AND ACTIVITY DURING DEPRESSION VS. DURING ESTROGEN USE

	DURING DEPRESSION	DURING ESTROGEN USE
Serotonin	↓	↑
Norepinephrine	↓	↑
Dopamine	↓ or ↑	↑
Adrenaline sensitivity	↓	↑
Endorphin	↓	↑

RULE OUT OTHER POSSIBLE CAUSES OF DEPRESSIONLIKE SYMPTOMS

If you're feeling sluggish, several other hormonal imbalances should be considered and can easily be ruled out. Two metabolic disturbances, hypothyroidism and diabetes, can be detected with a simple blood test (TSH, and glycosylated hemoglobin for diabetes). Together, these two blood tests can indicate whether your depression is an energy-hormone-related problem or a chemical imbalance in the brain.

Hyperparathyroidism is an oversecretion of the parathyroid gland, a group of four pea-size glands behind your thyroid. When they release too much parathyroid hormone, your bones release too much calcium. The elevated calcium levels can cause many of the same symptoms as depression, like weakness, fatigue, melancholy, constipation, aches, and appetite changes. Hyperparathyroidism is a fairly rare disorder that can be ruled out by a simple blood test to measure calcium levels.

Cushing's disease, the last hormone condition that can be confused with depression, develops from an excess production of the stress hormone cortisol. This is different from the excess cortisol that can actually cause depression because it's the result not of stress, but of a tumor that has developed. The tumor actually sends out signals to the adrenal glands to produce stress hormones. This is a very rare condition that can be difficult to diagnose, since elevated cortisol levels are also a sign of stress-related depression.

PERFECT BALANCE SOLUTIONS FOR DEPRESSION

Clinical depression is a major health problem and should be treated appropriately. Again, I am not suggesting that hormones be used to treat a case of severe depression or that clinical depression can be managed solely on the contents of this book. It can't. But these guidelines can help put you on the road to recovery and help prevent a relapse. From my experience, there is simply no doubt that falling levels of estrogen or testosterone are involved with a higher risk of depression.

To make recommendations that are most useful to you, I must first consider what hormones (if any) your ovaries are making. With that in mind, the natural balancing recommendations are based upon whether or not you are still experiencing menstrual cycles, at risk of becoming pregnant, or breast-feeding. This is especially important in the consideration of various herbs and supplements, since many of these BioUnknowns can reduce the effectiveness of contraception or may produce risks to your baby should you become pregnant.

Many doctors assume that women who are depressed are sexually inactive or that pregnant women don't get depressed because of their high estrogen levels. Neither of these assumptions is true. In a recent study of nearly 3,500 pregnant women, participants were asked to complete questionnaires midway through their pregnancy. The results showed that 20 percent of the expectant mothers had significant symptoms of depression, but few were being treated for it. Recent research shows that the elevated stress hormone levels in a pregnant woman can have lifelong effects upon the baby. Please review the following recommendations carefully and consult your health care provider to ensure you don't become pregnant unintentionally. If you are pregnant, seek treatment from your health care provider in addition to the natural balancing approach.

DIET

- Watch fats carefully. Omega-3 fatty acids (from flaxseed, soy, cold-water fish, beans, and walnuts) can improve depression by enhancing serotonin production. Too much omega-6 fatty acid (mainly from vegetable oils), on the other hand, can worsen it. Make sure to get at least 5 grams of omega-3s a day. One easy way to do that is to add 2 tablespoons (3.2 grams) of ground flaxseed or 1 tablespoon of flaxseed oil (6.6 grams) to various meals or juices. Getting enough omega-3 is especially important during pregnancy and while breast-feeding, since omega-3 (and, to a lesser degree, omega-6) is used by the developing brain of the fetus and newborn.

Although cold-water fish are a good source of omega-3, they're best consumed in moderation (no more than two 4-ounce servings per week), during pregnancy and breast-feeding to avoid any BioMutagens that could be passed on to your baby.

- For acute phases of depression, reverse the ratio of protein to carbs recommended in the Perfect Balance diet: This short-term (six to eight weeks only) high-protein/minimal carb plan is similar to the Atkins diet, but with much less concentration on animal fats. Make soy, fish, and whole grains your diet foundation during this time.

EXERCISE AND MIND-BODY BEST BETS

- Regular exercise will not only help resolve an existing bout of depression, but has been shown to reduce risk of recurrence. Try to get at least forty minutes or more of high-exertion aerobic exercise a day, since it boosts serotonin and lowers stress hormones. Yoga, tai chi, or other mind-centering exercise is also therapeutic. Seek out a class at least four days per week. The social interaction of a class situation—even if you don't utter a word to other class members—is always a good antidote for depression. And the physiological benefits—boosting the immune system and blood flow, lowering stress hormones, and promoting the relaxation response—are invaluable when recovering from a depressive episode or as an aid in its prevention.

- Get outside. Sunlight has been shown to markedly improve moods owing to the brain-boosting role of *melanocortin (MSH),* a hormone produced in your skin when exposed to ultraviolet light.

- Fill your home with bright white lights—preferably "full spectrum" lights of at least 6,000 lux—and make sure you're exposed to them for at least two hours in the early morning and two hours in late afternoon. They generally don't cost any more to operate than regular light bulbs, but they can be a big help in preventing depression, especially in the winter months when natural daylight fades early.

COMPLEMENTARY MEDICINE

- SAM-e (S-adenosyl-methionine), a metabolite found in all cells, is a popular supplement for depression. While the jury's still out on this one, its effectiveness is most likely due to its ability to serve as a building block for important neurotransmitters like dopamine and norepinephrine. It's usually taken as a 200 mg tablet two to four times a day (200–800 mg per day). Caution is advised for women susceptible to bipolar depression, as SAM-e can trigger a manic episode.

- Saint-John's-wort (botanical name *Hypericum*) may be effective for minor depression. I'm not a big fan of it, since it can possibly interfere with estrogen (by breaking it down in the liver). Women on birth control pills should be aware that Saint-John's-wort can decrease the pill's effectiveness and increase the risk of pregnancy. It's also been shown to interfere with medications that are used after organ transplantation and drugs used to treat HIV. To reduce mild depression, the recommended dose is 300–1,800 mg a day of a standardized formulation, taken for at least six to eight weeks.

BEST HORMONE TREATMENTS

Depression strikes at any age. Hormonal change, in addition to stressful life events, increases your susceptibility to depression. Therefore, my guidelines are dependent upon which hormone imbalance has participated in your condition. Most certainly we'll want to supplement your estrogen with a BioIdentical or BioSimilar estrogen to boost your serotonin production and stabilize your progesterone production at the lowest possible level. Our best strategies for meeting that twofold goal depend on how well your ovaries are functioning and whether or not you've had a hysterectomy. If you haven't, you'll need some progesterone to reduce your risk of vaginal bleeding (or pregnancy) and to reduce your risk of uterine cancer. Here are the options:

- Low-dose combination contraceptives. If you are still having menstrual cycles, even if they are irregular, you'll need to stabilize your estrogen and progesterone levels. My preferred methods are the Ortho Evra transdermal patch or the Nuvaring vaginal delivery system. Both of these products are commonly used for contraception. They provide continuous delivery of a fixed-dose regimen of BioSimilar estrogen and a very low dose of BioLimited progestin while suppressing any additional production of these hormones by your own ovaries. That leaves you with a totally predictable and stable hormonal status. The other advantage is that these preparations do not suppress your level of testosterone, another mood-improving hormone.

- An intrauterine progesterone device partnered with a BioIdentical estrogen patch. This very safe alternative to the low-dose combination contraceptives uses the Mirena intrauterine system. Mirena provides an ultraslow low dose of BioLimited progestin to prevent vaginal bleeding and endometrial cancer, but it does not raise progesterone to levels that could contribute to depressive symptoms. You can then supplement estrogen with BioIdentical patches such as Climara, Vivelle, Esclim, or Estraderm; a gel like EstroGel; a cream like Estrasorb; or a similar preparation produced in a compounding pharmacy. I recommend a dose of 0.1 mg (100 mcg) per day because this has been shown to be effective in about 70 percent of perimenopausal women.

ANXIETY

Anxiety is the feeling we get while watching a really scary movie or indulging in some heart-pumping, white-knuckle sport like bungee jumping or white-water rafting. We often actively seek out those "adrenaline" moments—wait in line, in fact, for our turn to get scared. Our attraction to these sensations is the sense of relief we get afterward when our brain is awash with "reward" chemicals like dopamine, prolactin, and oxytocin.

People who have an *anxiety disorder* don't have the ability to generate that sense of postanxiety relief; it's like an uncomfortable, ongoing, low-grade, unpleasant adrenaline rush. They live for prolonged periods of time with a growing sense of unease provoked by the chronic alert state of stress hormones. The unease is different from legitimate fear in response to a specific threat—it's more of an intrusive, persistent sense of foreboding that is not triggered by a particular event. When this prolonged state of worry is accompanied by the physiological response of fear—sweating, rapid shallow breathing, heart rate acceleration, and so forth—it's called *generalized anxiety disorder.* Over time, it tends to result in behavioral changes like avoidance and withdrawal, as if seeking a sense of safety through isolation. When this kind of anxiety state is sudden in onset, it is referred to as *panic disorder.*

Both anxiety disorder and panic disorder are essentially an imbalance of neurotransmitters. Just like the perfect hormone balance that maintains our general health, the perfect neurotransmitter balance allows us to remain alert without feeling anxious. When it's tipped too heavily in favor of inhibitory transmitters (such as GABA) and too light on the stimulatory neurotransmitters (such as glutamate and serotonin), we get anxious. Since serotonin is involved in libido, cognition, reward, and mood, when serotonin levels are low, our awareness of subtle changes going on in our bodies, from aches and pains to sweating and heart rate changes, is elevated—and this results in anxiety.

Women experience generalized anxiety disorder and panic disorder almost twice as much as men. The hormones you were exposed to during growth and development also influence your susceptibility to anxiety. If your mother had a bout of depression while you were in her womb, for instance, you're at higher risk for anxiety because of your exposure to high levels of cortisol and stress hormones during brain development. That's why symptoms often begin in childhood. Certain learned behaviors from childhood could also be a factor. A lack of nurturing, for instance, or the result of parents continually exacerbating natural childhood fears rather than assuaging them, can also lead to anxiety.

The severity of symptoms fluctuates, often with periods of remission; and it's rare to develop panic disorders after age fifty. In any given year, it's estimated that about 5 percent of the population experiences either general anxiety disorder or panic disorder. (Other anxiety disorders that are beyond our scope here are posttraumatic stress disorder, obsessive-compulsive disorder, and various phobias.) There are several signposts that tell you if your feeling of anxiety is actually bad enough to be considered a disorder.

You meet the diagnostic criteria for generalized anxiety disorder if . . .

- your anxiety consists of at least six months of excessive worry, typically related to actual-life situations like work, relationships, or finances.

- you find it difficult to control worry, or its related symptoms impair your ability to function in work or social situations.

Panic disorder is a sudden, unwarranted sense of intense fear that creates many physical symptoms like sweating and shortness of breath. You meet the criteria for panic disorder if . . .

- your onset of symptoms is abrupt and builds in intensity over ten to fifteen minutes, but typically doesn't last longer than thirty minutes.

- you have at least four of the following symptoms: sweating, palpitations, a sensation of choking, difficulty breathing, chest pain, nausea, dizziness, tingling sensations, and chills.

- you've had at least two attacks and have a fear of developing future attacks.

Basically, your estrogen-progesterone balance determines your neurotransmitter balance. Progesterone promotes GABA activity; estrogen promotes serotonin and norepinephrine activity. So any imbalance between estrogen and progesterone can trigger an imbalance between the neurotransmitters. If you're susceptible to anxiety, it's more likely to occur when your estrogen levels are high, because excess serotonin and norepinephrine stimulate neurons and can thus actually provoke your anxiety. A more common trigger, though, is the progesterone withdrawal we've talked about that occurs during the last week of a normal menstrual cycle or following childbirth.

PERFECT BALANCE SOLUTIONS FOR ANXIETY

Since at least an element of anxiety disorder is learned behavior, it can be unlearned. You can alleviate some of the symptoms that arise when the brain unnecessarily initiates the fear response by strengthening your "thinking response." In essence, you can retrain your brain to learn new techniques that may allow you to overcome anxiety without medication. Combining mind-centering exercises with hormone balance (consistent estrogen levels that are unaffected by changing progesterone levels) is one of the best ways to manage this common mood disorder.

DIET

- Avoid caffeine! Caffeine acts as a stimulant by blocking the "inhibitory" or relaxing response in the brain. This will make you more susceptible to anxious feelings and can provoke a panic attack.

- Eliminate Hormone Chaos Carbs from your diet. In many people, the "sugar rush" that follows exposure to large amounts of simple sugars can create a physiological response similar to that of an anxiety attack. If this should happen, the incoming signal to your brain can be misinterpreted by your amygdala and exacerbate anxious feelings.

- When you're feeling anxious, eat more foods high in tryptophan—eggs, tofu, peanuts, beans, and grains. Although there's not enough clinical research to be absolutely certain, there's a real possibility that tryptophan has a calming effect, since it's a precursor to serotonin. By providing more of the building blocks that go into making serotonin, you can overcome a minor serotonin deficiency without hormones.

EXERCISE AND MIND-BODY BEST BETS

- Remain active during periods of anxiety. It will help relieve stress hormones while boosting testosterone levels. Since some form of activity is your body's natural response to danger, continuing regular exercise helps reset your relaxation response. In effect, it retrains the brain not to trigger the stress response and actually makes new neural connections. However, don't work out to the point of exhaustion. Elevated levels of lactate—a by-product of extremely strenuous exercise—can provoke anxiety.

- Stay well hydrated. The rapid heart rate associated with dehydration can provoke an anxiety attack.

COMPLEMENTARY MEDICINE

- Slow deep breathing is crucial for anyone with anxiety. Focused deep breathing interrupts the abnormal fear reaction by giving your body the "all clear" sign and triggering the relaxation reflex. Studies have shown a success rate of over 60 percent in treating anxiety disorder with this simple, free treatment.

- Developing a relationship with a pet has been shown to relieve anxiety disorders. A study of 240 caring pet owners found not only that their stress levels were lower, but that their blood pressure and heart rates were lower when their pets were in the room with them.

- Biofeedback is a widely used technique for easing anxiety disorders. Inexpensive heart rate monitors can alert you of subtle changes in your pulse and indicate early changes associated with stress before the onset of a full-blown panic attack.

- Acupuncture (in which ultranarrow sterile needles are inserted in designated spots in your body) has been shown to be effective in reducing anxiety. In one study, acupuncture completely blocked anxiety reactions in a group of patients who were repeating tests that had previously raised their stress and tension levels. (No, it doesn't hurt, just tingles.)

• Kava kava has been proven to reduce a variety of anxiety disorders, but it's currently under investigation for possible liver damage. So talk to your health care provider before starting this herb. Limit duration of use to one month.

BEST HORMONE TREATMENTS

One of the best ways to control anxiety is to create stable hormone levels—most important, consistent estrogen levels that don't change on a daily basis and aren't influenced by changing progesterone levels.

• *If you haven't reached menopause:* I recommend the extended-cycle use of a BioSimilar birth control pill with a reduced estrogen dose. An extended cycle safely reduces your number of menstrual cycles to only four per year. Seasonale is the most convenient. As we discussed in chapter 3, this kind of menstrual regulation is now fairly common and has been found to be extremely safe.

• *If you are menopausal:* I recommend the use of one of the BioIdentical estradiol patches at a dose of 0.05 mg per day (50 mcg per day). This is one of the few situations where I recommend the addition of a BioIdentical progesterone (even if you don't have a uterus) to promote GABA and offset a possible estrogen-progesterone imbalance. Since everybody's response is different, I suggest you start with an oral tablet of Prometrium (100 mg) at bedtime. If you're still anxious in the morning, you can take another. Your physician will work with you to increase the dose gradually to the point where your mood is under control.

• *If you are postpartum:* Although depression is far more common in women who are breast-feeding, there are women who feel excessively anxious whether they breast-feed or not. I've prescribed BioIdentical progesterone in a few of these cases with great success. Typically, Prometrium in a dose of 100 mg once or twice a day is more than sufficient to produce a calming effect and relieve anxiety. (I have not found any creams to be as effective.) It's a good idea to get someone to help with child care while you're establishing your ideal dose, since progesterone can be highly sedating.

CHAPTER ELEVEN

HOT FLASHES AND NIGHT SWEATS

Hot flashes and night sweats have become the symbolic symptom of the menopausal transition in our Western culture, which isn't surprising since about 80 percent of women going through natural menopause and approximately 95 percent of women who undergo surgical menopause experience them. About 15 million women experience hot flashes and night sweats on a regular basis—and for 5 million of them, hot flashes are extremely severe. While some women can experience hot flashes during various phases of their menstrual cycles, postpartum, or while breast-feeding, the hot flashes and night sweats associated with menopause are by far the most frequent and bothersome. On average, these temperature fluctuations continue for about five years, but they can go on for as long as twenty.

Hot flashes are provoked by chemical-thermal and hormonal changes and are influenced (to various degrees) by genetic, climatic, and lifestyle factors—the cooler your surrounding temperature, for instance, the fewer hot flashes you'll experience. But the main hot flash factor, based on my research as well as other studies, is an energy imbalance triggered by sex hormone deficiencies. And rather than simply being the mere discomfort that many people believe them to be, they are in fact your brain's plea for help.

YOUR THERMOREGULATORY SYSTEM

To understand how hot flashes work, you need a little background on how your body handles temperature. All of us function best when our body temperature maintains a fairly constant 98.6 degrees Fahrenheit. At that temperature, all the body's chemical reactions occur at the proper rate, and all the vital elements that keep us healthy, such as our energy production, oxygen use, and cellular repair, stay well balanced.

Your brain is generally effective at maintaining your individualized ideal temperature. Throughout the day, it follows a fairly fixed pattern of variation called your *diurnal temperature,* which is a direct result of the hormones released by your brain at certain times of the day. Cortisol, for instance, produced in the morning to jump-start your day, helps bring up your temperature; melatonin, produced at night to help you sleep, likely lowers your temperature. Typically, your temperature peaks each day in the early evening at around 99.2 degrees. (A large dinnertime meal raises it even more because of the increase in metabolism necessary for digestion.) Your temperature is lowest (about 97.5 degrees) in the middle of the night during your deepest sleep, then begins to rise as your brain signals your morning cortisol production. While we all tolerate small temperature variations, our brain has its limits. At temperatures above 105.8 degrees, we go into convulsions; when they're below 96 degrees, our mental processes slow dramatically and approach a comatose state. The temperatures at which we thrive constitute the *thermoneutral zone.*

Your thermoneutral zone is your comfort zone. When your body temperature moves slightly above its set point, your brain sets things into motion to get rid of excess heat. It stimulates sweating, induces more rapid shallow breathing, and increases blood flow to your skin. If your temperature begins to dip down below your set point, your brain promotes heat production through shivering, increased metabolism, and decreased blood flow to your skin and limbs, and it prods you to get close to something warm or put on an extra layer of clothing. But as you get older, your thermoneutral range narrows, and you become less tolerant of temperature variations. During the years approaching menopause, the confluence of fluctuating estrogen levels, erratic progesterone production, falling testosterone levels, and lower tolerance for temperature change forms a perfect hormonal storm that creates the conditions for hot flashes and night sweats.

All three of the major sex hormones have an impact on temperature and can promote or reduce problems like hot flashes and night sweats. Estrogen regulates the temperature-sensitive area of your brain and essentially sets your internal thermostat. Progesterone raises your baseline body temperature. Testosterone plays a subtler role; aside from its ability to affect your brain through its conversion into estradiol, it regularizes your temperature by helping your muscles function more effectively, which makes it easier for you to stay in your thermoneutral zone. Your muscles produce most of the heat that keeps your body from cooling to room temperature. Chronically low testosterone levels cause muscle loss and thus less muscle-generated heat. That makes it more difficult to tolerate cooler temperatures. When you start to cool down, your body attempts to warm you up, overcompensates because of the low testosterone, and causes a hot flash. While attempting to regulate your body temperature, these three sex hormones interact with myriad other metabolic hormones, including thyroid hormone, leptin, and insulin.

ANATOMY OF A HOT FLASH

The onset of a hot flash is often announced with a feeling of pressure in the head, accompanied sometimes by heart palpitations or an urge to urinate. The hot flash itself is a sudden sensation of heat or burning that typically starts in the head and neck area and spreads in waves across the chest, neck, and back. Heavy perspiration sometimes follows. Hot flashes usually last two to three minutes and can occur every couple of hours, every couple of days, or anywhere in between, depending on your individual makeup. The intensity also varies from woman to woman. While they might be only mildly uncomfortable to you, your best friend could experience intense anxiety, fatigue, irritability, insomnia, forgetfulness, and sweating so severe that she'd rather avoid social situations than risk embarrassment. Hot flashes are a serious quality-of-life threat for many women.

When your estrogen level is very low, the "heat sensor" in your brain enforces temperature stability more strictly. So an increase (or decrease) in core body temperature of as little as 0.9 degree can trigger a series of blood flow changes geared to correct the temperature change. (While no one knows exactly why, my theory is that it's an evolutionary adaptation—the extreme low estrogen levels that follow childbirth trigger body heat production that helped keep newborns warm.) To initiate a temperature shift, your brain redirects blood flow. It sends more blood to your skin if you need to cool down and less if you need to conserve heat. The blood flow center of your brain and the region that controls your perspiration are adjacent to each other (in the hypothalamus), which allows for a coordinated effort.

When the temperature in the brain's hypothalamic region begins to rise, the brain sends out stress hormones that increase blood flow to the skin and promote sweating. Your skin temperature can increase by more than five degrees in a matter of minutes in response to these changes. Sometimes the higher blood flow continues for minutes, other times for hours. It's the increased blood flow that creates the characteristic flush that looks like embarrassment. Along with the flush, your brain initiates the forehead perspiration and shallow, rapid breathing that most of us interpret as anxiety. If the room you're in is cold enough, you might even start to shiver as your perspiration begins to evaporate and your core temperature drops.

Night sweats are basically hot flashes that occur during sleep. As you sleep, your temperature falls naturally, dropping by as much as three degrees as you begin to fall asleep. These nocturnal temperature depressions, which hit their lowest point in the middle of the night during your deepest sleep, often exceed the limits of the thermoneutral zone and bring on night sweats. Many women experience episodes of such profuse sweating that they wake up totally drenched and have to change their pajamas and sheets. Like hot flashes, night sweats are ineffective attempts by your body to correct a mild and previously tolerated normal temperature shift.

One of my biggest concerns about hot flashes (and night sweats) is the frequent brain-associated problems like forgetfulness and difficulty in concentrating. As discussed in chapter 2, my early studies found that blood flow to the brain decreases dramatically during a hot flash, especially in regions of the brain responsible for verbal memory and short-term memory. Many studies also show that hot flashes increase the production of damaging free radicals. More damage means more risk of nerve death, which can lead to brain conditions like Alzheimer's disease. The link between hot flashes and irreversible damage caused by free radicals is a compelling reason to take every step to fortify your brain health. While it's yet to be proven that preventing hot flashes helps prevent dementia, I've no doubt that such proof will come with time.

RULE OUT OTHER POSSIBLE HORMONAL CAUSES FOR HOT FLASHES

One of the most notable hormonal problems that can create hot flash–type symptoms is *hypoglycemia*—aka low blood sugar. The changes in blood flow patterns to your brain during hot flashes are the same as those experienced by diabetics when their blood sugar levels are dropping, so there's a connection. If you're in menopause or a similar low-estrogen state, you're more likely to experience hot flashes when your blood sugar levels are low than when they're high.

One way to tell if your hot flashes are related to hypoglycemia is to note how you feel after eating. If you have hypoglycemia, the hot flashes will get worse after a meal as a result of core temperature increases brought on by digestion (diet-induced thermogenesis). These kinds of hot flashes (often accompanied by reddening of the skin) are telling you that your blood sugar is getting low. If it seems that your hot flashes occur more often when you're hungry, have your blood sugar tested. (Normal blood sugar levels are 80–110 mg/dL unless you've eaten recently.) Also, ask your physician to do a *glycosylated hemoglobin level* blood test (also called a *hemoglobin A1C*). Although you might need additional testing, this one would provide a summary of your average blood sugar level for several weeks prior to testing.

You'll also want to rule out the other common hormonal problem that can mimic hot flashes: hyperthyroidism. This disorder occurs when the thyroid gland produces excessive amounts of thyroxine, which can make you intolerant to heat— that is, you always feel warm, and usually anxious and restless, as well. You'd also tend to have a rapid pulse, and your thyroid gland itself might be enlarged or even tender. The most differentiating symptom, though, is weight: Excessive amounts of thyroid hormone cause weight loss, whereas low estrogen and/ or testosterone levels are likely

ASK DR. GREENE

Q: DO ANY OF THE YAM CREAMS OR OTHER NATURAL PROGESTERONE CREAMS I'VE SEEN IN HEALTH FOOD STORES ACTUALLY REDUCE HOT FLASHES?

A: Not really. About the same percentage of women feel relief from these creams as they would from a placebo. Progesterone is very poorly absorbed through the skin. That's the reason "natural" progesterone creams are classified as cosmetics and don't require a prescription—they have a hard time getting through the skin to produce any kind of effect. Even if the progesterone in these creams could produce an effect, it would likely make things worse, since progesterone raises core body temperature.

to cause fatigue and weight gain. Also, if hyperthyroidism is your problem, rather than getting worse after ingesting food or drinking juice (as with hypo-glycemia), your hot flash spells will be relieved.

PERFECT BALANCE SOLUTIONS FOR HOT FLASHES

Since hot flashes are directly associated with hormone deficiencies, the best solutions involve correcting the deficiencies. The following will allow you to do that most effectively.

DIET

- Eat less. Since digestion always produces heat, a calorie-restricted diet lowers your metabolic rate and can provide some relief from hot flashes. You'd get the most noticeable effect if you consumed only 70 percent of your actual daily caloric need. You'd also drop some pounds, which would further lower your body temperature.

- Eat foods rich in phytoestrogens—soy, white and green teas, nuts, grains, and pomegranates are all best bets. Since phytoestrogens exert a weak estrogenlike activity, they may help regulate your internal thermostat, or they may stabilize blood vessels to diminish flushing. I don't recommend taking soy or other phytoestrogens in supplement capsule form, however, since they can actually *provoke* hot flashes through the rapid rise and fall in blood levels. When soy is consumed as food and part of a meal, on the other hand, the inherent fiber helps prevent rapid absorption. About 40–60 grams of soybeans or tofu a day is a good start—that's about $^1/_4$ cup of soybeans or one soy burger.

- Avoid spicy foods. They trigger perspiration, which can cause a drop in your core temperature. That can provoke an intense hot flash.

- Cut back on caffeine. Caffeine has been shown to increase heart rate and metabolism enough that it can disrupt your thermoneutral zone. If you drink coffee regularly, switch to tea at least part of the time. If you're going to get the caffeine, you might as well get the many health benefits of tea along with it. Green and white teas are best, since they have the antioxidants and phytoestrogens that help counter free radicals.

- Reduce your alcohol intake. Alcohol has been shown to trigger hot flashes in some women. This is likely due to the tyramine created by aging wines. This amino acid can provoke blood flow changes that result in a full-blown hot flash. The same holds true for other aged liquors like brandy and Scotch.

EXERCISE AND MIND-BODY BEST BETS

- Breathe! Whenever you feel a hot flash coming on, do some slow deep breathing. This has been widely studied and shown to be an effective means of interrupting hot flashes. You can anticipate about a 75 percent reduction in hot flashes with this simple technique. Not only does it interrupt the heart rate acceleration that precedes a hot flash, but it serves as a way of releasing some heat through your breath. It also promotes healthy circulation.

- Keep up your yoga. Hot flashes are often more frequent and intense during times of stress, so reducing stress helps reduce hot flashes. By practicing yoga, you'll get all the benefits of deep breathing with programmed stretches that will also lower your stress hormone levels.

- Meditation, reading, and anything that promotes relaxation has been shown to have some benefit. The possibilities are many, so don't rely on the research studies alone. Try anything that you find relaxing and test it for yourself.

- Go for a walk after dinner. It will lower your insulin level to help prevent weight gain, and it may reduce night sweats by promoting a slight increase in free testosterone. Lowering insulin resistance also prevents transient dips in blood glucose, removing another potential trigger of night sweats.

- Exercising in the middle of the day can help prevent the late afternoon metabolic changes that promote hot flashes. If you keep your metabolism revved up, your brain blood flow remains at a healthy level. One study showed that by doing at least forty minutes of aerobic exercise three times a week, a group of women reduced their hot flashes by about 50 percent compared with a similar group of women who remained sedentary. The benefits were measurable within the first few weeks of starting the program.

COMPLEMENTARY MEDICINE AND PRACTICAL SOLUTIONS

- Black cohosh is sold today primarily as an extract called Remifemin. The recommended dose is 40 mg taken twice daily. Results are gradual in onset, with peak relief reported at twelve weeks. While black cohosh has been considered fairly harmless, a recent study in lab rats with breast cancers found a much higher incidence of tumor metastasis to the lungs when rats were given comparable doses of this herb. I recommend using black cohosh with caution. If you've got breast cancer, discuss your options with your doctor.

- Red clover (Promensil), evening primrose, ginseng, vitamin E, and dong quai have all been studied, and while some benefits have been demonstrated, they haven't been consistent. Many women who come to me for advice have been disappointed by the inability of these BioUnknowns to relieve hot flashes; but since there is no evidence of any harm, they may be worth a try.

- The Chillow comfort device is a foam pillow insert that slips into your own pillowcase with your pillow. You add ordinary tap water just once, and the Chillow stays cool for months at a time. For many women, this $30 device can significantly reduce night sweats simply by keeping their head cool during sleep. (Available in most drugstores or at www.drugstore.com.)

- Obvious as it might sound, the right clothing counts. Your coolest fabrics are linen and cotton. Turtlenecks are deadly. And easily removable layers—vests, shawls, cotton cardigans—are the name of the game.

BEST HORMONE TREATMENTS

Restoring sex hormone equilibrium is the most consistent and reliable solution for relieving hot flashes and night sweats.

- If you're still having menstrual cycles, the easiest way to achieve this balance is through the use of a BioSimilar estrogen/BioLimited progestin hormone contraceptive. The Ortho Evra patch or the Nuvaring is ideal because neither will lower your testosterone the way a birth control pill will. In fact, if you're on an oral contraceptive pill and having hot flashes, switching to one of these may relieve your symptoms.

- If you're in menopause, I recommend BioIdentical estrogen via a patch, cream, or gel. It will maintain a stable blood level—even in the middle of the night—and won't suppress your already reduced testosterone level. This is the only treatment many women need. Start with a low dose of 0.3–0.5 mg per day and request that your doctor increase the dose in six to eight weeks if your hot flashes or night sweats persist. Many women also respond well to BioSimilar estrogen tablets, so if you're on one of these or aren't keen on transdermal delivery, it isn't necessary to switch; these preparations are also safe and effective. For some women, especially those who have had their ovaries removed, hot flashes will persist on estrogen. If this happens, talk to your doctor about adding testosterone to your regimen.

- BioIdentical testosterone is often the missing piece to continued relief, since it stabilizes the testosterone receptors in the temperature regulatory region in your brain. It can be made by a compounding pharmacy as a transdermal gel, vaginal cream, or lozenge to dissolve under your tongue. Start on a 2 mg dose, then begin to increase the dose by 1 mg every three months until symptoms are under control. My patients have rarely had to exceed 5 mg. Rest assured, side effects like excess hair growth or deepening voice don't occur at doses under 50 mg per day.

- If you've got cancer, you may be on a BioLimited estrogen or a BioAntagonist. These can often make hot flashes worse or increase their intensity. Discuss your discomfort with your doctor. Many new regimens, like the ones in the following list, may be able to relieve your symptoms while you complete your treatment. Additionally, a greater number of physicians are now willing to consider (and will discuss with their patients) the continuation of estrogen therapy during breast cancer treatment.

For those of you who stick with the mainstream treatment for your cancer (BioLimited estrogen or a BioAntagonist), many emerging nonhormonal remedies are worth considering:

- Several **antiseizure medications** seem to provide significant relief for hot flashes. Though they don't reach the 90–95 percent effectiveness of BioIdentical estrogens, they might reduce your symptoms to a tolerable level. The two drugs in this category that have been tested most thoroughly for hot flashes are Neurontin and Topamax. With either one, your doctor should start you on a low dose and increase it gradually until you experience symptom relief. An added benefit is that these medications often relieve chronic pain, as well.

- **Antidepressants** that target serotonin and norepinephrine are effective at reducing hot flashes and night sweats, since these two key neurotransmitters are used by the thermoregulatory region of your brain. The specific brands that have been used most widely for this purpose are Effexor, Prozac, and Paxil. The success rates are typically about 70–80 percent reduction in symptoms, and they have the added benefit of reducing depression. With time, I am certain that this list will grow, because there are other medications that promote similar actions in the brain.

- Certain **"antianxiety" medications** have been shown to have some benefit in reducing hot flashes. This, too, makes sense, since as previously described, hot flashes are abnormal blood flow responses. The one that is oldest and most widely used is clonidine. It's effective in 40–60 percent of women and is typically prescribed at doses of 0.05–0.15 mg per day. Other medications that have also been tested include Bellergal, Iofexidine, and veralipride. Generally, the side effects of each can be pretty difficult to manage, and there is a potential for addiction. I've found their use to be markedly declining since the other treatments are so well tolerated and effective.

CHAPTER TWELVE

SLEEP, FATIGUE, AND INSOMNIA

Sleep is a very busy time and a crucial aspect of hormone brain health. It gives your brain the break it needs from receiving incoming information so that it can perform its own maintenance. It gives it time to organize newly acquired thoughts, memories, and knowledge. And it allows your twenty-four-hour hormonal clock to reset so that your body's functions are coordinated. So sleep is essential; you simply can't function without it. After only seventeen hours without sleep, most people operate as if they had a blood alcohol level of 0.05 percent. After a few more sleepless hours, their impairment is equivalent to having a blood alcohol level of about 0.1 percent. When you consider that a commercial truck driver can receive a "driving under the influence" for a blood alcohol level of 0.04, you get an idea of just how dysfunctional that is.

That makes sleep disturbances more than just a minor annoyance; they can be serious health hazards. When they create distress or impairment, or otherwise exert a negative impact on your quality of life, they qualify as medical problems. As a woman, thanks in part to your fluctuating sex hormone levels, you're at least 30 percent more likely to experience a sleep disturbance than a man your age. The most common of those disturbances by far is *insomnia* (difficulty falling or staying asleep or having non-restorative sleep that leaves you tired). Since the Perfect Balance solutions for insomnia and other sleep disorders depend largely on the way hormones influence the brain—and vice versa—let's take a quick look at the connection and how it works.

HEALTHY SLEEP

Our circadian rhythm—alternating periods of high and low activity over a twenty-four-hour period—is guided by light exposure first, then by the environment and our conscious ability to modify it. This natural inner clock is set by a pair of light-sensitive, pea-size nerve clusters in the hypothalamus called the *suprachiasmatic nucleus,* which promotes a natural state of sleepiness twice daily, usually between 11:00 p.m. and 6:00 a.m. and between 1:00 p.m. and 4:00 p.m. The suprachiasmatic nucleus receives incoming data, coordinates the information, and sends a hormonal signal to the pineal gland, which then releases melatonin. Light inhibits the production and release of melatonin, which is why melatonin levels are low during the day and rise in the evening—and why if we wake up in the middle of the night and turn on bright lights, it's harder to get back to sleep. As we turn *on* the lights, we turn *off* our melatonin production. As we get older and our melatonin production declines naturally, we have a greater tendency to develop insomnia.

Other hormones affect sleep patterns, too. Estrogen promotes the deep dream sleep state and, as you've seen, stabilizes temperature, which protects you from sleep-interrupting night sweats or chills; progesterone acts as a hormonal sedative; and testosterone promotes the deep sleep that fosters dreaming. One of the most important chemicals involved in sleep is the metabolite *adenosine.* Throughout the day, adenosine builds up in the brain in proportion to brain activity—the more you use your brain, the more adenosine builds up. As it accumulates, it slows down the rate at which nerves fire, which makes you sleepy. Adenosine also increases the blood flow to the brain so that the brain can restore itself more efficiently throughout the night. During sleep, your brain recycles the adenosine to use during your next day's activity. If you don't sleep long enough to reprocess your supply of adenosine, you create a sleep debt that continues to make you feel sleepy until the debt is "paid off" by getting a good night's sleep and clearing the residual adenosine. Since we all accumulate and process adenosine at a different rate, some of us need more sleep than others.

As you sleep and your brain organizes everything you've learned on any given day, it designates some information for long-term storage, other information for deletion, and some for retention and reconsideration during your next sleep cycle. Essentially, the only way your brain can accomplish such a full agenda every night is for your sleep to be organized into stages. The sleep stages—often referred to as *sleep architecture*—starts with a very light, easily interrupted sleep, moves gradually into deeper, more restorative, slow-wave sleep, and culminates in the dream phase, known as *REM (rapid eye movement)* sleep. The longer you're in the deeper, more restorative, slow-wave stages (which is when adenosine is most aggressively recycled), the more refreshed you'll feel when you wake up.

Since a good part of sleep is dedicated to processing information, as you get older you need less sleep. You simply don't need as much time to process information, since you've already stored a good solid information base and are therefore learning less on a day-to-day basis. A newborn baby sleeps for up to twenty hours each day. By age four, she'll need about twelve hours. By age ten, she'll feel rested after about ten hours of sleep, and from there her need for sleep will decline gradually so that by the time she's eligible for Medicare, she'll need only about six hours. Although these patterns are fairly predictable, we still all vary in our need for sleep. Here's a simple test that will help you determine if your sleep needs are being met.

SLEEP RISK ASSESSMENT QUESTIONNAIRE

Use the numerical scoring to indicate how likely you are to fall asleep in the following situations. Base your answers on your current normal routine. This test is meant to help you access how sleepy you get during the day, which can indicate a sleep disorder. Use the following scale to choose the most appropriate number for each situation:

SLEEP LIKELIHOOD SCALE

0—fully alert, no chance of sleep

1—might fall asleep

2—would be fighting to stay awake

3—likely to nod off

IF I WERE ...	MY CHANCE OF FALLING ASLEEP
1. Having a daytime conversation	_____
2. At work during early afternoon	_____
3. Watching a favorite TV show	_____
4. Reading a great book	_____
5. Waiting in the car, midafternoon	_____
6. Sitting in a movie theater	_____
7. The passenger in a two-hour car ride	_____
8. Getting a haircut	_____
9. Resting midday	_____
10. Driving your car for an hour at sunset	_____
TOTAL	_____

*Modified from the Epworth Sleepiness Scale

TOTAL UP YOUR SCORE. HERE'S THE BOTTOM LINE:

0–9   You're meeting your sleep needs.

10–12   You're pushing yourself.

13–20   You're sleep deprived.

21–30   Your sleep deprivation puts you at risk of injury.

SLEEP PROBLEMS RELATED TO YOUR MENSTRUAL CYCLE

Your circadian rhythm directs the release of your sex hormones by your ovaries. The sex hormones in turn have an impact on your sleep quality. So to rectify hormonally induced sleep problems, you need to factor in just what your hormones are up to when you're experiencing the problems, and that means matching the solutions to the key stages of your hormonal life: when you're menstruating, pregnant, or in or around menopause.

As an adult woman, you're much more likely to have sleep disturbances related to your menstrual cycle if you experience PMS. It probably takes you longer to fall asleep, and you most likely wake up more frequently throughout the night. That leads to decreased sleep quality and sleep efficiency—that is, you spend less time in the deep, restorative stages of sleep, and less time in bed is actually spent sleeping. So the cycling of your sex hormones affects your restorative sleep and thus indirectly influences the way you feel and function when you're awake.

During menstruation, normal sleep patterns are disrupted by low estrogen and progesterone levels, adenosine builds up and creates a sleep debt, and you end up feeling tired. During the first few weeks of your cycle, the rising estrogen levels restore the normal sleep architecture, which revitalizes your energy. These healthy, normalized sleep patterns continue to improve as progesterone levels rise.

For some women, and we're not certain why, the sedative properties of progesterone induce an abnormally deep sleep, almost like a stupor, rather than the normal beneficial increase in slow-wave sleep. If you're one of these women (and again, you're more vulnerable if you have PMS), your own biological progesterone can provoke an erratic pattern of excessive sleepiness and insomnia. Before and during the first few days of your menstrual cycle, when your progesterone levels decline, your non-REM (light) sleep is compromised, and your body isn't able to recycle serotonin properly. That makes it more likely that your insomnia will get worse, that you'll experience increased irritability and restlessness, and that you will not sleep very soundly until around day five, when your estrogen levels start to rise again.

RULE OUT OTHER POSSIBLE HORMONE CAUSES

The most common hormone-related problem that creates similar erratic variations in energy and sleep patterns is *Hashimoto's thyroiditis* (autoimmune thyroid disorder). The earmarks of the disease are periods of alternating high and low thyroid hormone levels and an enlarged, tender swelling in the front of the neck (not always present). Diagnosis is easily established by blood tests for thyroid hormones and thyroid antibodies. When experiencing sleep disturbances and low energy together, you also want to rule out depression. If you feel depression is a possibility, consider an assessment by a health care provider. In addition to ruling out depression, your health care provider can help determine if any medications you are on might be contributing to your sleep difficulties.

PERFECT BALANCE SOLUTIONS FOR FATIGUE AND INSOMNIA

DIET

- Eat high-protein breakfasts, low-protein dinners. To maximize your day-time energy level and minimize evening restlessness, consume your major protein early in the day and gradually introduce Hormone Power Carbs in subsequent meals. Since protein digestion is metabolically similar to light exercise, it tends to raise your temperature and can provoke sleep-interrupting night sweats. Eating Power Carb–based meals slows sugar absorption and lowers insulin levels, which helps avoid fatigue-producing hypoglycemia and keeps stress hormones stabilized, thereby improving your sleep patterns.

- Avoid caffeine after 3:00 p.m. Caffeine perks you up by blocking the effects of sleep-inducing adenosine on your brain. Since the adenosine is still building up when the caffeine wears off six or seven hours later, you've built up a sleep debt, which will make you even sleepier later. Caffeine also causes brain blood vessels to constrict, so when the caffeine wears off and the blood vessels dilate, it can provoke a headache, which needless to say is not conducive to a good night's sleep. (Many headache medications actually add caffeine to their preparations to keep the vessels constricted.)

- Eat foods that contain tryptophan (one of the essential amino acids) in the evening. It helps your body produce niacin, the B vitamin that the brain converts to serotonin, and can naturally facilitate sleep. It's absorbed better when consumed as part of a Power Carb–based meal than one concentrated in high protein. Best-bet tryptophan foods (in order of highest tryptophan content) are spinach, seaweed, peanuts (with skin), sesame seeds, tofu, mushrooms, lobster, crab, turkey, lentils, and bananas.

- Avoid more than two glasses of wine or one serving of hard liquor. Alcohol induces sedation, especially if you have a sleep deficit. But as your blood alcohol level drops, there's typically an increase in stress hormone levels that can promote rebound insomnia in the early morning hours and interrupt your sleep.

EXERCISE AND LIFESTYLE BEST BETS

- High-intensity aerobic exercise often promotes melatonin release. Though this can be great for promoting sleep on the day you're exercising, it often causes a twelve-to-twenty-hour delay in serotonin release the next day. As a result, you may have a more difficult time sleeping on the next night.

The solution: Exercise at the same time each day, ideally around 3:00 or 4:00 p.m. to boost melatonin levels before bedtime; this produces a consistent signal to your brain to synchronize hormonal release.

· Certain other behavioral patterns and environmental influences promote sleep and can have a subtle influence upon your circadian rhythm. To boost your natural rhythm, try to adopt the following habits:

Wake at the same time each day to "set" your biological clock.

Minimize daytime napping to build up adenosine levels in your brain.

Eat larger meals early in the day; keep evening meals light.

Move your alarm clock away from your bed, so it doesn't become a source of distraction. If you're too focused on time, it can further disrupt sleep.

CASE IN POINT

When I first met Hillary, she was a sixteen-year-old student at a nearby school for troubled teens. She was very lethargic, had a history of lashing out unpredictably, and had been going through alternating phases of chaotic behavior and severe fatigue, which had culminated with her falling asleep at the wheel and having an auto accident.

As we reviewed her history, I found out Hillary had been having erratic menstrual cycles for about three years. She said that although her periods were unpredictable, she could easily tell they were coming because she'd go into "hibernation mode"—she'd get extremely tired and fall asleep in class, even after ten hours of sleep. About ten days later, she'd be so energized that her parents thought she was using drugs. She was also gradually gaining weight.

I placed her on the birth control pill Yasmin, a BioLimited pill that suppresses natural progesterone production while regulating the cycle with a nonsedating progestin and stable levels of estrogen. Next I set her up on a meal plan that emphasized high-fiber Power Carbs and more protein early in the day. When I saw her ten weeks later, the difference was already noticeable. Her skin had cleared, she was far more alert, she had lost weight, and she reported that her menstrual cycles were very mild. On her follow-up visit two months later, Hillary had lost more weight, was playing soccer on a regular basis, and scored above average in all her classes. Best of all, she was planning to return home in a few months, much to the delight of both her and her parents.

Use your bed only for sleep and sex—no reading, TV, or lounging.

Keep your bedroom quiet, cool, and dark to reinforce your hypothalamic brain center's ability to dial in to the day-night cycles of the sun.

COMPLEMENTARY MEDICINE

Herbal products for sleep improvement are some of the most popular on the market. But remember, some are safer than others, and just because herbal products don't require a prescription doesn't mean they're not potent. There's actually been a recent spate of traffic citations issued for "driving under the influence" of medicinal herbs. If you need to use any of these herbs more than two weeks out of any month, I recommend that you have an assessment by a sleep specialist to determine if your sleep problem is symptomatic of a more serious medical problem. Following are the herbs that I feel are safest and most effective.

- Valerian *(Valerian officinalis).* The roots and rhizome of this tall, perennial flowering herb have been used as a tranquilizer for more than one thousand years and are still widely used in Europe. In the United States, the FDA categorizes it as "generally recognized as safe." Aside from its use as a tranquilizing agent, it lowers anxiety levels and induces a sedative state. Recommended doses are between 400 and 900 mg. At these doses, it has been shown to improve normal EEG patterns as well as "sleep efficiency." Most probably safe with limited use.

- Kava kava *(Piper methysticum)* is a large shrub cultivated in the Pacific Islands whose roots and rhizome are used to treat the anxiety, restlessness, and stress often associated with insomnia. It's worth noting that in some parts of the world, kava kava is available by prescription only. When you want to use kava kava for sleep, doses of 180–210 mg are considered most effective—start out with the low dose and increase if needed. Do not take this herb if you've been drinking alcohol. The FDA is investigating the toxicity of kava kava because there have been reports of liver damage. So consult your health care provider before using, and limit use to no more than one month.

- Passionflower *(Passiflora incarnate).* Though there aren't many studies on its effectiveness, passionflower is an ingredient in many pharmaceutical sedative products sold in Europe. Herbalists in the United States recom-

SLEEP, FATIGUE, AND INSOMNIA

mend it for insomnia—most usually as a tea made from 4–8 grams of the herb. Since side effects seem minimal, this may be one of the safest herbs to try as a sleep aid.

- Hops *(Humulus lupulus)*. This perennial climbing vine with some estrogenlike properties has been recommended for centuries to aid with intestinal problems as well as sleep. Its calming effects are reported to have a natural onset twenty to forty minutes after ingestion, typically in the form of a 0.5 g dose of the dried herb or a comparable dose of a plant extract.

BEST HORMONE TREATMENTS

- The most effective hormonal treatment for sleep disorders during your fertile years is a BioSimilar combination birth control pill. If insomnia is part of your premenstrual syndrome, I recommend you try one of the new birth control pills with a BioSimilar estrogen and BioLimited progestin. Yasmin, for instance, has been shown to reduce nighttime awakenings dramatically for many of my patients without causing daytime fatigue. Another excellent option is Ortho Tri-Cyclen. I recommend that you take either pill about two hours before bedtime. (While there's no formal research on the timing, this is what has worked best for my patients.) You'll probably find that by suppressing your body's natural progesterone surge, you no longer experience the premenstrual sleep problems that are a natural consequence of progesterone withdrawal.

- Seasonale is another good alternative. It's packaged in a three-month extended-use regimen designed so that you have one menstrual cycle per season. This kind of menstrual regulation is totally safe and preferred by a great many women for its convenience and predictability. Use caution when combining any of these birth control pills with herbal remedies. Some herbs, such as Saint-John's-wort, have recently been shown to *decrease* the effectiveness of birth control pills. If you combine therapies, a backup method of contraception, such as condoms, is recommended.

- If you're trying to get pregnant, supplemental estrogen is a good viable option. By using BioIdentical estrogen during the second half of your menstrual cycle, you'd be able to improve sleep quality because of estrogen's ability to normalize sleep patterns. If your sleep disturbance is significant enough to impact your ability to function, the benefits would clearly outweigh the small potential risk. I recommend sticking with a standardized formulation like the Climara or Vivelle patch (0.1 mg per day) during the last two weeks of your menstrual cycle.

• If you're experiencing severe insomnia, I recommend trying BioIdentical progesterone about two hours before bed. Though not a good idea on a regular basis, this is safer and probably as effective as an occasional use of prescription sleep aids. Discuss with your doctor using the BioIdentical progesterone sold as Prometrium at doses of 100–400 mg before bedtime, but be certain that you have at least six to eight hours available for sleep.

SLEEP DISORDERS DURING PERIMENOPAUSE AND MENOPAUSE

Over 90 percent of women who visit menopause clinics cite fatigue as a prominent symptom, and over 75 percent complain of insomnia. Not being able to stay asleep is, in fact, the most common symptom brought on by the hormone shifts of perimenopause and the low hormone levels of menopause and beyond. The low estradiol levels, absence of sleep-inducing progesterone, and progressive decline of testosterone typical of menopause all contribute to diminished sleep quality, and as you get older your risk of sleep disturbances increases even further.

Remember, one of estrogen's many jobs is to regulate your body temperature. So when estrogen levels are low, your normal temperature fluctuates, resulting in lighter sleep stages—and often night sweats, to boot. Also, since estrogen increases REM sleep cycles, when levels are low you tend to dream less, which leaves you tired and may even contribute to some memory loss about recent events. The bottom line: Estrogen establishes normal sleep patterns and promotes a more restful sleep.

Another factor: Cortisol levels change in menopause. This stress hormone normally peaks in the early morning hours and, like a cup of coffee, helps boost morning energy levels to start your day. During menopause, the spike in cortisol tends to shift to earlier hours and promotes earlier awakenings. Plus, as noted previously, as you age you produce less of the melatonin that helps you stay asleep. Add the melatonin and cortisol factors to the sex hormone shifts and you've got a winning trifecta of sleeplessness.

Although testosterone doesn't seem to have any isolated effect on sleep, many of my patients have reported that their dreaming increased when they start testosterone supplementation. I find this interesting but haven't seen any studies to support that finding. On the other hand, numerous studies show that testosterone can dramatically reduce fatigue through its ability to improve muscle metabolism and growth.

RULE OUT OTHER SLEEP PROBLEMS

If you've been told that you snore a lot, request an evaluation by a sleep specialist. Snoring is often a sign of *sleep apnea* (interrupted breathing during sleep). This condition, which results in low oxygen levels in your blood, unfortunately increases significantly during menopause and may put you at elevated risk of heart attack. Bladder-related problems can also be a source of compromised sleep quality. *Nocturia*—the need to urinate frequently during the night—is a common sign of chronic interstitial cystitis. This condition is easily treated, so if you're getting out of bed to empty your bladder more than once per night and it's having an impact on your sleep quality, talk to your OB/GYN or a urologist about it.

PERFECT BALANCE SOLUTIONS TO SLEEP DISORDERS IN AND AROUND MENOPAUSE

If you're experiencing hot flashes or night sweats, your chances of improving your sleep quality are already compromised. Review the solutions in chapter 11 and take steps to minimize your symptoms and optimize your sleep efficiency. Following are some additional solutions that are more specific to sleep disturbances.

COMPLEMENTARY MEDICINE AND LIFESTYLE

- Short naps of only twenty or thirty minutes can give you a temporary energy boost. Avoid sleeping for longer periods of time to prevent interference with your late night sleep.

- Some data suggest that you may benefit from taking a melatonin supplement. It's more likely to help you stay asleep than to let you simply fall asleep. No studies indicate clear dosing guidelines, but I'd recommend between 0.3 and 5 mg. As always, it's best to start with a low dose and increase the amount gradually as needed. Seek out supplements that don't use "bovine pineal gland" as their source, to minimize your risk of Bio-Mutagens as well as mad cow disease.

- Also remember to avoid eating too much after 6:00 p.m.; try to wake up at close to the same time every day; and keep your bedroom quiet, cool, and dark to reinforce your brain sleep patterns.

BEST HORMONE TREATMENTS

- If you're not already on hormone therapy, I highly recommend BioIdentical hormone supplementation. It's far safer and more effective at restoring healthy sleep patterns than the commonly prescribed sedatives or herbs. Start with estrogen first. If you're not having hot flashes or night sweats, start with a very low dose (Climara and Vivelle patches both come in a dose of 0.025 mg per day). Increase the dose gradually every three to four weeks until your normal sleep function returns. If you reach a dose of 0.1 mg per day and your sleeping still hasn't improved, talk to your doctor about adding progesterone.

- If you do add progesterone, start with a 200 mg dose of Prometrium, the BioIdentical progesterone sold as a capsule. Take it about an hour before bedtime so that it wears off by morning. You can double the dose every one to two weeks as needed to induce sleep (don't exceed more than a 600 mg dose). This product has a peanut oil base, so don't use it if you're allergic to peanuts; discuss alternatives with your doctor.

- Finally, if you find that you still have daytime muscle fatigue, I suggest adding in BioIdentical testosterone. It not only will boost your daytime energy level, but will increase REM sleep time in the evening. As you'll see in the next chapter, increasing REM sleep time will also improve your memory.

CHAPTER THIRTEEN

MEMORY AND COGNITIVE HEALTH

Having the cognitive ability to remember things that are important to us and to learn new information and skills is our most valuable asset. That's why any loss or decline in these vital brain functions is terrifying. Nearly 5 million people in the United States have Alzheimer's disease, and the majority of them are women. As our population ages, another 360,000 people will join those ranks annually; that's another 980 cases per day, or 40 per hour. As a woman, your risk of developing Alzheimer's is two to four times higher than that of your male contemporaries, and your risk doubles every five years after you turn sixty. So it's of utmost importance for you to take preventive measures to ensure your brain health.

After you enter menopause, one of the most effective strategies for reducing your risk of dementia is hormone therapy. Sufficient levels of estradiol and the other hormones, like testosterone and stress hormones, help you get enough glucose and oxygen to your brain so that it can function properly. They also work to preserve neural connections and reduce free radical damage to your brain. It's actually the higher estrogen levels in aging men that afford them the added protection from many brain-related illnesses. Since estrogen levels decline in women, not men, hormone deficiency plays a greater role in contributing to dementia in women.

MEMORY AND HORMONES

In the most basic terms, memory is stored information. You have three essential types of memory: long-term, short-term, and working memory. Long-term memory relies on neuron growth in your brain and creates the memories that remain with you over a lifetime (we now know that we have the ability to grow new neurons all our life). Short-term memory is formed from brief connections in your hippocampus and allows you to store information for a few days at a time. And working memory is your ability to hold information in short-term storage while applying it to something you're doing at the moment. Adding numbers, for instance, requires you to grab the numbers with your working memory, hold the new numbers in your short-term memory while accessing the rules of addition, and then join the two to solve the problem.

Each of these different types of memory serves a vital role in cognitive health, and all are dependent upon estrogen. Working memory is especially estrogen sensitive, which is why when your estrogen is low, you may experience the "whachamacallit" syndrome (that feeling of not being able to find the correct word is essentially an inability to access old information to feed into the new situation). Healthy cognitive functioning is what allowed you to fix yourself breakfast this morning, take a shower, check your e-mail, and then read this book.

If cognitive health becomes compromised from a lifetime of neglect, the damage is hard to reverse. Nothing can actually stop the brain-aging process. The best treatments we have to offer today are effective only at slowing down the changes that occur as the brain ages—and sex hormones can help significantly in that regard. They promote the formation of new neuron connections and prime the existing connections to work harder. Sex hormones, in fact, rank at the top of the "best things to do for your brain" list. They might not improve IQ points, but they can preserve memory and intelligence while preserving your ability to learn.

Your history and any symptoms you may now be experiencing can help determine whether or not you're protecting your cognitive health and memories or increasing their rate of decline. The following questionnaire will let you know how you're doing and establish the current level of your cognitive health.

COGNITIVE HEALTH QUESTIONNAIRE

The questions listed here are designed to gather your past history and your present-day complaints. Circle either "Yes" or "No," then score the test by giving yourself one point for every question to which you answered "Yes." The grading scale is listed at the end.

1.	Do you have hot flashes or night sweats?	Yes	No
2.	Have you ever had a severe head injury?	Yes	No
3.	Do you have diabetes?	Yes	No
4.	Have you ever had a bout of major depression?	Yes	No
5.	Do you eat a high-fat diet (more than 30% of total calories)?	Yes	No
6.	Do you have high blood pressure?	Yes	No
7.	Do you have osteoporosis?	Yes	No
8.	Do you frequently forget what you were going to say?	Yes	No
9.	Did you drop out of high school before graduation?	Yes	No
10.	Are you a cigarette smoker?	Yes	No
11.	Is your waist greater than thirty-five inches?	Yes	No
12.	Do you have a family history of dementia?	Yes	No
13.	Have you had your ovaries removed?	Yes	No
14.	Are you over eighty years of age?	Yes	No
15.	Do you have trouble remembering where you parked?	Yes	No
16.	Do you spend most of your time alone?	Yes	No
17.	Do you get lost more than most people you know?	Yes	No
18.	Have you lost your sense of smell?	Yes	No
19.	Do you have high cholesterol levels?	Yes	No
20.	Are you a "couch potato"?	Yes	No

TOTAL NUMBER OF QUESTIONS YOU ANSWERED "YES": _____

SCORE

0–3	Excellent! You're at low risk of cognitive decline.
4–7	Not bad, but you should make changes to reduce your risk of cognitive decline.
8–10	The symptoms you're ignoring may be causing you harm.
11–14	Make radical changes while you still can.
15 or higher	Consult a health care professional and request testing for mild cognitive impairment.

AGING NATURALLY

There's a lot of talk about "aging naturally," but there's some question as to what that actually means. There's no doubt our society as a whole is aging; the problem is we're not necessarily aging well. Over half of all American women over the age of eighty-five are cognitively impaired on some level. The reason for that is that as women are living longer, they are living more than half their lives *after* their ovaries have stopped producing brain-protecting sex hormones.

EARLY REVERSIBLE COGNITIVE DECLINE

Estrogen (estradiol) is the most important hormone in terms of your cognition. Estradiol improves nerve functions and boosts hearing, vision, and even your sense of smell—your information-gathering tools. They provide multiple means to take in information. So you need estradiol to keep your senses sharp and help you gather information to process later into memory. Estradiol affects the formation of memories by strengthening nerve connections and increasing neurotransmitter production. It's also important in guiding your emotions. The hippocampus (the central brain region), which is the initial storage bin for incoming information, also processes memory and emotion and is densely populated by estrogen receptors (the links that make emotionally charged information so much easier to remember). Most of us remember our first kiss and recall exactly where we were and what we were doing when we learned of the 9/11 tragedy. During these highly emotional moments, sudden elevations of stress hormones etch the memories deep into neural networks. It's the job of estrogen to give these memories permanence and keep them from fading.

Of all our various types of memory, visual, spatial, experiential, and so on, verbal memory (the ability to remember words and meanings) is one of the first to become compromised when estrogen levels begin to drop—and, fortunately, the one that responds most readily to estrogen therapy. In fact, brain-imaging studies (including my early research) show that when menopausal estrogen levels are restored to healthy levels, brain blood flow increases more on the left side of the brain, where verbal memory is processed and stored.

There's another dimension to estrogen's role in memory. As we've seen, when estrogen levels are low, you're more susceptible to chronic stress—and chronic stress impairs memory. If stress hormones are chronically elevated, the neuron branches become so overgrown that your brain can't access stored information quickly. Eventually the neuron forest can become so thick with connections, it chokes itself off. That can result in neuron loss measurable in brain images as shrinkage of the hippocampus. This is the basis of most early age-related memory problems. The stunted growth of these connections doesn't allow information to be stored properly in short-term memory, so it gets lost before it can be reinforced. Without adequate amounts of estradiol, the problem is exacerbated, and the effectiveness of the information-processing and -collection system is compromised.

Progesterone can interfere with memory formation by increasing fatigue and blunting the sensory neurons, which slows the rate at which incoming information is processed and dilutes some aspects of memory storage and recall. Though progesterone's effects are minimal for most women, if you're especially sensitive to monthly elevations in progesterone, you can feel a significant decline in cognitive performance—a sort of foggy or spaced-out feeling. The bottom line is that healthy cognitive functioning is all about being able to take in information and storing it in short-term

THE POWER OF HORMONAL BALANCE

A nurse practitioner recently told me one of the most dramatic stories I've ever heard about the cognitive-boosting abilities of estrogen. Her sister, Carol, has Down syndrome and had had such profound cognitive difficulties that she was nonverbal, needed constant supervision, and had been placed in a group home when she was in her late teens. While in the home, Carol began having severe problems with menstrual bleeding and pain. Her doctors decided to do a hysterectomy with removal of her ovaries. Immediately after surgery, they started her up on a Bioldentical estrogen patch. Remarkably, within weeks she began speaking. Her parents were so enthused, they hired special tutors to work with her in the group home. A few months later, Carol had improved so dramatically that she started occupational therapy to learn job skills. Within a year, she was doing so well that she was able to relocate to an apartment and live on her own with minimal supervision. It was a dramatic transformation, but in some ways not that surprising. Her improvement was brought on by the stable levels of Bioldentical estrogen, combined with the *absence* of progesterone, which may have been impeding her learning. It's also possible that her testosterone levels had been too high before her ovaries were removed. She may have been just on the border of becoming functional and independent when these hormonal changes took place at puberty. Whatever the case, the transformation was undoubtedly inspiring.

memory until your next REM sleep period, when it can be converted into long-term memory. Estrogen helps these stages of this process, and progesterone has the potential to hinder them.

RULE OUT OTHER POSSIBLE RELATED CAUSES FOR COGNITIVE DECLINE

Several problems not related to estrogen loss can also interfere with memory. Chronic elevations of stress hormones due to depression, anxiety, or insomnia are some of the most common causes of memory disturbance. (Refer to chapter 11.) *Attention deficit hyperactivity disorder (ADHD)* can also result in memory problems, since it shortens attention span, and distraction prevents information from being taken in accurately and processed effectively. People with ADHD describe their world as watching a television with channels that change at random. If you feel that your ability to concentrate is compromised, or that you're so easily distracted that it interferes with your ability to function, seek out additional information at one of the online self-screening tests to determine if you may have this chemical imbalance (see, for example, content.health.msn.com/content/article/84/98192.htm). Your doctor should also be able to diagnose or refer you to a local provider if you think this may be your problem.

Hypothyroidism is another hormonal problem associated with reversible memory problems. This can be ruled out as part of a yearly exam. The exam should also assess blood pressure (for stroke risk) and diabetes risk, as well as other problems that can cause memory loss.

ASK DR. GREENE

Q: CAN ANTIOXIDANT VITAMINS HELP BRAIN HEALTH?

A: Yes. But to successfully counter the damaging effects of free radicals, antioxidants (vitamins C and E) have to be present at the exact time the free radical is forming. Since free radicals form naturally during digestion, antioxidant supplements are effective in terms of free radical reduction only if they're taken at mealtime. That's why getting antioxidants *in* your food rather than in vitamin supplements is much more effective. Free radicals are present for only a fraction of a second, and the antioxidants have to be there at that exact moment to counter their damaging effects. So by the time you have your next vitamin, it could be too late; the damage might have been done already.

PERFECT BALANCE SOLUTIONS TO COGNITIVE DECLINE

DIET

- The Perfect Balance diet plan is designed for ultimate brain health as well as hormone balance. It helps counter most common obstacles to lifelong brain health—high blood pressure, vascular problems, diabetes, and free radicals. So it's even more important to follow the principles if you're suffering from memory loss.

- Avoid excessive alcohol consumption. Too much alcohol can interfere with your ability to take in information; it will also interfere with your REM sleep, resulting in reduced conversion of memory from short-term to long-term storage.

- Combine caffeine and complex carbohydrates to improve attention and memory. One study showed that a regular breakfast including an 8-ounce cup of coffee with 1 cup of oatmeal significantly improved short-term memory in a group of elderly women.

EXERCISE AND LIFESTYLE BEST BETS

- Aerobic exercise is especially important if you've been experiencing memory problems. Not only does exercise stimulate brain blood flow, it also lowers free radical production. It does this in two ways. First, exercise stimulates your muscles to produce more antioxidants. Second, exercise promotes the production of red blood cells by boosting testosterone levels, thereby increasing the amount of oxygen your blood can actually carry. Recent studies have also shown that the lactic acid produced by your muscles during exercise actually improves brain functioning by acting as an alternate fuel source. So boosting your exercise really strengthens your mind.

- Chew gum. It can actually improve brain functioning. One study found that chewing a stick of gum when studying or taking a test improves short-term and long-term memory by 35 percent! This could work because the chewing increases your pulse by about five or six beats per minute, supplying more glucose and oxygen-rich blood to your brain. Sugarless gum works as well, but without the extra calories.

- When you have something you really want to remember, say it out loud. That will keep it in your working memory longer and also allow you to store the information in two ways, visually and auditorily.

- Create memory links. Attaching new important information to something that's familiar to you increases the chance that you'll remember it. If you meet somebody new named Stanley, for instance, and want to remember his name, link it to somebody or something else named Stanley, like the Stanley Cup, for instance.

- Listen to music. Music has the ability to boost both memory retrieval and creative thinking by stimulating the right side of your brain, the side opposite that responsible for verbal memory information. Music also lowers stress hormone levels and heightens your level of alertness.

COMPLEMENTARY MEDICINE

- *Choline,* also called lecithin, is one of the B vitamins used to make the memory storage neurotransmitter acetylcholine, which is crucial for memory formation. It's present in eggs (about 200 mg per yolk), nuts (about 70–100 g), and meats (about 80–100 g). Though it would be unusual to have a nutritional deficiency of choline, in some studies, men and women in their mid-sixties performed better on recall, attention, and concentration tests after increasing their consumption of choline. Typical studies used 500–1,000 mg per day.

- *Ginkgo biloba* extracts have been touted for centuries as a means of boosting memory. The leaves contain a variety of chemicals, but the key ingredients are broken down into two groups, flavonoids and terpenes, both very powerful antioxidants. Since there are conflicting studies with ginkgo, I recommend a safe, reasonable approach. Start with 120 mg daily for four weeks to see if you notice a difference. If you don't notice an improvement, it's probably not worth continuing.

- *Salvia lavandulaefolia* (Spanish sage) has been shown to improve verbal memory. The phenomenon may be sage's ability to promote the production of acetylcholine, the neurotransmitter associated with memory. Standardized dosage recommendations are not yet available, but 1–4 grams of sage leaf in food or as a tea is reasonable. To avoid risks of seizure or hypoglycemia, consult your doctor first if you have diabetes, high blood pressure, or epilepsy.

- *Ginseng* is thought to improve brain functioning. Its strength probably lies in its ability to reduce blood clotting and thus increase blood flow to the brain. As a precaution, when taking ginseng make sure that you're not using any other medication that acts as a blood thinner.

BEST HORMONE TREATMENTS

Estrogen promotes a variety of cognitive functions, primarily those related to verbal memory and short-term memory, as well as the performance of feats related to speed and formulation of complex plans. Testosterone may further improve nonverbal memory and problem solving. And again, progesterone can oppose some of estrogen's benefits (though each woman's response is variable). The goal is to produce the most favorable estrogen-to-progesterone ratio—one that optimizes your estradiol level and minimizes your progesterone. So the trick is to shift your hormone balance so that it's estrogen dominant without creating negative side effects like breast tenderness and bloating. Here are the ways I achieve that balance:

- *Menstruating women:* If you're between ages sixteen and fifty and experiencing memory problems during your menstrual cycle, the BioSimilar/BioLimited contraceptive Seasonale has a favorable estrogen-to-progesterone ratio. This pill is packaged to create only four menstrual cycles per year, which means that there are only four times during the year when your estrogen levels drop low enough to contribute to memory problems. In other words, this pill can create a brain-hormone balance that is preferable in terms of memory to the variable hormone levels of a natural menstrual cycle.

- *Menopausal women:* I recommend BioIdentical estrogen on a continuous regimen. (Remember, estradiol is the only estrogen I recommend. No bi-est or tri-est creams, since they contain the weak estrogens that can diminish the benefits of estradiol.) Patches, rings, or gels are preferred. It's important that you use doses high enough to suppress hot

ALZHEIMER'S AND DEMENTIA

Dementia, in general, refers to any condition that leads to mental deterioration. Alzheimer's disease is only one form of dementia, but it's the most common form affecting women, and women are two to four times more likely to develop it than men. By their eighty-fifth birthday, at least half of all American women have Alzheimer's.

flashes. Don't exceed 0.1 mg per day unless instructed by your doctor. It's unlikely you'd get any additional benefits, and you could get side effects like breast tenderness and fluid retention. If you prefer pills, I recommend the BioSimilar pill called Cenestin. It's in a timed-release capsule, so it's more likely to work throughout the day without bottoming out before your next dose is due, making it more convenient as a once-a-day dose regimen. Start with 0.3 mg and work your way up to a maximum of 1.25 mg daily if needed. (This regimen may have better antioxidant effects than the transdermal, but we don't know yet whether or not the difference is significant. Stay tuned.)

ALZHEIMER'S DISEASE

Alzheimer's is the degenerative brain disease marked by progressive loss of mental ability. It was first described in medical literature in 1906 by German physician Dr. Alois Alzheimer. He reported finding very unusual lesions, which he called "tangles and plaques," in the brain of a woman who had died after a struggle with progressive and unusual memory loss. The "tangles and plaques" are actually nerves that have died. As we've discussed, when a nerve dies, the memories it was involved in preserving are lost forever. The plaques become a potent source of free radical production, adding insult to injury.

Alzheimer's disease is like a gradual unlearning of your own life—the most recent stored information is lost first; childhood memories tend to be preserved until nearly the end. Rarely does anyone die of Alzheimer's, but there's no cure for the disease nor any effective treatment.

Blood flow to the brain is one of the most important issues when it comes to Alzheimer's disease. When blood flow is compromised, damaging free radical production increases. One of the crucial findings of my early studies is that hot flashes create a significant decrease in brain blood flow. This is serious business, because hot flashes also increase free radical production. So hot flashes and night sweats may increase the risk of developing Alzheimer's disease. While having a few hot flashes now and then isn't significant, if you have many hot flashes per day, day after day, year after year, they can add up to the long-term changes that result in dementia.

Since I first presented that hypothesis, other research supporting it has grown stronger. Some studies have shown that women who have their ovaries removed—a condition that increases the frequency and intensity of hot flashes—not only tend to develop dementia sooner, but also have a more rapidly progressive decline in their cognitive abilities. Also, to date over thirty studies have demonstrated that women who don't take estrogen in menopause have a much higher risk of developing dementia than those who do.

FREE RADICALS AND BRAIN AGING

Unfortunately, no one knows for sure what triggers brain deterioration, but most researchers agree that free radical production is the biggest culprit. Free radicals are the leading obstacle to healthy brain aging. Since free radicals are made from oxygen, any part of the body that uses more oxygen than another generates more free radicals. Neurons use huge amounts of oxygen to function, and the number of free radicals produced in the process is astounding. (That's why the brain is at higher risk from free radical damage than the liver or lungs, which use less oxygen.) As these free radicals whiz around, they strike and damage proteins, DNA, and nerve membranes. When the damage occurs faster than it can be repaired, nerve cells die; and when enough die in a specific region of the brain, memories are lost forever.

When neurons die, they leave various chemicals behind that act like brain pollutants, accelerating damage to the remaining nerves. As we aim to correct the problem, nobody's sure which of these brain-polluting chemicals should be targeted first. Already, at least three proteins are the focus of a vaccine to clean up the pollution: beta-amyloid protein (BAP), tau protein (TAU), and alpha-synuclein (SYN). I believe that with time we'll garner a greater understanding of these brain pollutants and discover how to prevent and treat them.

PERFECT BALANCE SOLUTIONS TO
ALZHEIMER'S DISEASE PREVENTION

First, get a checkup. There are many physiological changes that can cause memory problems. If you've noticed your memory getting worse, get a complete physical examination from a skilled health care provider. If you're sixty-five or older, ask for a Mini Mental State Examination, which is a brief questionnaire for screening against dementia. You may want to get even more detailed cognitive function testing, administered by a clinical psychologist. Getting an early diagnosis is the best way to prevent an irreversible process from advancing. The following solutions will help boost brain health for all women, but especially for those over fifty, who naturally have lower estrogen levels, and those who already have mild cognitive impairment or Alzheimer's disease. They not only help maintain brain health, but can also help slow progressive brain injury.

DIET

- Experiment with various fresh herbs and spices—most are great antioxidants. This could significantly improve your day-to-day functioning as well as memory.

- Drink green tea. It's relatively low in caffeine and loaded with potent antioxidants as well as other chemicals that promote brain health. The caffeine combats the fatigue often associated with the early stages of Alzheimer's disease. I recommend three to five cups a day before two in the afternoon, preferably of an organic variety. If you continue drinking tea later in the day, switch to decaffeinated to avoid sleep problems.

- Soy is great for brain health if eaten in moderation. But don't consume more than 200 grams a day; if your estrogen levels are low, soy can actually compete with estradiol and block its brain-protecting effects. Also, don't expect soy capsules to be a viable alternative to estrogen therapy when it comes to preventing Alzheimer's disease.

EXERCISE, LIFESTYLE, AND MIND-BODY BEST BETS

- Take up dancing. Aging adults participating in dance classes demonstrate much better memory retention. The combination of aerobic exercise, complex movements, music, and human interaction makes for a perfect prescription for brain health.

- Exercise daily. Retirement means more time for more various activities: Garden, sail, swim, fly a kite, take your grandchildren for walks. Your brain loves variety. Your body benefits from the challenge, as well.

- Use it, don't lose it. Crossword puzzles and other games that activate your brain provide added protection against brain deterioration. Word games are beneficial because they challenge the verbal region of the brain, which really needs the exercise. Jigsaw puzzles are terrific, too, since they tap into your visual and spatial skills.

- Write things down to help you remember the small stuff. Post-it notes in appropriate places are excellent memory triggers. This should also reduce stress, another important goal of healthy brain aging.

- Photo albums and scrapbooks are great tools to trigger memories. As you create a scrapbook, you store the information in a new and unique way—visually. Each time you review your artistic work, you reinforce those memories.

- Put things in obvious places to trigger memories. Leave

ASK DR. GREENE

Q: MY MOTHER HAS ALZHEIMER'S DISEASE AND IS IN A PERMANENT CARE FACILITY. THE ANTIPSYCHOTIC DRUGS THE DOCTORS HAVE PUT HER ON TO COUNTER HER COMBATIVENESS HAVE TURNED HER INTO "A LIVING STATUE." CAN ESTROGEN HELP HER?

A: While nothing can reverse the kind of neuron loss your mother has already suffered, some medicines can reduce the rate of progression of memory loss, and estrogen has been shown to increase the length of the medicine's effectiveness. Estrogen also helps to reduce the aggressive behavior typical of severe Alzheimer's disease—so much, in fact, that many patients can be taken off antipsychotic medications. In several studies, Bioldentical estrogen has been found to be as effective as some of the standard medicines, with fewer side effects.

your reading glasses by your book, your bedtime pills by your toothbrush, and your umbrella by the door. These simple memory ploys can prevent a lot of confusion and frustration—another strike against stress.

COMPLEMENTARY MEDICINE

- Juvenon, a blend of L-carnitine and lipoic acid, is a great supplement for brain health and memory. It's more than an antioxidant; it actually encourages your cells to use energy more efficiently, markedly reducing free radical production. It works within the "powerhouse" of each nerve, the mitochondria, where you actually burn calories, so that you do so more efficiently. And it's well supported by research in addition to its biological plausibility. Dose is one tablet twice daily. For more information, call 1-800-588-3666, or go online to www.juvenon.com.

- Since vascular changes often contribute to declining brain function, aspirin is a good prevention strategy. Aspirin helps keep blood vessels dilated and optimizes blood flow to the brain. I recommend a low children's dose (81 mg) once a day. If you have a sensitive stomach, enteric-coated tablets will help reduce your risk of heartburn. (The coating delays the pills from dissolving until they're well past the stomach and into the colon, so it prevents gastrointestinal irritation.) Make sure if you're on other medications that your doctor knows you're taking a regular course of aspirin.

BEST HORMONE TREATMENTS

Because of the many studies demonstrating that estrogen can reduce the risk of Alzheimer's disease, I recommend estrogen therapy for any woman in menopause who is having hot flashes. Despite the confusion that arose from the Women's Health Initiative Memory Study, I continue to counsel women on the benefits of estrogen, as do most of the other leading researchers in this field. I do, however, have greater concerns about Provera, the highly synthetic progestin used in that study. There is evidence that it had an adverse effect, whereas there is no such evidence from BioIdentical progesterone.

- If you have symptoms of memory or cognitive problems indicative of Alzheimer's, you should seriously consider estrogen replacement—ideally with a BioIdentical formulation. Again, I feel that transdermal preparations are best. Start with the lowest doses available if you've been off estrogen for longer than a year, and increase the dose about every ten weeks as needed to provide symptom relief. You shouldn't have to exceed a dose of 0.1 mg per day. If you choose an oral BioSimilar preparation such as Cenestin or Premarin, you are likely to achieve symptom relief with a dose of 0.625 mg per day (you can go as high as 1.25 mg per day).

• This is one of the rare instances where I recommend a blood test even if you have no symptoms. Several studies have shown that the risk of dementia may be related to having a very low blood estradiol level. If you've been in a hormonally depleted state like menopause for a long time, it's possible that your ovaries are producing dangerously low levels of estradiol, putting you in the serious risk category. If your blood estradiol levels are less than 20 pg/mL, I recommend you consider a small dose of BioIdentical estrogen replacement. Start with the lowest dose available—Menostar 0.014 mg per day. This new formulation is such an ultralow dose that it has been approved for use without progesterone, even if you have not had a hysterectomy. Consider it like any other vitamin or supplement that you use to improve your health.

CHAPTER FOURTEEN

BALANCE AND COORDINATION

Various aspects of movement are closely connected to hormones. Because of the hormonal impact on the brain, shifts in sex hormone levels play a pivotal role in balance and coordination, and because of that connection, a hormonal imbalance can put you at higher risk for fall-related injuries and certain movement disorders. Since the ability to move freely and with confidence is a key factor in maintaining lifelong independence, this can have a huge impact on your quality of life, now and in the future.

When your sex hormones are balanced, the nerves in the motor and sensory regions are able to perform the complex tasks of coordination and balance much more efficiently. *Balance* is essentially your ability to maintain your body in an upright position. *Coordination* refers to your ability to move your arms, legs, and body through a complex set of movements. To maintain balance and coordination, your brain has to integrate information from your eyes, ears, muscles, and vascular system. The term used to describe the combined efforts involved in balance and coordination is *executive motor functioning*—the executive in charge being your brain. When any aspect of your executive motor functions is impaired, you can experience problems with movement.

Coordinated movements, no matter how automatic they seem, are always initiated by your thoughts. Though the initial thought to move can begin almost anywhere on the surface of your brain, it has to be processed by the motor and sensory regions, a narrow strip that arches across the crown of your head, before any action takes place. To move with the fluidity that most of us take for granted, the muscles involved in movement have to receive precisely timed signals and adjustments from these regions in terms of the type of movement and the appropriate strength that will be necessary to accomplish the act. So a simple action like walking across the street requires your brain to consider the forces of gravity, the firmness of the walking surface, any obstacles that may be in your way, and any dangers that may be approaching and to integrate that information with your muscles. And it does it all effortlessly, in the blink of an eye. Estrogen helps make all that possible. The difference between your smooth movements and a child's somewhat uncoordinated effort is that your brain has matured under the influence of sex hormones and continues to be influenced by them.

BALANCE AND COORDINATION QUESTIONNAIRE

This questionnaire will give you an idea where you stand in terms of movement problems. Answer the following questions by circling either "Yes" or "No." Then score the test by giving yourself one point for every question to which you answered "Yes."

1. Do you ever become dizzy?	Yes	No
2. Have you fallen within the last year?	Yes	No
3. Do you notice worsening fatigue?	Yes	No
4. Have you developed a tremor?	Yes	No
5. Are you over sixty-five years of age?	Yes	No
6. Have you experienced a loss of strength?	Yes	No
7. Is your vision failing?	Yes	No
8. Do you have osteoporosis?	Yes	No
9. Are you in your third trimester of pregnancy?	Yes	No
10. Have you fallen within the last month?	Yes	No

SCORE

0–1   You're at low risk of having a movement disorder or injury.

2–3   You need to take some preventive steps against injury.

4–10   You need to make an appointment with your health care provider.

DIZZINESS IS YOUR GREATEST RISK FACTOR FOR INJURY

In the United States, about 5 million emergency room visits a year are due to dizziness, and more than half of those patients are women. Although serious illness is involved only about 5 percent of the time, the risk of injury due to falling is substantial. The most important variable with respect to these kinds of injuries—even more important than bone strength—is the hormone-brain connection. Light-headedness, typically caused by a sudden decrease in blood flow, and vertigo, a false sense of motion that makes you feel as if the room is spinning, are associated with changes in sex hormone levels at least 50 percent of the time.

As women get older, their risk of fracturing a hip rises steadily. At age fifty, the risk of hip fracture doubles, and it continues to double every five to six years, so that by age ninety you're more likely to have had a hip fracture than not. The explanation for that is that aging women are simply no longer able to react as quickly when they stumble and thus land on their hip rather than an outstretched arm. Within one year of a hip fracture, the risk of death is 25 percent. That ranks it as more lethal than most serious diseases, including breast and ovarian cancer. That's why even though most dizziness isn't an indication of a serious illness,

ASK DR. GREENE

Q: WHAT'S THE CORRELATION BETWEEN DIZZINESS AND HORMONAL BALANCE?

A: The most common cause of vertigo is estrogen deficiency. Since low estrogen levels can slow your reaction time and nerves that carry messages to and from your brain are slower to process information, slower reaction signals result. Fluid volumes in the inner ear may also shift, contributing to the sensation of dizziness. And during a fall, because reaction time is much slower, you're less likely to catch yourself. When estrogen levels are low, your reaction time can be reduced by almost half a second, which could mean the difference between breaking a fall with your hand or breaking a hip.

DIZZINESS AND PREGNANCY

Many pregnant women experience frequent episodes of light-headedness, especially when standing. During pregnancy, high progesterone levels stimulate the respiratory centers in the brain, which makes breathing faster and more shallow. That alone can cause light-headedness. But as pregnancy progresses, the developing fetus decreases the return of blood flow to the heart; as a result, there is a slight delay getting blood to the brain when you stand up. The added abdominal weight in the third trimester also shifts the center of gravity forward by several centimeters, which makes for further unsteadiness. This combination of factors significantly increases the risk of falling late in pregnancy.

it does represent a serious risk to health.

RULE OUT OTHER POSSIBLE CAUSES FOR DIZZINESS

Low blood sugar (hypoglycemia) can cause dizziness, alerting you to the need to eat. Hyperthyroidism (excess thyroid hormone production) can also initiate light headedness, as can problems of fluid imbalance. Retention of fluid in the ears can contribute to balance disturbances like Ménière's disease or benign positional vertigo. See your health care provider for an evaluation; though not serious, these are all easily diagnosed and treatable. Other possible causes of dizziness are migraine headaches, hyperventilation, various changes in your blood circulation, low blood pressure (which prevents the proper transportation of oxygen to the brain), and some medications. If all of these problems are ruled out and you're not experiencing a hormone-related problem, you may need to see a neurologist to rule out one of the more rare causes of vertigo like Parkinson's disease or multiple sclerosis. These two serious neurological disorders are often diagnosed many years after initial symptoms. So don't ignore your symptoms if they persist. Seek an evaluation by a neurologist.

PERFECT BALANCE SOLUTIONS FOR IMPROVED BALANCE AND COORDINATION

Many of these recommendations are aimed at strengthening your bones and improving muscle function. Taking these steps should reduce not only your risk of falling, but also your risk of injury if you do fall.

DIET

- Get enough calcium and vitamin D. If you don't have enough calcium to maintain bone strength, you end up with progressively weaker bones, which can ultimately lead to osteopenia (early bone loss) and osteoporosis. The current recommendation for calcium is 1,000 mg per day for nineteen-to-fifty-year-olds and 1,500 mg per day for women fifty and older. Low-fat yogurt, fortified soy, and fortified orange juice are great sources. Take an over-the-counter supplement with your meals if your dietary calcium is low. Vitamin D is vital for absorbing calcium. Recommendations for vitamin D are 200 IU daily for women ages nineteen to fifty and 400 IU daily for women ages fifty-one to sixty-nine. Best sources are fortified milk, cereals, and supplements.

- Avoid high doses of vitamin A (retinoic acid) because it stimulates *osteoclasts,* the cells that break down bone. Additionally, it counteracts the benefits of vitamin D so that you don't absorb calcium. Keep your intake below 500 IU per day.

- Eat plenty of protein to preserve bone strength. The calcium in your bone is actually applied to *osteoid,* a protein matrix that helps keep cracks from growing through the hard portions of bone. Without osteoid, cracks move like a panty hose run—very quickly, until they run completely end to end.

EXERCISE AND MIND-BODY BEST BETS

- Strength training is critical because it stimulates the cells that build bone. So exercises that build muscle, such as weight lifting or power yoga, will make your bones stronger. One hour of combined balance and resistance training two or three times per week (along with a fall-safe home environment) has been shown to reduce the risk of falls by almost 50 percent.

- Practicing tai chi for thirty minutes three or four times a week has been shown to markedly improve balance and confidence in walking without falling. Hatha yoga is another best bet.

PRACTICAL TIPS

- Fall-proof your home. Adjusting furniture so there are no dark corners, uneven easy-trip rugs, or narrow passages between furniture can reduce your chance of falling.

- Try extrasensory stimulation. Currently under investigation is a vibrating gel insole that you can slip into your shoe. So far, it's been shown to improve balance and reduce falling in young and old alike. When the soles vibrate intermittently, they provide additional sensory information to the brain regarding the positioning of the feet. Since vibrating insoles are not yet available, consider using acupressure insoles that press gently on healing spots on your feet as you walk. They cost less than $15, and even if they don't help, they'll feel good. (Call 1-800-438-8143, or go online to www.massager-machines-and-more.com/acupressure-insoles.htm.)

COMPLEMENTARY MEDICINE

- Ginkgo biloba is recommended for dizziness because it may help inner ear disturbances as well as problems related to circulation. The amount generally recommended is 120 mg per day, split into 60 mg doses taken twice a day. If you want to continue it beyond six weeks, make sure you discuss it with your doctor.

- B_6 is one of the most important vitamins for producing healthy neurotransmitters, and it also helps manufacture red blood cells, reduce anemia, and improve your brain's ability to function. Studies show that 10–25 mg per day can be helpful in reducing problems associated with dizziness. The best sources are bananas, lentils, grains, and turkey. My recommendation: 25 mg per day.

- Ginger has been reported to reduce dizziness. It's been used in Chinese medicine for 2,500 years. General recommendations are 500–1,000 mg per day. You can get 500 mg by consuming two pieces of crystallized ginger candy or a half-inch piece of peeled ginger.

BEST HORMONE TREATMENTS

The best tool for preventing dizziness is BioIdentical estrogen therapy. By improving the speed with which your nerves can transmit information, estrogen improves the way your brain resolves conflicting spatial information. Continuous stable BioIdentical estrogen supplementation will help alleviate dizziness and coordination problems now, while also lowering your risk of problems later.

- The transdermal patches are the most thoroughly studied, but the newer gels and creams should be equally as effective. Climara or Vivelle are two popular patch regimens, while Estrasorb and EstroGel are newer formulations that are absorbed through the skin. I recommend a minimal dose of 0.05 mg per day. At least thirty studies to date (including the WHI's) have found that long-term estrogen use helps reduce hip fracture risk. In fact, if you combine estrogen with a bone-strengthening agent like Fosamax or Actonel, your bones will get harder than if you took these medicines without estrogen.

- If you prefer BioSimilar replacement regimens, Cenestin is a BioSimilar preparation with a slow, steady absorption pattern designed for gradual release. Premarin and Estrace, on the other hand, are absorbed quickly and can make dizziness a bit worse because of their rapid entry into the bloodstream. If you're on them and doing well, don't worry, they're working for you. But if you're having trouble with balance, it's a good idea to switch to a more stable regimen.

ASK DR. GREENE

Q: SINCE PARKINSON'S DISEASE INVOLVES A MOVEMENT DISORDER, IS THERE A CONNECTION BETWEEN PARKINSON'S AND HORMONES?

A: Yes, and it's a very important connection. Estrogen has been shown to reduce symptoms of Parkinson's and slow the progression of the disease. It indirectly promotes dopamine production, which helps improve nerve function, and is extremely beneficial in terms of maintaining the structural integrity of the remaining nerves. Some studies suggest that Parkinson's patients who stay on estrogen replacement have an 80 percent reduction in the risk of developing dementia. For my Parkinson's patients, I recommend BioIdentical estrogen therapy by means of patch, cream, or gel because it promotes steady blood levels of estrogen and doesn't interfere with the absorption of any Parkinson's medications. Although BioIdentical testosterone hasn't been formally studied in women, it has been shown to reduce Parkinson's symptoms in men. I recommend it for my patients to keep muscles strong and provide an additional source of estradiol for the brain. (Interestingly, some recent findings show that both BioIdentical estrogen and testosterone may be beneficial for patients with multiple sclerosis.)

• Finally, I want to mention concerns regarding the BioLimited preparations that are often recommended to "lower breast cancer risks." These synthetic drugs commonly exacerbate symptoms of vertigo. They're often prescribed because of their ability to "protect your bones," but they are not nearly as effective as BioIdentical estrogen. So if you're on Evista (raloxifene) or Nolvadex (tamoxifen) and are experiencing vertigo, discuss this issue with your doctor to determine if the benefits are outweighing the risks of falling as a result of feeling unstable.

CHAPTER FIFTEEN

YOUR PHYSICAL APPEARANCE

Through discussions with my patients, I've learned just how important various aspects of appearance are for women. They've taught me that for most women, looking good is about putting their best foot forward, feeling good about themselves, and having more self-confidence. And those certainly are important quality-of-life factors.

There are also some biological reasons behind our general desire to look good. Strong white teeth, lustrous hair, beautiful skin, and many of the other qualities we associate with a stellar appearance are, for the most part, signs of good health, which explains, at least on a base biological level, why most of us are attracted to beauty. In the days when we roamed the plains as hunters and gatherers, it would have been a sign of a good potential mate, since the health and fertility of our partners ensured survival of the clan. So maybe beauty isn't just skin deep after all. All this considered, it's not surprising that hormones play a vital role in many aspects of appearance, including skin, hair, teeth, and eyes.

The skin is one of the primary sites where testosterone is converted to the potent androgen *dihydrotestosterone (DHT)*. The rate and amount of the conversion is determined genetically and plays a major role in the oiliness of your skin as well as the thickness and distribution of your hair. The variation in these genetic traits explains why some of us are more susceptible to acne and excessive hair growth or hair loss than others. But while genetics is a significant factor, there are measures you can take to slow the signs of skin aging and control acne, hair thinning, hirsutism, and even tooth loss.

SKIN AGING

Four main factors contribute to skin aging: sun damage (aka photodamage), smoking, environmental BioMutagens, and the naturally occurring age-related changes in skin cells.

Sun damage causes skin pigment changes and wrinkles that are much coarser than the fine wrinkles characteristic of normal aging. It also creates free radicals that damage DNA and collagen and promotes skin cancer. (While Caucasian women, particularly those with fairer skin, are more vulnerable to sun damage, women with darker skin are also susceptible to skin aging as a result of photodamage.) Estrogen can reduce sun damage by promoting cell turnover in the skin, so that if a DNA mutation occurs, the cell can be sloughed off before it can divide and become a cancer. And because estrogen is a great antioxidant, it may be able to prevent some of the free radical damage that can promote cancer formation.

Smoking presents different problems. It decreases oxygen delivery to the skin and cumulatively lowers estrogen levels, making skin look sallow. While you're puffing on a cigarette, blood flow to your skin decreases by about 30 percent owing to constriction of the blood vessels in your face. In addition, chemicals in cigarettes contain numerous free radical–producing chemicals that can overwhelm your natural antioxidant protection and cause DNA damage. The nicotine in tobacco also causes your body to convert some of your beneficial estrogen, estradiol, into a nasty metabolite of estrogen called a *catechol* estrogen. Catechol acts as a BioAntagonist and possibly as a BioMutagen, inhibiting beneficial actions of estradiol and promoting changes in DNA that increase cancer risks. Environmental BioMutagens can interfere with estrogen's ability to promote cell turnover in the skin, encouraging the formation of wrinkles and making skin appear dry and less vibrant.

During your youth, it normally takes a skin cell about thirty days to "turn over"—to migrate from the base of your epidermis to the surface of your skin.

That turnover keeps skin in tiptop shape by quickly sloughing off dead cells and provides effective protection from the environment. The turnover process tends to take twice as long by the time you reach age forty. Having a slower cell turnover time makes your skin look dull and leaves pores susceptible to becoming plugged and more prominent. It also allows for toxic buildup and reduces water content in your skin, which contributes to wrinkling.

Loss of collagen also contributes to age-related skin wrinkling. The dermal layer of your skin—the layer directly below your epidermis, or top layer—is about 85–90 percent collagen. Women lose an average of 30 percent of that collagen during the first five years of menopause, then continue to lose about 2 percent a year up until around age seventy. With the loss of collagen comes a depreciation of skin elasticity and a reduction in skin moisture, which results in fine lines and wrinkles.

ASK DR. GREENE

Q: ARE THERE ANY HORMONAL BENEFITS TO TANNING?

A: Actually, yes. When sunlight hits your skin, it delivers energy that is absorbed by the skin. The sun's ultraviolet rays injure the skin cells and induce them to produce the hormone melanocortin. MSH, in turn, promotes production of the melanin that causes you to tan. MSH also enters the bloodstream and feeds information back to the brain, which prompts it to boost your libido and suppress your appetite. So though it isn't healthy to tan, there may be health benefits associated with having higher levels of this tanning hormone.

The good news is that estrogen helps improve both conditions. Studies have found that estrogen replacement reduces the risk of developing wrinkles by at least 30 percent. Estrogen causes your skin to form new collagen fibers by stimulating the collagen-producing cells (improving skin tone) and helps to speed up the cell turnover time, which promotes the kind of healthy, vital skin changes associated with youth. And there's a good chance that testosterone plays a role in promoting more rapid turnover of skin cells, too, though we'll need additional research to confirm that.

In addition to the natural aging process, some cosmetics may actually contain BioMutagens that can further damage your skin. Some can damage DNA, promoting cancer formation. Others simply block the hormone receptors, jamming the signals from the brain that trigger DNA repair; adjust skin moisture level; or even promote release of oils or perspiration. Lanolin, for instance, is often contaminated with the potent pesticide DDT, and there's good evidence that the commonly used preservative parabens may promote breast cancer—especially when it's added to underarm deodorants, which, of course, is frequently applied immediately after shaving. Although many cosmetic companies talked about terminating use of these chemicals, switching to safer preservatives is expensive, so it's anybody's guess when and if this will happen. I've listed several of the most common toxins in cosmetics in the BioMutagen chart in chapter 7.

ASK DR. GREENE

Q. CAN HORMONE IMBALANCE CAUSE DRY OR RED EYES?

A: Yes. The longer your estrogen levels are low, the greater your chances of developing dry eyes (aka *Keratoconjuntivitis sicca*). Estrogen dilates the blood vessels in the tear ducts so they can effectively keep your eyes moist. I recommend non-prescription eye drops and topical estrogens (patches, creams, or gels) for my patients. Compounding pharmacies can also create eye drops made with Bioldentical estrogen (recommended dose is 0.005 mg of estradiol in 20 ml of sterile ophthalmic saline).

PERFECT BALANCE SOLUTIONS FOR SKIN AGING

DIET

- Staying hydrated is your best defense against wrinkles. Make sure that you get at least eight to ten glasses of fluid per day. Include several glasses of high-antioxidant green tea in that count.

- Eat lots of Hormone Power Carbs. They have the ability to bind water so that it remains in the dermis—the layer beneath the skin. Without enough carbs, you're not able to bind as much water. One of the things that keeps young, healthy skin wrinkle-free is its elasticity. If you're not getting enough water or carbohydrates to maintain this elasticity, your skin begins to feel leathery and your cheeks appear sunken. Veggies, fruits, and whole grains are packed with water and nutrition.

• Eat more omega-3-packed foods such as walnuts, flaxseed, and fish. Omega-3 fatty acids can markedly improve skin quality because their potent antioxidants aid in the repair of damaged skin.

BEST HORMONE TREATMENTS

• BioIdentical and BioSimilar estrogen replacement products are among the only treatments that have demonstrated objective improvements in skin quality. To minimize wrinkles, use BioIdentical estrogen. I recommend 0.05–0.1 mg per day, administered by a patch delivery system (Climara, for instance). As an alternative to the tried-and-true patch, I recommend BioIdentical estrogen compounded as a cream. (Keep in mind that this can be applied to trouble spots as a localized treatment instead of, or in addition to, the patch. This is unlikely to provide much benefit if you're in your twenties or early thirties, since any skin wrinkles at that age are more likely to be the result of sun damage than natural loss of your skin's wrinkle resistance.) Another option is a promising new formulation, Estrasorb cream. It may be applied to the areas you're most concerned about. Although estrogen hasn't been studied for administration this way, there's no reason to believe it wouldn't be effective.

• Retinoic acids (tretinoin) are synthetic formulations similar to vitamin A. These drugs, sold under names like Renova and Tazorac, work by enabling the collagen in your skin to form new bonds, essentially tightening up the skin. They're very effective, but they can be irritating to your skin. If you use these products, you should also be aware that they significantly increase your susceptibility to sun damage, so a good sunscreen is vital. (Also, effective contraception is a necessity since they can cause mutation if you become pregnant while you are using them!) While these products can give skin a more youthful appearance by causing stretched collagen fibers in your skin to form crosslinks with one another, only estrogen works by stimulating the body's natural response, so these other products should be reconsidered as adjunct treatments.

ACNE

Acne is the most common skin disorder in the United States. It affects at least 85 percent of all teenagers and many young adults and in some cases can last into adulthood. It can contribute to depression, anxiety, loss of self-esteem, and even social isolation.

Acne is primarily a hormonal imbalance that is the result of heredity—what it means is that you've inherited too much of the enzyme in the skin that converts testosterone to DHT instead of estradiol. Acne can also be caused by an imbalance of your estradiol-to-testosterone ratio (it's tipped too far toward the androgens). Certain bacteria in the skin or chronic irritation to the skin can also contribute to acne by inciting oil-producing pores to become inflamed and blocked.

This hormonal imbalance usually happens when you hit puberty. Rising testosterone levels stimulate the oil glands at the base of hair follicles to increase their production rate. The glands effectively form an "oil slick," clogging your pores as skin cells are sloughed off. The combination of dead skin cells, increased oil, and blocked pores makes for an excellent breeding ground for bacteria. This sets off a cascade of inflammatory changes that result in acne lesions, especially on your face, back, and upper chest. And stress can exacerbate the acne by boosting stress hormone levels, which decreases the rate of skin cell turnover.

The hormonal changes of menstruation can cause or worsen acne, too. As your estrogen level increases and promotes the production of more carrier proteins

ASK DR. GREENE

Q: DOES GREASY FOOD CAUSE ACNE?

A: Food doesn't cause acne per se, but high-fat, calorie-dense foods with lots of simple sugars can trigger a hormonal imbalance that can make it worse. In general, anything that increases oil production by your skin or skin cell loss can contribute to acne. Here are some of the things that can do that:

- Use of greasy skin or hair products containing animal fats

- Airborne pollutants (including those created by frying foods) and dust

- Scrubbing your skin too vigorously during cleaning

- Hormones or medicines that generate an imbalance of sex hormones, such as lithium and prednisone (which, in effect, deactivates some of your testosterone), your free testosterone level declines, providing your skin with a brief break from the acne-producing chemicals in your skin. But as your estrogen levels fall again before the next cycle, and your testosterone becomes more dominant, the process starts anew, resulting in the kind of cyclic acne experienced by so many women. Since testosterone levels gradually decline starting in the early twenties, as you get older you have much less chance of developing a testosterone-dominant hormonal balance and thus much less chance of having acne.

When both estrogen and testosterone are high, pores are far more likely to become blocked because of the increase in cell turnover promoted by estrogen and the testosterone-driven oil production. The combination promotes both infection and pimples. Stress can further exacerbate acne by boosting stress hormone levels, which causes detrimental changes in skin cell turnover. Your best bet for clear skin is to shift your estradiol-to-testosterone ratio toward estradiol and to keep your stress hormones low and stable.

PERFECT BALANCE SOLUTIONS FOR ACNE PREVENTION

COMPLEMENTARY MEDICINE

- Tea tree *(Melaleuca alternifolia)* essential oil has many antibacterial properties and is a potent antioxidant that can help prevent acne. You can find many mild soaps, hair products, and organic skin cleansers containing tea tree extracts in health food stores.

- Basil *(Ocimum basilicum)* has been reported to improve skin lesions. Eat fresh basil and try steeping a handful of leaves in 1 cup of water for fifteen minutes. Let it cool to room temperature, then apply the liquid to your face with a cotton ball.

- Witch hazel *(Hamamelis virginiana)* astringent helps balance your skin's oil production. Apply after cleansing your face.

BEST HORMONE TREATMENTS

- The single best hormone-balancing treatment for minimizing acne is the birth control pill, but only the pills that contain BioSimilar estrogen and BioLimited progestin. The one I recommend based on findings from chemical testing is the birth control pill Yasmin. It blocks the enzyme that converts some testosterone to DHT, which protects your skin from

ASK DR. GREENE

Q: IS THERE A HORMONE CONNECTION IN TERMS OF TOOTH LOSS?

A: Yes. Low levels of estrogen cause calcium loss and ultimately bone loss in your jawbone. When the bone at the root of a tooth is gone, the tooth becomes loose; inflammation can set in and accelerate eventual tooth loss. There's a strong diet connection, too. A poor diet combined with decreased blood flow to the gums and decreased immune functioning during menopause significantly raises the risk of tooth loss. So be sure to watch your diet and keep up adequate levels of calcium (at least 1,500 mg per day) and vitamin D (200–400 mg daily). Finally, consider Bioldentical estrogen therapy. (Various research studies have found that menopausal women on estrogen have a 20–30 percent reduction in tooth loss.) If you have no other symptoms of hormonal imbalance and your teeth are in excellent condition, I recommend a minimal dose of 0.025 mg per day. This will serve as a preventive measure, not just for teeth, but for your bones and brain, as well. If you've already experienced problems with your teeth, I recommend 0.05 mg per day up to 0.1 mg per day.

the androgenic affects of excess testosterone and lowers testosterone levels (which promotes healing of acne lesions). Ortho Tri-Cyclen and Ortho-Cyclen are also effective at reducing the severity of acne.

HIRSUTISM

We are born with about 5 million hair follicles covering every surface on our body except the palms of our hands, the soles of our feet, and our lips. (Approximately one hundred thousand of them are on our scalp.) We don't form any new hair follicles after birth, but rather spend our life cycling the follicles we're born with. The cycle passes from a growth phase *(anagen),* to a transitional phase *(catagen),* followed by a resting and shedding phase *(telogen).* How often the hair follicles move through these phases is influenced by sex hormones and their impact on hair growth and hair loss.

Hirsutism is excessive hair growth—a thickening of hair follicles. In women it occurs in testosterone-sensitive regions of the body, such as the face, neck, chest, and abdomen. It's a problem for between 5 and 10 percent of women in the United States—

about 41 million women. Nearly 50 percent of American women wax or pluck facial hair on at least a weekly basis.

Two factors determine hirsutism: a hormonal imbalance (specifically excess levels of testosterone) and genetics. Hair follicles are one of the key regions of the body where testosterone, instead of being converted into estradiol, is converted to its potent androgenic form, DHT. DHT is the hormonal stimulant that converts soft, fine, barely noticeable hair (vellus hair) into thick, coarse hair that is hard to ignore. Bottom line: When you have excess levels of testosterone, it is converted into DHT in the hair follicles and promotes excess hair growth in the wrong places.

There are a couple of scenarios that can promote an excess of testosterone. Your ovaries may be producing too much of it—only about 25 percent of the women with hirsutism have this problem. Or you could be taking a form of testosterone or other drugs that binds to the testosterone receptor and stimulates follicle growth. That's often the case when using a non-BioIdentical form of testosterone to treat a testosterone deficiency. Since synthetic testosterone simply can't be converted into estrogen the way BioIdentical testosterone can, it often results in hirsutism and acne. That's why I rarely prescribe synthetic forms of testosterone.

But by far the most common cause of hirsutism is genetics. When you're genetically predisposed to hirsutism, as many Hispanic and Mediterranean women are, it's not that you have too much testosterone per se, but that your skin is simply more sensitive to it. That causes excess hair growth—even when your testosterone levels are normal.

RULE OUT OTHER POSSIBLE CAUSES OF EXCESSIVE HAIR

Excessive release of the stress hormone prolactin can promote surplus hair growth, although at this time we're not certain why. High levels of insulin—which, as we've discussed, is common in the United States—can also promote excess hair growth. Both excess insulin and prolactin can be detected through blood tests (a fasting morning prolactin level and fasting morning insulin level with simultaneous glucose testing).

PERFECT BALANCE SOLUTIONS FOR HIRSUTISM

- My preferred hormone-balancing recommendation for excessive hair growth is the combination oral contraceptive Yasmin, which has a fixed

ASK DR. GREENE

Q: WHAT DO YOU RECOMMEND TO COUNTER HAIR LOSS AND PROMOTE GROWTH?

A: The Perfect Balance diet will provide you with the nutrients you need. For hormone treatments, you'll need a stable amount of estrogen (which prompts your hair to stay in its growth phase) and testosterone (which promotes normal amounts of oil production). Bioldentical estrogens like Climera, Estrasorb, or EstroGel should do the trick. (Hair loss after pregnancy, incidentally, is very common, but rest assured it *will* grow back.)

dose of BioSimilar estrogen with a BioLimited progestin that blocks the testosterone receptor in the skin, thus reducing excess hair growth. Of all the oral contraceptives, Yasmin is most effective for this purpose. Ortho Tri-Cyclen is also a great alternative.

• In addition to the use of a BioSimilar combination hormone, I recommend a diuretic called Aldactone (or the generic spironolactone), which has properties similar to a mild BioAntagonist. It binds and blocks the testosterone receptor in the skin. Aldactone is typically prescribed in tablet doses of 25–50 mg once or twice per day, depending on the severity of the problem. It also has the added benefit of slightly reducing blood pressure, a common need for many women.

• Finally, there is a new topical medication that is actually not a hormone at all. This medication, called Vaniqa, blocks the enzyme responsible for hair follicle growth. It doesn't come in a fixed dose; rather, you apply a small amount to the area you wish to treat each morning and night. It is remarkably well tolerated; even patients with sensitive skin are rarely bothered. You can apply any makeup after it has been absorbed.

Note: With all hair growth reduction regimens, it can take eight to twelve weeks before you see results, so be patient.

CHAPTER SIXTEEN

CANCER PREVENTION

Since cancer is so prevalent in our society and so many women are concerned about the relationship between hormones and cancer, in this chapter I'll sort out some of the confusion, examine the truth about the way hormones affect the chances of developing cancer, and explore the best cancer-prevention strategies.

First and foremost, hormones, including the much-maligned estrogen, do not cause cancer. Estrogen's reputation as a cancer-causing agent is completely unfounded, based on loose associations, misinformation, and our all-too-human desire to ascribe blame to something concrete and specific. The only thing that estrogen can do in terms of cancer is promote its growth if it already exists in your body. As we've seen, estrogen stimulates activity in the DNA of healthy cells that have estrogen receptors. Since the estrogen can't differentiate between normal cells and cancer cells, it stimulates both equally; if cancer is in a cell, it will grow. So what we want to do here is reduce your risk of developing cancer in the first place. That means minimizing the *true* cancer risks, especially exposure to carcinogenic BioMutagens in your life that are linked with

Q: IS CANCER GENETIC?

A: Contrary to popular thinking, most cancers are not the result of genetic inheritance. In fact, only about 2 percent of all cancers are related to risks embedded in your genetic code. Cancer-promoting damage to the gene DNA can occur in one of two ways: by accident as cells are going through their normal patterns of division or by the accumulation of BioMutagens we're exposed to throughout our life. Either way, the damage doesn't kill cells per se, but rather transforms them into rogue cells that ignore the normal rules of cellular growth. To prevent an abnormal cell from becoming a full-blown tumor, your immune system has to be able to identify, isolate, and remove these cells.

cancers of the breast, colon, ovaries, and uterus.

WHAT IS CANCER?

A cancer forms when cells in some part of your body begin to grow in an uncontrolled manner. Normally your cells grow, divide, and die in a systematic fashion. But cancer cells continue to grow and divide in an abnormal way. They live longer and divide more often than normal cells. These cancer cells form tumors and sometimes spread to other parts of the body through the blood or lymphatic system. To initiate this sort of uncontrolled growth and maintain it, the cell has to go through genetic changes. So cancer is, in effect, a disease of the genes, and in order to cause cancer, an agent must have the ability to induce change in gene DNA. No hormone that your body makes has demonstrated an ability to do that.

WHAT IS YOUR RISK OF DEVELOPING CANCER?

Risk assessment is a numbers game. Nobody can accurately predict whether or not you will get cancer. Risk factors reflect your chances of getting cancer, but having a risk factor for cancer doesn't mean you'll get it. Some risk factors—your age, gender, and family medical history—are *nonmodifiable* risk factors. You have to look at those risk factors carefully. Your family history, for instance, doesn't reflect just genetics—remember, that's estimated to put you at only a 2 percent increased risk—it also reflects diet, lifestyle, and BioMutagen exposures. If your dad smoked five packs of unfiltered cigarettes a day and died of lung cancer, that's part of your family history, but it doesn't necessarily affect you much, especially if your parents were divorced and he lived a thousand miles away (not even a secondhand smoke risk factor there). On the other hand, if your mom and siblings were exposed to BioMutagens sprayed in nearby fields as you were growing up, chances are you were, too. Your age is a risk factor for at least two reasons. First, as you get older, your immune system becomes less effective at identifying and neutralizing any cancer cells that develop. Second and most important, many of the damaging effects of BioMutagens you've been exposed to throughout your life accumulate and concentrate in muscle and fat cells. The more you're exposed to these environmental carcinogens, the more you store, and the more you're at risk of developing cancer.

Other risk factors are *modifiable*—you can do something about these now. They include current lifestyle choices, physical activity, and exposure to BioMutagens. These modifiable risk factors account for nearly 75 percent of all cancers. You can lower your risk factor for cancer by the double digits by modifying these factors. For example, obesity increases your risk of breast cancer fourfold. Reducing your future exposure to BioMutagens, a serious modifiable risk factor, is a central focus of our program, as is getting plenty of exercise. So you have a certain amount of control over your exposure risk factors—you can actually reduce your risk of cancer now and in the future.

CARCINOGENS VS. BIOMUTAGENS

A *carcinogen* is a chemical that has been well documented to trigger cancer. The fact that you can be exposed to a carcinogen and *not* develop cancer suggests to me that the term *carcinogen* is somewhat inaccurate. That's why I coined the term *BioMutagen*. A BioMutagen is anything that can disrupt normal hormonal response and therefore has the *potential* to cause cancer. In contrast with the current regulatory guidelines for chemicals "presumed safe until proven dangerous," when it comes to potential disruption of hormone signals, I recommend a more cautious attitude of "at risk until proven safe." BioMutagens can alter your normal cellular activity, cause the premature death of a cell (a real problem if it kills an immune cell that might otherwise fight off a cancer), injure a cell in a way that makes it less functional, or transform a cell so that it resists your body's signals to stop growing or moving beyond a certain border (which can turn normal cells into cancerous ones).

Some BioMutagens actually masquerade as hormones, which fools receptors into allowing them to enter a cell. For example, DDT (found in fish and lanolin) mimics estrogen and interferes with the function of testosterone. Our exposure to these disruptors comes mostly through food and lifestyle. There are a growing number of chemicals in the air we breathe, the water we drink, and the food we eat, all of which are able to alter our body's normal hormone responses. They can also amplify the body's normal response to a hormone signal—and that's what I believe is the most likely link between sex hormones and most of the cancers in which they've been implicated.

BREAST CANCER

Breast cancer is the most common cancer diagnosed in women. Fortunately, when the cancer is detected early, the survival rate is high—over 90 percent. This is your actual risk of being diagnosed with breast cancer on a decade-by-decade basis:

From thirty to forty years old, your risk of breast cancer is 1 in 257

From forty to fifty: 1 in 67

From fifty to sixty: 1 in 36

From sixty to seventy: 1 in 28

From seventy to eighty: 1 in 24

You'll remember that after the results of the WHI study—which found that the estrogen/progestin formulation Prempro increased the risk of breast cancer by 26 percent—were grandly presented to the media and followed up by a series of scathing indictments against "hormone therapy," a second publication from the same study was quietly presented to the medical community, this one reporting that women who were on estrogen alone experienced no increased breast cancer risk at all. In fact, their risk decreased and was actually lower than the risk of women who had been taking a placebo.

My personal theory is that the *reduction* in breast cancer seen in the women taking BioSimilar estrogen may be due to estrogen's ability to promote normal immune functions and improve overall health (exactly how that happens is still under investigation). In other words, the women in the estrogen-only phase of the study may have been able to prevent breast cancer by boosting their own immune system with the help of estrogen, enabling it to kill cancer cells before they could develop into a tumor and thus countering the immune system failure that is most likely a factor in cancer. And BioIden-

Gloria, fifty-five, first came to see me when she was undergoing postsurgical treatment for breast cancer. She had been taking tamoxifen to block estrogen activity in case some breast cancer cells lingered after her surgery. Gloria had been first-chair concert violinist when she was first diagnosed and felt her musical abilities were deteriorating rapidly—though no one could figure out exactly why. The idea that she could no longer continue with her greatest passion was causing her great anguish. She had been moved to third-chair violin and was contemplating stopping the tamoxifen when her oncologist referred her to me.

Since tamoxifen has been shown to improve breast cancer survival, I strongly recommended that Gloria stay on it if possible. But I also suggested she begin taking methyltestosterone; this, I felt, had an excellent chance of improving her condition, since stimulating testosterone receptors in the brain could help restore some of her lost dexterity. And since methyltestosterone is a BioLimited form of testosterone that cannot effectively be converted to estrogen, the health risks would be minimal. Her oncologist gave the go-ahead. Four months into treatment, Gloria noted a significant improvement! Her violin skills returned to a level she was comfortable with—and her hot flashes diminished, as well. Gloria, her oncologist, and I mutually agreed that she would be a candidate to resume estrogen therapy once her cancer treatment was completed.

tical hormones may be even safer than the BioSimilar estrogen used in the study for all the reasons we've been talking about throughout—they promote normal healing and repair, lower stress hormone levels, and foster the brain's ability to monitor everything going on both in and around you.

As for the oft-heard argument that a higher lifetime exposure to estrogen (as the result of early onset of menses or delayed menopause) results in a higher risk of developing breast cancer—it's just not true. One pregnancy exposes a woman to several years' worth of estrogen, and there is no correlation between having a higher number of pregnancies and a higher risk of breast cancer. In fact, some data suggest that pregnancy reduces the risk.

BIOMUTAGENS: MORE LIKELY CAUSES OF BREAST CANCER

So much for estrogen. Now let's look at the more likely cause of breast cancer—BioMutagens. The toxins in the environment put you at far greater risk of developing breast cancer than estrogen ever could. As our society has

ASK DR. GREENE

Q: WILL USING A TESTOSTERONE SUPPLEMENT INCREASE MY RISK OF BREAST CANCER?

A: No, in fact, there's a good chance that it might decrease your risk. While estrogen and progesterone increase the growth of normal breast cells, testosterone actually decreases breast cell growth. Several recent studies have shown that testosterone probably has the same effect on most breast cancers, as well.

become more and more exposed to BioMutagens, breast cancer rates have gone up tremendously. Parabens, for instance (also listed as ethylparabens, methylparabens, propylparabens, or butylparabens) a BioMutagen used as a preservative to prevent bacterial growth in beauty and hygiene products—almost 80 percent of commercial women's cosmetics contain parabens. While parabens might keep bacteria down, it's a hormone disruptor and probable carcinogen.

Parabens was briefly in the news in 2004 when correlations were made between deodorants that contained them and breast cancer. Although U.S. regulatory agencies dismissed the connection because they said that parabens doesn't pass through the skin easily, they failed to consider that women often apply deodorant *after* shaving their underarms, which abrades the skin and opens the door to toxic absorption. Subsequent studies found that women in geographical regions where frequent underarm shaving is de rigueur have higher breast cancer incidences. And did I mention that breast cancers occur most commonly in the upper, outer quadrant of the breast, the region closest to the underarm? One of the most compelling arguments regarding this particular BioMutagen was presented in 2003 in a study that appeared in the *European Journal of Toxicology*. The study found that parabens not only displaces and binds the estrogen receptor about one thousand to ten thousand times more tenaciously than BioIdentical estrogen, but was also present in a large percentage of the breast cancer tumors that were examined. While scientists in Europe are lobbying to ban the use of parabens altogether, it remains on the FDA's list of approved chemicals and additives. Obviously it's better to be safe than sorry. My advice: Read labels and avoid any products that contain parabens.

Even though each deodorant application is small, we now know that BioMutagens have a *bioaccumulation* effect. That is, many of them build up and create cumulative damage over time. This finding is supported by what we know about breast cancer. As we've seen, no matter what you do or don't do, or whether you're on hormone therapy or not, your risk of breast cancer increases as you get older. That's very different from tobacco's connection to lung cancer. Quit smoking, and after five years your risk of lung cancer is back to that of a non-smoker (provided you were cancer-free when you quit, of course). So tobacco is a BioMutagen, but it does not accumulate. Hormone-disrupting BioMutagens, on the other hand, amass in your body and continue to bombard your system. And, of course, their effects are irreversible.

ASK DR. GREENE

Q: WHAT ARE THE MOST IMPORTANT DIETARY GUIDELINES FOR PREVENTING BREAST CANCER?

A: Eat organic fruits and vegetables, and if you eat meat, remember to buy organic products. Meat consumption increases breast cancer rates by two to six times compared with vegetarian fare. Countries like China and Japan where dietary animal fat intake is less than 20 percent have the lowest incidence of breast cancer. (While no data are yet available on the cancer risks associated with consuming organic meats, my guess is that the risk would be lower than that for commercial beef, since the animals consume and thus bioaccumulate fewer toxins.)

EARLY DETECTION—SCREENING TESTS FOR BREAST CANCER

- Mammography is currently the most readily available technique and is recommended every one to two years for women between ages forty and fifty and then annually each year after that. As most of you know, mammography consists of creating an image of the internal anatomy of the breast by passing X-rays through from top to bottom and then side to side in a search for any changes in tissue density suggestive of cancer. It's believed to be sensitive enough to diagnose about 86 percent of all breast cancers.

- Breast ultrasound is frequently needed in addition to a mammogram to get additional information if you're on hormone therapy or if you're still

ASK DR. GREENE

Q: DO BIRTH CONTROL PILLS INCREASE THE RISK OF BREAST CANCER?

A: No. Based on over forty years' worth of data, birth control pills do not seem to increase or decrease breast cancer rates. This opinion is shared by a host of international expert panels that seem to be free of bias. Even the most recent, best-designed studies in the United States support this conclusion. There just isn't a biologically plausible way that birth control pills could promote breast cancer.

having menstrual cycles. It uses sound waves to create images similar to mammograms, but with better detail of the breast's fluid components. By combining ultrasound with mammography, almost 97 percent of breast cancers are accurately detected. MRI scanning, which clearly shows abnormal growths, will no doubt be the next generation of screening techniques, though we probably have a way to go before costs will allow it to replace current technologies. Stay tuned.

COLON CANCER

Colon cancer is the third most common cancer in women. It's also one with a far higher mortality rate than breast cancer when it develops before sixty-five years of age. The good news is that it can be detected by early screening—and by supplementing with estrogen, which has been shown to lower the risk of colon cancer by a consistent and dramatic margin. More than twenty research studies have found that hormone therapy lowers the risk of colon cancer by 20–50 percent. Even BioSimilar birth control pills lower the risk of colon cancer by over 40 percent. Specifically, we know that precancerous colon polyps often have estrogen receptors that suppress the growth of these benign tumors before they can become cancers. Although the reason for this is not entirely understood, the observed cancer reduction is well documented.

SEX HORMONES, DIET, AND COLON CANCER PREVENTION

Colon cancer is clearly linked to our highly processed low-fiber, low-carb, high-fat, high-protein diets. When dietary fiber is low, it allows insulin levels to climb, promotes constipation, and increases the amount of time the intestinal lining is exposed to the BioMutagens in food. Not only does the typical American diet promote free radical formation, but the prevalence of so many additives and chemicals in the food increases the chance of DNA damage that can trigger cancer growth.

Hormone therapy used during menopause or as contraception lowers these risks of colon cancer in several ways. First, the hormone balance established by BioIdentical and BioSimilar estrogen improves your insulin sensitivity, making it possible for your insulin levels to drop. This insulin reduction is important in lowering colon cancer risks because insulin promotes cell division, which can be dangerous if a cell has already undergone abnormal changes. Insulin reduction also helps reduce *hyperplasia*—the overgrowth of cells—by turning off the growth signal within cells. Second, it increases intestinal activity, which in turn prevents constipation. Third, it promotes the production of bile acids to eliminate toxins. Hormone therapies most likely have other cancer-fighting properties, including an ability to absorb free radicals and possibly even improve the body's natural immune response.

The insulin connection may actually end up being one of the key reasons for the association between colon cancer and obesity. In 2004, two studies involving over ninety thousand women found that foods that cause the highest insulin levels increase the risk of colon cancer six times above average. That's a 600 percent increase compared with women following the sorts of dietary recommendations we offer in our Perftct Balance diet plan. Other studies have shown that women with insulin resistance are ten times more likely to die from colon cancer. Clearly, reducing insulin resistance is one of the best strategies for reducing the risk of colon cancer. As the research continues, I believe we'll discover even more ways that sex hormones help protect against colon cancer.

HORMONE STRATEGIES TO LOWER COLON CANCER RISK

Because of the compelling evidence linking estrogen to colon cancer risk reduction, I recommend using a BioSimilar hormone contraceptive during your reproductive years (if you're not looking to conceive). It's been estimated that the associated 40–50 percent reduction in colon cancer risk continues for between five and fifteen years after you stop taking the pill. Since colon cancer risk increases with age, and the benefits of hormone use in menopause are even more firmly established than they are for use in contraception, it would be a good idea to continue hormone-balancing treatments into menopause for as long as you have symptoms.

ASK DR. GREENE

Q: IF I TAKE BIRTH CONTROL PILLS FOR A SIGNIFICANT PERIOD OF TIME, WILL IT BE MORE DIFFICULT TO BECOME PREGNANT IF I DECIDE TO CONCEIVE?

A: No. In fact, the first few months after stopping birth control pills is statistically a period highly conducive to conception. That's because birth control pills cause the ovaries to go into a resting state, so when you're ready to conceive they are primed to respond. In my work as a fertility specialist, I typically start women on a birth control pill for the month or two before advanced fertility treatments like in vitro fertilization to improve the success of the treatment.

EARLY DETECTION— SCREENING TESTS FOR COLON CANCER

Screening tests for colon cancer are terribly important—and too often overlooked. The Centers for Disease Control and Prevention (CDC) estimates that only 40 percent of U.S. citizens follow the recommended screening guidelines. When screening tests are used, however, studies show that over 90 percent of colon cancers are curable. Here's what you should do:

• Fecal occult blood testing measures microscopic blood in your stools. It's readily available at many drugstores (it generally costs less than $20). Though it is considered close to 100 percent accurate for detecting blood from your colon, don't be alarmed if the test is positive. Many benign conditions such as hemorrhoids and polyps can also cause blood in your stool. If your test is positive, make an appointment with your health care provider to discuss a more involved test. Fecal occult blood testing should be performed annually after age fifty.

• A colonoscopy is recommended about every five years after age fifty, and it's especially important for women, since colon cancers in women are located at the opposite end of the large bowel and can't currently be detected by any other examination method. If you have a family history of colon cancer, your health care practitioner may recommend more aggressive early screening.

OVARIAN CANCER

Ovarian cancer is a relatively rare cancer—your lifetime risk is only about 1–2 percent—but because diagnosis is typically delayed, the disease is often deadly. That fact is a big scare factor and often drives women to have their healthy ovaries removed as a preemptive measure. It's estimated that in 2005 alone, approximately four thousand women in the United States will have both ovaries routinely removed at the time of hysterectomy to prevent cancers that would probably never occur. I feel most of those surgeries are unnecessary and often lead to a decreased quality of life. Though ovarian cancer kills an estimated seven thousand women per year in the United States, the rate continues to go down thanks to the popularity of birth control pills and new screening tests.

OVARIAN CANCER AND HORMONES:
HORMONE STRATEGIES TO LOWER YOUR RISK

If you've had a close relative (mother or sister) with ovarian cancer, your risk of developing the cancer increases from about 1.5 percent to about 5 percent. So even if your risk is statistically high, it's probably lower than you may have thought it was. But it's still important to do all you can to lower it further.

Besides consuming less meat and avoiding toxic BioMutagens, anything that you do to reduce the number of times you ovulate during your lifetime lowers your risk. (Pregnancy and breast-feeding reduce frequency of ovulation naturally.) Ovulation frequency increases your risk because each time you ovulate, your ovary ruptures a tiny bit to release the egg. Nearby cells repair the rupture by dividing and growing. Because these cells divide rapidly to repair the small rupture, there's more chance of a genetic accident that could result in a mutation. Simply put, the more cycles of ruptures and repairs, the more of an ovarian cancer risk. You can reduce the cumulative number of ovulations throughout your lifetime with hormonal contraception—birth control pills effectively stop ovulation. That's a viable way to go if you choose not to have children or want to limit your brood to one or two. Birth control pills are certainly a better route than having healthy ovaries removed—which incidentally still leaves you with about a 0.5 percent risk of ovarian cancer.

Studies have shown that with only one year of using BioSimilar combination oral contraceptives, your risk of ovarian cancer is reduced by about 12 percent. After five years of continuous use, your risk is reduced by at least 50 percent. Some studies suggest that longer use further reduces ovarian cancer risk while also reducing the risk of colon cancer and endometrial cancers. Best of all, it seems that the risk reduction lasts for at least ten to fifteen years after you stop an oral contraceptive. The bottom line: BioSimilar hormones decrease ovarian cancer risk if they're taken at doses high enough to suppress ovulation.

Whether or not BioIdentical or BioSimilar hormone use in menopause increases ovarian cancer risk is still under investigation. Research so far is conflicting, which suggests that if there is a relationship, it is minimal. If there is an increase in risk, it is most likely to be much like breast cancer risk. That is, hormones may stimulate the cancer to grow more rapidly if it is already there, but they do not cause the cancer. That's why screening tests are particularly important.

EARLY DETECTION—SCREENING TESTS FOR OVARIAN CANCER

- Currently, the most accurate blood test, CA-125, is about to be replaced. The CA-125 can create unnecessary fear because it detects many benign conditions, including endometriosis, that can produce misleading results. Plus it can miss about 20 percent of ovarian cancers. The new blood test, OvaCheck, looks for various proteins—called *biomarkers*—that indicate ovarian cancer. Early studies show that it is accurate in detecting about 95 percent of ovarian cancers. The cost is likely to run between $100 and $200 per test after it receives final approval from the FDA.

- Ultrasound is currently the best screening test we have for ovarian cancer. It's generally not necessary in most situations unless your ovaries feel enlarged during an annual examination. The sensitivity of this test is nearly 100 percent, but it can be costly if not covered by your insurance.

UTERINE CANCER

Uterine cancer is the fourth most prevalent cancer in women and is very curable. Endometrial cancer, the most common kind of uterine cancer, refers to an overgrowth of the lining in the uterus (the endometrium). Typically, it manifests as unusual vaginal bleeding (either heavy or irregular) and should not be ignored in its earliest, most treatable stages. Uterine cancer is the only cancer in which estrogen seems truly to play an adverse role—and that can happen only when the sex hormones are out of balance with one another.

One of the functions of the sex hormones is to prepare the endometrial lining for the implantation of a fertilized egg. Estrogen promotes cell division only in this lining; it essentially builds a veritable cushion for an embryo to nest in. Progesterone slows down this estrogen-stimulated growth, thus preventing accelerated cell growth and reducing the chance that an endometrial cell will have a genetic accident during division that would allow it to become a cancer.

If your endometrial lining has been exposed to estrogen for a prolonged period of time without progesterone, it's had a continuous signal to grow and divide. Continued growth of the lining means fewer, if any, periods. And more growth means more chance for DNA damage and mutation. So balancing estrogen to progesterone alleviates the risk of cancer that occurs naturally through menstrual bleeding. When a pregnancy doesn't occur, the estrogen and progesterone levels fall and the endometrial lining is shed in the menstrual bleeding.

Another way to achieve the same kind of cancer protection is by using continuous combined BioSimilar hormones in a balanced regimen. It eliminates the menstrual cycle and creates a balanced regimen with enough progesterone to offset the effects of the estrogen. So even though you're not having regular menstrual bleeding, you're taking enough progesterone to prevent overgrowth of the uterine lining. This is a safe alternative to having a monthly menstrual cycle.

Obesity can increase your risk of endometrial cancer more than almost any other risk factor, since fat tissue creates estrone—the "bad" estrogen that promotes endometrial growth. Estrone is also the reason that overweight or obese women have higher rates of abnormal bleeding, typically periods of very heavy flow mixed with none at all. Anything that weighs down the estrogen-progesterone seesaw on the estrogen side will increase your risk of endometrial cancer.

BioMutagens that bind and stimulate the estrogen receptor so aggressively that progesterone is dominated are called *estrogenic*. They also increase your risk of endometrial cancer. Some of the BioLimited estrogens that are designed to remain active in your uterus, such as tamoxifen, also increase your risk. While tamoxifen, used to treat breast cancer, blocks estrogen activity in your breast (and, unfortunately, your brain), it remains active in your uterus.

The problem is that tamoxifen is generally not prescribed with progesterone the way estrogen is, so the cell division continues and can promote overgrowth of the uterine lining. This is a concern I would suggest discussing with your oncologist.

HORMONAL STRATEGIES TO LOWER ENDOMETRIAL CANCER RISK

The use of BioSimilar hormone contraceptives reduces your risk of developing endometrial cancer by ensuring a balanced hormone profile within your uterus. Women who use birth control pills in their forties actually lower their risk of endometrial cancer by more than 50 percent for at least ten years. The reason this is so effective is that many women don't ovulate on a monthly basis during their forties and as a result are more likely to have high estrogen levels. The use of a birth control pill essentially prevents the high estrogen level by suppressing the ovaries, while at the same time providing progesterone to control vaginal bleeding.

If you're in menopause, it's important to consider at least occasional use of progesterone to avoid uterine cancer—whether you're on estrogen replacement or not. If you have no menopausal symptoms and you're not on estrogen therapy, you're probably producing enough estrogen on your own. But in menopause you won't be producing *any* progesterone. (Remember, you produce progesterone only when you're ovulating.) So you may need occasional progesterone to stay balanced. As a self-test, ask your doctor for 200 mg of BioIdentical progesterone (Prometrium) that you can take at bedtime for two weeks. If you have menstrual bleeding after you finish the progesterone, it means your body is producing estrogen in sufficient quantities to promote endometrial hyperplasia (a precancerous cancer) and you need to balance the estrogen with regular, or at least occasional, progesterone to offset the possible growth. To do that safely, repeat the Prometrium regimen at least four times per year. More than four times a year won't create any increased benefit, but if it improves your peace of mind, there's no reason not to induce a faux cycle every month.

If you are taking estrogen regularly, you should also make sure that you are on a balanced monthly regimen with progesterone or at least the intermittent regimen of progesterone that I just described. One regimen is not better than another here; it's more a matter of which one you feel best on. So use your symptoms to guide your treatment and dosage choices.

EARLY DETECTION—SCREENING TESTS FOR UTERINE CANCER

- Ultrasound imaging of your uterus is considered the recommended screening test for uterine cancer, but it's generally not necessary unless you've experienced unusual vaginal bleeding. This technique does provide the additional benefit of screening for ovarian cancer at the same time. If the lining of your uterus is measured and is thicker than 5 mm, an endometrial biopsy may be recommended. This is considered sensitive enough to detect about 96 percent of uterine cancers.

- Endometrial biopsy—also called endometrial aspiration—is necessary to rule out cancer if your endometrial thickness is greater than 5 mm. This technique is believed to approach 100 percent in its accuracy. Be prepared, however: It can cause discomfort that's generally compared to a severe menstrual cramp.

DIET AND LIFESTYLE PREVENTION STRATEGIES FOR ALL CANCERS

DIET

- By eating organic foods, you eliminate your exposure to a large percentage of BioMutagens. Pesticides are some of the most damaging hormone disruptors that we're exposed to, and each pesticide that has already been banned was reported as safe right up until the day its use was prohibited. Many pesticides are now being used that will no doubt be proclaimed dangerous in the near future. Don't wait for the official word to take action.

- If you eat fish, poultry, and animal products, remember to buy organic products whenever possible rather than those that are industrially farmed. Meat, fish, and poultry consumption increases breast cancer rates by two to six times compared with eating vegetarian fare.

- Get a water filter for your drinking and cooking use. The Environmental Protection Agency (EPA) monitors at least forty BioMutagens that are common in our water supply, and many of them have been closely linked with various cancers, including breast cancer. Most water filters remove contaminants through a simple activated charcoal filter. The charcoal filter should be changed on regular basis (follow manufacturer's guidelines).

LIFESTYLE

- Avoid exposure to personal hygiene products that contain high levels of BioMutagens, especially if you apply them to skin that has just been shaved or abraded. In addition to parabens, watch out for lanolin. It's in myriad skin care products and is frequently applied to babies' skin or used by pregnant women to soothe sore nipples. It's commonly contaminated with DDT as well as other BioMutagens.

- Don't forget to exercise. Many studies have consistently shown that moderate aerobic exercise on a regular basis reduces the risk of developing breast, endometrial, and colon cancers. Estimated risk reductions vary from 20 to 60 percent!

- Avoid polycyclic aromatic hydrocarbons and other airborne BioMutagens. Over two hundred of these are formed when you burn coal, gasoline, tobacco, or garbage. These have been shown to induce breast tumors in laboratory animals. You can avoid exposure to these by disposing of petroleum products through approved means, minimizing your consumption of smoked meats/cheeses, avoiding charred foods, and not burning chemicals or trash in poorly ventilated areas. Consider carpooling, using public transportation, or getting a hybrid vehicle to minimize fuel emissions.

CHAPTER SEVENTEEN

THE FINAL STEP TO PERFECT BALANCE: WORKING *WITH* YOUR DOCTOR

We've covered a lot of ground here. But you will absolutely find it's been worth the ride. You now have a firm grasp of one of the most important health factors in your life and the tools and solutions to take smart, appropriate actions that will allow you to feel your best every day and enjoy your life to its fullest—right into your golden years.

Just as important, you're now in a position to be an equal partner with your health care provider. While you can easily implement diet and lifestyle changes on your own, if you feel that your symptoms warrant any of the prescription hormones or medications suggested here, you'll need the help of a good health care provider. As a well-informed patient, your opinions count and should be seriously considered, so who you choose for this role is very important. You want someone who is open to your input and will respect your ideas and opinions; someone who is on your wavelength and will serve as a compassionate guide to restoring your hormone balance. If you already have someone who fits the bill, that's terrific. Stick with him (or her). If you don't, here are a few tips on what to look for in a good health care provider:

- **Credentials.** Consider your potential doctor's background, and make sure you're comfortable with the doctor's knowledge, not just his or her charm.

- **Good listening skills.** You deserve someone who is completely engaged in assisting you. When something important comes up for you, you want to make sure that your distress signal will be heard.

- **Holistic perspective.** Holistic care includes the ability to write a prescription when it's indicated. If a health care provider is not able to offer you this service, it's far more likely the provider will have you try everything else rather than offer you what you may really need. The use of BioIdentical and BioSimilar hormones requires a prescription.

- **Unbiased by preconceived notions.** Few hormone-balancing problems have only one solution. Since each hormone affects every other one, there are usually many possible solutions. It's all right to have strong beliefs on the best solution, but if you decide to choose an option other than that of your health care provider, your doctor should respect your decision. Don't be offended if the doctor suggests a second opinion to back up his or her point of view, and insist on one yourself if you're uncomfortable with the advice you receive.

- **Values quality of life, not just the absence of disease.** To put it simply, you want a doctor who is willing to speak about "off label" medication uses. As I mentioned, the FDA approves prescription medications for a specific purpose. Often the same medicine is shown to be useful for many other uses that may be important to you. Only in rare situations does the FDA labeling focus on a quality-of-life issue. As long as recommendations are safe and well supported by current research, it is within your rights to request these treatments. Simply assure your health care provider that you understand the benefits as well as the risks (even the smallest ones). In other words, collaborate in your decision making. As the director of your own hormone-balancing program, that's your prerogative.

CAUTION: THESE HEALTH CARE PROVIDERS COULD BE HAZARDOUS TO YOUR HEALTH

So how can you tell what kind of health care provider you're talking to? Well, there are a few telltale signs that give you a pretty good idea a particular health care provider isn't going to suit your purposes. Personality types reveal a lot about practice style. Here are ones you should avoid:

- **The Dictator** takes the "Do as I say because I've got your best interest in mind" approach. He or she knows everything, and you know nothing. This type is the boss; you're not. He or she leaves you feeling patronized and marginalized. Not good. You shouldn't have to play second fiddle or convince someone that your symptoms are real, nor should you ever feel discounted.

- **The Salesman** pushes you too hard to accept his or her modus operandi. Whether the doctor has a conflict of interest or simply a lack of knowledge is less relevant than the fact that he or she may not be able to meet your needs.

- **The Reactionary** treats first and asks questions later. Watch out for somebody who's too fast on the draw with *the* solution. Whether you're discussing medication, herbs, surgery, or a medical procedure, don't invest your money or waste your time jumping into treatment without first considering all your choices. You deserve to be fully informed of various options before starting anything.

- **The Genius** is a total know-it-all. You deserve a health care provider who is confident enough to seek outside advice, not hide behind false bravado.

While those red-flag-type health providers should be avoided, there are a few others with whom you can work effectively, but it might require greater initiative from you. So proceed with caution with these kinds of doctors.

- **The Pill Pusher** has a pill for everything. Not every problem requires a prescription. You want someone with a broader vision. Your health care provider should be able to discuss intelligently dietary and lifestyle suggestions, as well.

- **The Historian** takes the "I've always done it this way" approach. Medicine is a very dynamic science. You deserve the best and most current treatments available. So if you bring in an idea, he or she should be agreeable to doing a little extra research.

- **The Five-Minute Manager** has one hand on the doorknob. It may just be a busy day, or it may be a warning sign that this is someone who's not going to give you his or her full attention.

- **The People Pleaser** just wants to be nice and give you whatever you want. You want an adviser, not someone who can offer only affirmations. Sometimes "people pleasers" lack a strong knowledge base or may be more concerned with your happiness than in giving you good sound advice.

If you think you need to modify your current relationship with your health care provider, start by making an appointment to "discuss revising your hormone balance." If the doctor isn't receptive to that, then it's time to start looking elsewhere. Don't be afraid to "fire" someone who's not meeting your needs. I think you'll find that most health care providers will welcome your proactive role as long as he or she is not caught off guard. You want your doctor's full attention for a period of time that is proportional to your problem and medical history.

FIVE STEPS TO INITIATING YOUR HORMONE-BALANCING PLAN

In order to be truly proactive from this point forward, it's best to form an action plan. Now that you've got a good idea of the type of person you'd like to work with, let's consider the best way to proceed. Time is a commodity that few good health care providers have today, and you should plan your appointment time wisely.

STEP 1: GET A COPY OF YOUR MEDICAL RECORDS

Take the time to review your medical records to make sure there aren't any inaccuracies. This is especially important if you're starting care with a new provider or if your needs haven't been met in prior visits with your current one. New regulations require that your chart be made available and that you be allowed to amend any inaccuracies or discrepancies with which you don't agree. Don't be intimidated. Most health care professionals encourage the interest and participation of their patients. Ask the new doctor you'll be seeing if he or she would like to see your records.

STEP 2: PRIORITIZE YOUR TROUBLESHOOTING LIST

Don't try to take on too many problems at one time. As you've learned, you can often solve several hormone-related symptoms with one solution. To avoid creating an overcomplicated plan or diluting what's really bothering you, choose the top two or three problems on your list. Write down any additional concerns that you may have so that if you have more time, you can use it effectively. Set the agenda based upon the amount of time that you're scheduled for so you can direct and control the flow of your meeting. By taking control, you'll not only earn the doctor's respect, but also demonstrate your knowledge of the situation. These are vital keys to achieving your goals of excellent health and individualized care.

STEP 3: BRING COPIES OF PERTINENT QUESTIONNAIRES FROM THIS BOOK TO YOUR APPOINTMENT

I've designed the questionnaires in this book to facilitate a discussion of your problems with your health care provider. After you complete them, make a photocopy to bring with you to your appointment. That will simplify the process of explaining the symptoms you're experiencing and help you avoid any communication glitches. The questionnaires will also save time and make it possible for the doctor to focus his or her attention on getting any additional information that may be necessary.

STEP 4: BRING THIS BOOK TO YOUR OFFICE VISIT

If certain treatment options mentioned here sound right to you, request them. It will be up to the doctor to explain to you whether or not he or she would recommend the same advice in your situation—and if not, why. Reserve judgment, but remember that it's your doctor's obligation to explain his or her assessment to you. All the recommendations in this book are supported by today's science. I've also included a detailed reference list in appendix 5, so that your doctors can review the pertinent studies if desired, and they can also contact me via my website if they need further information.

STEP 5: SCHEDULE A FOLLOW-UP APPOINTMENT

Before leaving the office, schedule a follow-up visit. Not only will it help motivate you to follow through with the developed plan, it will also provide you with an opportunity to fine-tune and adjust your hormone-balancing plan later on. Ideally, you'll have fully implemented the Perfect Balance hormone-balancing strategies before your first office visit. If you had trouble putting any of these plans into action, one of the first things you should discuss is alternative methods for achieving hormone balance without medications. Your needs may change and require new strategies to reestablish balance.

New studies may come along, and new products are always being tested. One of these may encourage you to modify your plan. Now you've got the power to do that.

Share this information with your friends—both men and women. By increasing their understanding of the hormone-brain connection, they'll not only better understand your experiences, but develop better insight into their own well-being. We all want to live a long, happy life and feel our best each and every day. It's my sincere desire that this book will help you do that, now—and far into the future.

APPENDIX 1

PERFECT BALANCE HORMONE BIOSYSTEM™ TREATMENT RECOMMENDATIONS

Many hormone therapies are available today, and undoubtedly more will be released in the future. Following are some of my favorite commercially manufactured treatments in each category. All are available through any pharmacy. I've indicated dosages available to assist you in communicating your wishes to your doctor and your pharmacist. If your needs are not met by one of these, a compounding pharmacy can create a preparation (creams, gels, eye drops, etc.) tailored to your individual requests.

BIOIDENTICAL HORMONES

BIOIDENTICAL ESTROGEN: I prescribe BioIdentical estradiol in cases where women have an estradiol deficiency. Supplementation can relieve hot flashes, improve sexual functioning and cognition, and provide tremendous relief for migraine sufferers. All BioIdentical estradiols are chemically the same and produce the same results; it's the application method that differs from one product to another. Patches come in various sizes and doses, and creams and gels are also available. Whichever application method you choose, start with the lowest (or second lowest) dose available. If your symptoms aren't completely relieved by the eighth week, talk to your doctor about increasing the dose or switching to another method if you're experiencing any other problems. I don't recommend bi-est (estradiol with estrone or estriol) or tri-est (which contains all three estrogens), because the addition of either estrone or estriol diminishes the benefits of estradiol. In fact, if you swallow a estradiol tablet, about half is converted to estrone, in effect, making it bi-est. That's why tablets are my least preferred form of BioIdentical estrogen.

BIOIDENTICAL PROGESTERONE: I prescribe this in cases of progesterone deficiencies. BioIdentical progesterone can improve sleep quality, regulate menstrual bleeding, and help reduce anxiety for some women. It comes in pills and vaginal gels. Pills should be taken at bedtime to avoid daytime sleepiness. Using a vaginal gel reduces the risk of depression, which some women experience as a side effect of progesterone because applying the gel near the uterus dramatically reduces the dose needed to prevent vaginal bleeding.

BIOIDENTICAL HORMONES

HORMONE	BRAND NAME	HOW IT'S USED	AVAILABLE DOSES
Estradiol	Climara	Skin patch: weekly	0.025 mg/day
			0.0375 mg/day
			0.05 mg/day
			0.06 mg/day
			0.075 mg/day
			0.1 mg/day
	Vivelle DOT	Skin patch: twice a week	0.025 mg/day
			0.0375 mg/day
			0.05 mg/day
			0.075 mg/day
			0.1 mg/day
	Menostar	Skin patch: weekly	0.014 mg/day
	Estrasorb	Topical lotion: daily	0.025 mg/packet
	EstroGel	Topical gel: daily	0.75 mg/pump
	Estring	Vaginal ring: 3-month	0.0075 mg
	Femring	Vaginal ring: 3-month	0.05 mg/day
			0.1 mg/day
	Vagifem	Vaginal tablet: daily	0.025 mg
	Estrace	Vaginal cream: daily	0.01%
Progesterone	Prometrium	Oral capsule: daily	100 mg
		Oral capsule: daily	200 mg
	Crinone	Vaginal gel: daily	4%
			8%
Testosterone	Micronized gel available through a compounding pharmacy		

BIOIDENTICAL TESTOSTERONE: I prescribe this for problems such as low libido and fatigue and to correct symptoms of estrogen imbalance such as breast tenderness. As of this writing, BioIdentical testosterone is available only through compounding pharmacies. I recommend you have the pharmacy prepare a gel that can be applied daily to the skin. There is a BioIdentical testosterone patch currently being evaluated by the FDA that will be made available following approval.

BIOSIMILAR HORMONES

BIOSIMILAR ESTRADIOL: I prescribe these for the same problems for which I prescribe BioIdentical formulations: hot flash relief, improved sexual functioning, memory problems, improved balance, and other symptoms associated with estrogen deficiency. Some women prefer these to BioIdentical preparations because they can be taken in pill form. Doctors are familiar with them since they've been around for a long time. There is no BioSimilar progesterone or testosterone.

BIOSIMILAR HORMONES

HORMONE	BRAND (AND GENERIC) NAME	HOW IT'S USED	AVAILABLE DOSES
Estradiol	Cenestin (synthetic conjugated estrogen)	Oral tablet: daily	0.3 mg 0.625 mg 0.9 mg 1.25 mg
	Premarin (conjugated equine estrogen)	Oral tablet: daily	0.3 mg 0.625 mg 0.9 mg 1.25 mg
		Vaginal cream	0.625 mg
	Menest (esterified estrogen)	Oral tablet: daily	0.3 mg 0.625 mg 1.25 mg 2.5 mg

BIOLIMITED HORMONES

BIOLIMITED ESTROGENS: These are commonly called SERMs (selective estrogen receptor modulators). They're a synthetic form of estrogen designed to bind the estrogen receptors in specific parts of your body while blocking estrogen activity in others. As a result, they've become widely used for treating cancers that are sensitive to estrogen, like breast cancer. They are able to improve your cholesterol and preserve bone strength like a normal estrogen, but they are not active in the brain. Many women have bothersome side effects from BioLimited estrogens that dramatically limit their usefulness.

BIOLIMITED PROGESTERONES: These have been very successful as treatments for heavy vaginal bleeding and contraception. Because they're not as readily recognized by the brain, their side effects are minimal.

BIOLIMITED HORMONES

HORMONE	GENERIC NAME	BRAND NAME	HOW IT'S USED
Estradiol	Raloxifene (BioLimited estrogen)	Evista	Oral tablet: daily
	Tamoxifen (BioLimited estrogen)	Nolvadex	Oral tablet: daily
Progesterone	Levonorgestrel (BioLimited progestin)	Mirena	Intrauterine system: 5-year
	Norethindrone (BioLimited progestin)	Micronor	Oral tablet: daily

BIOANTAGONIST HORMONES

BioAntagonists are used to artificially lower the hormone levels in your body. Since hormones can't be simply removed, these medications are used either to prevent your body from producing them or to block their activity. Since BioAntagonists actually create a hormone imbalance, they're used only to treat serious illnesses like painful endometriosis, severe excess facial hair, premature puberty, and breast cancer. Because they create many side effects, I recommend that they be used for the shortest period of time possible to obtain the desired benefit. There should always be a defined dosage and end point to treatment established between you and your doctor, and you should have a serious discussion about side effects before initiating these BioAntagonists.

BIOANTAGONIST HORMONES

BRAND (AND GENERIC) NAME	HOW IT'S USED
Femara (Letrozole)	Oral tablet: daily
Synarel (Nafarelin)	Nasal spray: twice daily
Lupron (Leuprolide acetate)	Injection: usually monthly or every 3 months (used daily for infertility treatments)
Propecia (Finasteride)	Oral tablet: daily
Chimax (Flutamide)	Oral tablet: daily

COMBINATION PRODUCTS

Combination products are readily available, and most health care providers are familiar with them. Each product contains either a BioSimilar estrogen with a BioLimited progestin or a BioSimilar estrogen with a BioLimited androgen in a fixed-dose regimen. Every woman responds differently to the hormone mixtures, but for the most part they're well tolerated. These are designed for women still experiencing menstrual cycles as well as menopausal women (who have or have not had a hysterectomy).

BIOSIMILAR/BIOLIMITED CONTRACEPTIVE COMBINATIONS

For women still having menstrual cycles, more potent combinations are required to suppress the signal from the brain to the ovaries while also providing a high enough dose to prevent symptoms. Each of these combinations provides specific "off label" benefits beyond their ability to prevent pregnancy. The products listed here are the ones I prescribe most often because so many of my patients find them to be the "best fit."

BRAND (AND GENERIC) NAME	HOW IT'S USED
Ortho Evra (Ethinyl estradiol/norelgestromin)	Skin patch: weekly
NuvaRing (Ethinyl estradiol/etonogestrel)	Vaginal ring: monthly

Advantages: These provide stable blood levels, reducing chances of migraine headache or upset stomach, and have the added benefit of not requiring you to take them every day.

Ortho Tri-Cyclen (Ethinyl estradiol/norgestimate)	Tablet: daily
Ortho Tri-Cyclen Lo (Ethinyl estradiol/norgestimate)	Tablet: daily

Advantages: Few side effects and well-established benefits in improving acne and reducing excess facial hair. Ortho Tri-Cyclen Lo is simply a lower-dose version that can reduce symptoms of estrogen excess for women who have bloating and breast tenderness on the standard Ortho Tri-Cyclen.

Mircette Ethinyl estradiol/desogestrel	Tablet: daily

Advantages: Shorter menstrual periods. Most birth control pills have seven days of placebo pills, which cause extremely low levels of estrogen. Mircette has only two days, which extends the high-estrogen, feel-good period of your cycle.

Yasmin Ethinyl estradiol/drospirenone	Tablet: daily

Advantages: Has a BioLimited progestin uniquely able to minimize symptoms of PMS and PCOS, making it my preferred recommendation for women with those problems.

Seasonale Ethinyl estradiol/levonorgestrel	Tablet: daily

Advantages: Allows women to reduce the number of their menstrual cycles to only four per year, a desired outcome for many women who are bothered with menstrual pain or other problems during the time of menstrual bleeding.

BIOIDENTICAL/BIOLIMITED COMBINATIONS FOR MENOPAUSE

For women in menopause, there are several convenient combinations that are generally well tolerated. Two pill formulations contain BioIdentical estrogen: Prefest and Activella. Since these are taken orally, some of the estrogen is converted to estrone, decreasing its effectiveness, but the dosage is high enough that many women feel quite well while on these tablets. Climara Pro or CombiPatch are both patches that combine BioIdentical estrogen with a BioLimited progestin to control uterine bleeding. (The BioLimited progestin, unlike the BioIdentical form, has been modified so it can be absorbed effectively through the skin.)

BRAND (AND GENERIC) NAME	HOW IT'S USED
Prefest Estradiol/norgestimate	Tablet: daily
Advantages: Contains a very low dose of BioLimited progestin, which helps progesterone-sensitive women avoid depression and fatigue.	

Activella Estradiol/norethindrone acetate	Tablet: daily
Advantages: Same as Prefest, but contains a different progestin that may be better suited for some women.	

Climara Pro Estradiol/levonorgestrel	Skin patch: weekly
CombiPatch Estradiol/norethindrone	Skin patch: twice weekly
Advantages: These patches make for a continual absorption of BioIdentical estrogen and BioLimited progestin that promotes stable hormone blood levels—a great help when it comes to controlling migraines.	

BIOSIMILAR/BIOLIMITED COMBINATIONS FOR MENOPAUSE

Estratest is the only pill available for menopausal women that combines a BioSimilar estrogen with a BioLimited testosterone. It comes in two doses, the lower designated as HS for "half strength." This preparation has been available for many years and is generally prescribed for women with low libido or other signs of androgen deficiency. It is readily available to women who don't have access to a compounding pharmacy that can prepare BioIdentical testosterone (my treatment of choice).

BRAND (AND GENERIC) NAME	HOW IT'S USED
Estratest Esterified estrogen/methyltestosterone	Tablet: daily
Estratest HS Esterified estrogen/methyltestosterone	Tablet: daily
Advantages: The only pills on the market to contain testosterone.	

APPENDIX 2

COMPOUNDING PHARMACIES

There are many excellent compounding pharmacies located across the country. However, just as the best recipes still depend on the skill of the chef, the success of our compounded recommendations depends on the skill of your pharmacist. I can personally recommend the following:

Owens Compounding Pharmacy
2025 Court St., Suite B
Redding, CA 96001
1-530-244-8669
www.owenshealthcare.com

Hillcrest Atrium Pharmacy
6670 Mayfield Rd.
Mayfield Heights, OH 44124
1-444-605-1611
www.hillcrestatriumpharmacy.com

If you would like to work with a pharmacy closer to home, contact the agency below (it certifies the pharmacies). By contacting this agency, you can provide your zip code and obtain a list of nearby pharmacies to meet your needs.

International Academy of Compounding Pharmacists
P.O. Box 1365
Sugar Land, TX 77487
1-800-927-4227
www.iacprx.org

APPENDIX 3

RECOMMENDED READING

These are some of the books I frequently recommend to my patients.

Jennifer Berman, Laura Berman. *For Women Only.* New York: Henry Holt & Co., 2001—a self-help book on female sexual dysfunction written by an acclaimed pair of clinicians.

Greg Critser. *Fat Land.* Boston: Houghton Mifflin Company, 2003—exposé on how dietary changes in America have changed and the politics as well as health consequences involved.

Victor W. Henderson. *Hormone Therapy and the Brain: A Clinical Perspective on the Role of Estrogen.* New York: Parthenon Publishing, 2000—a brief but readable summary of some of the research that has revolutionized hormonal studies of the brain.

Sheldon Krimsky. *Hormonal Chaos.* Baltimore: Johns Hopkins University Press, 2000—an alarming yet real summary of how hormone-disrupting pollutants are influencing our health and future.

Marianne J. Legato. *Eve's Rib.* New York: Harmony Books, 2002—excellent introduction to the emerging field of gender-based medicine and how women's needs have not been met.

Andrew Newberg, E. D'Aquili. *Why God Won't Go Away.* New York: Ballantine Books, 2001—a fascinating, nondenominational exploration using brain imaging to determine how religion and meditation are experienced in the mind.

Lesley Rogers. *Sexing the Brain.* New York: Columbia University Press, 2001—scientific but very readable summary of how hormones shape the mind.

Robert Sapolsky. *Why Zebras Don't Get Ulcers.* New York: Henry Holt & Co., 2004—an excellent summary of how stress hormones influence your health, with practical advice on how-to prevention.

Suzanne Somers, *The Sexy Years.* New York: Crown Publishing Group, 2004—empowering personal experience of a celebrity's path to maintaining her health and wellness through hormone balance, even during breast cancer treatment.

APPENDIX 4

WEBSITES AND RESOURCES

The Internet is a treasure trove of information, but it should be accessed with caution: Many venues make inaccurate or exaggerated claims. The following websites represent excellent sources for further exploration and clarification of the information covered in this book. I have arranged them to follow the order of the topics referred to in the chapters.

INTRODUCTION

Society for Women's Health Research
1025 Connecticut Ave. N.W., Suite 701
Washington, D.C. 20036
Phone: 1-202-223-8224
Fax: 1-202-833-3472
E-mail: info@womenshealthresearch.org
www.womenshealthresearch.org

CHAPTER 1

The Public Education Affiliate of the Endocrine Society
8401 Connecticut Ave., Suite 900
Chevy Chase, MD 20815-5817
Phone: 1-800-HORMONE
www.hormone.org

American Society for Reproductive Medicine
1209 Montgomery Highway
Birmingham, AL 35216-2809
Phone: 1-205-978-5000
Fax: 1-205-978-5005
www.asrm.org

Polycystic Ovarian Syndrome Association
P.O. Box 3403
Englewood, CO 80111
Phone: 1-877-775-7267
www.pcosupport.org

CHAPTER 2

The Brain Connection Web Site
www.psycheducation.org/index.html

CHAPTER 3

Turner Syndrome Society of the United States
14450 TC Jester, Suite 260
Houston, TX 77014
Phone: 1-800-365-9944
Fax: 1-832-249-9987
www.turner-syndrome-us.org

Optimum Performance Institute—a place for empowerment and growth
Phone: 1-866-358-2395
Fax: 1-847-954-0201
www.optimumperformanceinstitute.com

The North American Menopause Society
P.O. Box 94527
Cleveland, OH 44101
Phone: 1-440-442-7550
Fax: 1-440-442-2660
E-mail: info@menopause.org
www.menopause.org

CHAPTER 4

Center for Science in the Public Interest
1875 Connecticut Ave. N.W., Suite 300
Washington, D.C. 20009
Phone: 1-202-332-9110
Fax: 1-202-265-4954
www.cspinet.org

Food News
1436 U St. N.W., Suite 100
Washington, D.C. 20009
Phone: 1-212-667-6982
www.foodnews.org

Physician's Committee for Responsible Medicine
Vegetarian Starter Kit
5100 Wisconsin Ave. N.W., Suite 400
Washington, D.C. 20016
Phone: 1-202-686-2210

E-mail: pcrm@pcrm.org
www.pcrm.org/health/VSK/starterkit.html

CHAPTER 5

Healthy People 2010
www.healthypeople.gov/default.htm

America on the Move:
The Partnership to Promote Healthy Eating and Active Living
44 School St., Suite 325
Boston, MA 02108
Fax: 1-617-367-6899
E-mail: sani@americaonthemove.org
www.americaonthemove.org

CHAPTER 6

Yoga Journal
2054 University Ave.
Berkeley, CA 94704
Phone: 1-510-841-9200
Fax: 1-510-644-3101
www.yogajournal.com

The Wild Divine Project
P.O. Box 381
Eldorado Springs, CO 80025
Phone: 1-866-594-WILD (9453)
Fax: 1-303-499-3688
E-mail: takeoff@wilddivine.com
www.wilddivine.com

CHAPTER 7

Chemical Body Burden
www.chemicalbodyburden.org/home.htm

CHAPTER 8

The Alexander Foundation for Women's Health
1700 Shattuck Ave., Suite 329
Berkeley, CA 94709
E-mail: info@alexanderfoundation.net
www.afwh.org/about

CHAPTER 9

The American Council for Headache Education
19 Mantua Rd.
Mt. Royal, NJ 08061
Phone: 1-856-423-0258
Fax: 1-856-423-0082
www.achenet.org

Interstitial Cystitis Network
ICN Administrative Offices
4983 Sonoma Highway, Suite L
Santa Rosa, CA 95409
Phone: 1-707-538-9442
Fax: 1-707-538-9444
www.ic-network.com

The Endometriosis Association
8585 N. 76th Pl.
Milwaukee, WI 53223
Phone: 1-414-355-2200
Fax: 414-355-6065
www.endometriosisassn.org

National Vulvodynia Association
P.O. Box 4491
Silver Spring, MD 20914-4491
Phone: 1-301-299-0775
Fax: 1-301-299-3999
www.nva.org

CHAPTER 13

Alzheimer's Association
225 N. Michigan Ave., Fl. 17
Chicago, IL 60601-7633
Phone: 1-800-272-3900
Fax: 1-312-335-1110
www.alz.org

CHAPTER 16

Union of Concerned Scientists
National Headquarters
2 Brattle Square
Cambridge, MA 02238-9105
Phone: 1-617-547-5552

Fax: 1-617-864-9405
www.ucsusa.org

CHAPTER 17

Society for Reproductive Endocrinologists
1209 Montgomery Highway
Birmingham, AL 35216-2809
Phone: 1-205-978-5000
Fax: 1-205-978-5005
www.socrei.org

APPENDIX 5

REFERENCES
INTRODUCTION AND CHAPTER 1

Anderson, G., M. Limacher, et al. "Effects of Conjugated Equine Estrogen in Post-menopausal Women with Hysterectomy: The Women's Health Initiative Randomized Controlled Trial." *JAMA,* vol. 291, iss. 14 (2004): 1701–12.

Azziz, R., L. A. Sanchez, et al. "Androgen Excess in Women: Experience with over 1000 Consecutive Patients." *J Clin Endocrinol Metab,* vol. 89, iss. 2 (2004): 453–62.

Brower, V. "A Second Chance for Hormone Replacement Therapy [in process citation]?" *EMBO Rep,* vol. 4, iss. 12 (2003): 1112–15.

Corbould, A. M., S. J. Judd, et al. "Expression of Types 1, 2, and 3 17{beta}-Hydroxysteroid Dehydrogenase in Subcutaneous Abdominal and Intra-Abdominal Adipose Tissue of Women." *J Clin Endocrinol Metab,* vol. 83, iss. 1 (1998): 187–94.

Flood, C., J. Pratt, et al. "The Metabolic Clearance and Blood Production Rates of Estriol in Normal, Non-Pregnant Women." *J Clin Endocrinol Metab,* vol. 42, iss. 1 (1976): 1–8.

Graaf, C. D., W. Blom, et al. "BioMarkers of Satiation and Satiety." *Am J Clin Nutr,* vol. 79 (2004): 946–61.

Gruber, C. J., W. Tschugguel, et al. "Production and Actions of Estrogens." *N Engl J Med,* vol. 346, iss. 5 (2002): 340–52.

Haskell, S. "After the Women's Health Initiative: Postmenopausal Women's Experiences with Discontinuing Estrogen Replacement Therapy [in process citation]." *J Women's Health (Larchmt),* vol. 13, iss. 4 (2004): 438–42.

Kiecolt-Glaser, J., C. Bane, et al. "Marriage and Divorce: Newlyweds' Stress Hormones Foreshadow Relationship Changes." *J Consulting and Clinical Psychology,* vol. 71, iss. 1 (2003): 176–88.

Lovas, K., G. Gebre-Medhin, et al. "Replacement of Dehydroepiandrosterone in Adrenal Failure: No Benefit for Subjective Health Status and Sexuality in a 9-Month, Randomized, Parallel Group Clinical Trial." *J Clin Endocrinol Metab,* vol. 88, iss. 3 (2003): 1112–18.

McLachlan, J. "Environmental Signaling: What Embryos and Evolution Teach Us About Endocrine Disrupting Chemicals." *Endocrine Reviews,* vol. 22 (2001): 319–41.

Nilsen, J., and R. D. Brinton. "Divergent Impact of Progesterone and Medroxyprogesterone Acetate (Provera) on Nuclear Mitogen-Activated Protein Kinase Signaling." *PNAS,* vol. 100, iss. 18 (2003): 10506–11.

Rittmaster, R. "Androgen Conjugates: Physiology and Clinical Significance." *Endocr Rev,* vol. 14, iss. 1 (1993): 121–32.

Roca, C. A., P. J. Schmidt, et al. "Differential Menstrual Cycle Regulation of Hypothalamic-Pituitary-Adrenal Axis in Women with Premenstrual Syndrome and Controls." *J Clin Endocrinol Metab,* vol. 88, iss. 7 (2003): 3057–63.

Saez, J. "Leydig Cells: Endocrine, Paracrine, and Autocrine Regulation." *Endocr Rev,* vol. 15, iss. 5 (1994): 574–626.

Sharpe, R., and D. Irvine. "How Strong Is the Evidence of a Link Between Environmental Chemicals and Adverse Effects on Human Reproductive Health?" *BMJ,* vol. 328 (2004): 447–52.

Stokstad, E. "BIOMONITORING: Pollution Gets Personal." *Science,* vol. 304, iss. 5679 (2004): 1892–94.

Turgeon, J., D. McDonnell, et al. "Hormone Therapy: Physiological Complexity Belies Therapeutic Simplicity." *Science,* vol. 304 (2004): 1269–73.

Vrblkova, J., D. Cibula, et al. "Insulin Sensitivity in Women with Polycystic Ovary Syndrome." *J Clin Endocrinol Metab,* vol. 89, iss. 6 (2004): 2942–45.

CHAPTER 2

Arnold, A. P., J. Xu, et al. "Minireview: Sex Chromosomes and Brain Sexual Differentiation." *Endocrinology,* vol. 145, iss. 3 (2004): 1057–62.

Bishop, J., and W. Simpkins. "Role of Estrogens in Peripheral and Cerebral Glucose Utilization." *Reviews in the Neurosciences,* vol. 3, iss. 2 (1992): 121–37.

Cutter, W., R. Norbury, et al. "Oestrogen, Brain Function, and Neuropsychiatric Disorders." *J Neurol Neurosurg Psychiatry,* vol. 74, iss. 7 (2003): 837–40.

De Vries, G. J. "Minireview: Sex Differences in Adult and Developing Brains: Compensation, Compensation, Compensation." *Endocrinology,* vol. 145, iss. 3 (2004): 1063–68.

Diaz, B. R., S. Chen, et al. "The Women's Health Initiative Estrogen Replacement Therapy Is Neurotrophic and Neuroprotective." *Neurobiol Aging,* vol. 21, iss. 3 (2000): 475–96.

Greene, R., and W. Dixon. "The Role of Reproductive Hormones in Maintaining Cognition." *Obstet Gynecol Clin N Am,* vol. 29 (2002): 437–53.

Greene, R. "Cerebral Blood Flow." *Fertil Steril,* vol. 73, iss. 1 (2000): 143.

———. "Measurement of Estrogen's Effects on the Brain Using Modern Imaging Techniques." *Menopausal Medicine,* vol. 7, iss. 4 (1999): 9–11.

Hochberg, Z. E., K. Pacak, et al. "Endocrine Withdrawal Syndromes." *Endocr Rev,* vol. 24, iss. 4 (2003): 523–38.

Inoue, T., J.-I. Akahira, et al. "Progesterone Production and Actions in the Human Central Nervous System and Neurogenic Tumors." *J Clin Endocrinol Metab,* vol. 87, iss. 11 (2002): 5325–31.

Kruijver, F., J. Zhou, et al. "Male-to-Female Transsexuals Have Female Neuron Numbers in a Limbic Nucleus." *J Clin Endocrin Metab,* vol. 85 (2000): 2034–41.

Mazziotta, J. C. "Imaging: Window on the Brain." *Arch Neurol,* vol. 57, iss. 10 (2000): 1413–21.

McEwen, B. "Estrogen Actions Throughout the Brain." *Recent Prog Horm Res,* vol. 57, iss. 1 (2002): 357–84.

Nilsen, J., and R. Brinton. "Impact of Progestins on Estradiol Potentiation of the Glutamate Calcium Response." *Neuroreport,* vol. 13, iss. 6 (2002): 825–30.

Osterlund, M., J. Gustafsson, et al. "Estrogen Receptor Beta (ERbeta) Messenger Ribonucleic Acid (mRNA) Expression Within the Human Forebrain: Distinct Distribution Pattern to ERalpha mRNA." *J Clin Endocrinol Metab,* vol. 85, iss. 10 (2000): 3840–6.

Swaab, D. F., M. A. Hoffman. "Sexual Differentiation of the Human Hypothalamus in Relation to Gender and Sexual Orientation." *Trends Neurosci,* vol. 18, iss. 6 (1995): 264–70.

CHAPTER 3

Backstrom, T., A. Andersson, et al. "Pathogenesis in Menstrual Cycle–Linked CNS Disorders." *Ann N Y Acad Sci,* vol. 1007 (2003): 42–53.

Greene, R. "Estrogen and Cerebral Blood Flow: A Mechanism to Explain the Impact of Estrogen on the Incidence and Treatment of Alzheimer's Disease." *Int J Fertil Women's Med,* vol. 45, iss. 4 (2000): 253–37.

———. "Aging and the Brain: Restoring Neurologic Functioning Through HRT." *Clinical Courier,* vol. 17, iss. 17 (1999).

Hughes, C., and W. Foster. "Some Potential Health Effects of Endocrine-Disrupting Chemicals Across the Lifespan of Adult Women." *Menopausal Medicine,* vol. 9, iss. 2 (2001): 7–12.

Smith, Y., and J. Zubieta. "Neuroimaging of Aging and Estrogen Effects on Central Nervous System Physiology." *Fertil Steril,* vol. 76, iss. 4 (2001): 651–59.

Wong, C., T. Bottiglieri, et al. "GABA, Gamma-Hydroxybutyric Acid, and Neurological Disease." *Ann Neurol,* vol. 54, suppl. 6 (2003): S3–12.

CHAPTER 4

American Meat Institute. Fact Sheet: *Organic Meat Products* (2003).

Bajaj, M., S. Suraamornkul, et al. "Decreased Plasma Adiponectin Concentrations Are Closely Related to Hepatic Fat Content and Hepatic Insulin Resistance in Pioglitazone-Treated Type 2 Diabetic Patients." *J Clin Endocrinol Metab,* vol. 89, iss. 1 (2004): 200–06.

Bray, G. "Low-Carbohydrate Diets and Realities of Weight Loss." *JAMA,* vol. 289, iss. 14 (2003): 1853–55.

Castillo-Martinez, L., J. Lopez-Alvarenga, et al. "Menstrual Cycle Length Disorders in 18- to 40-yr-old Obese Women." *Nutrition,* vol. 19, iss. 4 (2003): 317–20.

Crespo, C. J., E. Smit, et al. "Hormone Replacement Therapy and Its Relationship to Lipid and Glucose Metabolism in Diabetic and Nondiabetic Postmenopausal Women: Results from the Third National Health and Nutrition Examination Survey (NHANES III)." *Diabetes Care,* vol. 25, iss. 10 (2002): 1675–80.

Cummings, D., D. Weigle, et al. "Plasma Ghrelin Levels After Diet-Induced Weight Loss or Gastric Bypass Surgery." *N Engl J Med,* vol. 346, iss. 21 (2002): 1623–30.

Cummings, D. E., R. S. Frayo, et al. "Plasma Ghrelin Levels and Hunger Scores in Humans Initiating Meals Voluntarily Without Time- and Food-Related Cues." *Am J Physiol Endocrinol Metab,* vol. 287, iss. 2 (2004): E297–304.

Davies, K., R. Heaney, et al. "Calcium Intake and Body Weight." *J Clin Endocrinol Metab,* vol. 85, iss. 12 (2000): 4635–38.

Davy, B., and C. Melby. "The Effect of Fiber-Rich Carbohydrates on Features of Syndrome X." *J Am Diet Assoc,* vol. 103, iss. 1 (2003): 86–96.

Duffy, R., H. Wiseman, et al. "Improved Cognitive Function in Postmenopausal Women After 12 Weeks of Consumption of a Soya Extract Containing Isoflavones." *Pharmacol Biochem Behav,* vol. 75, iss. 3 (2003): 721–29.

Gann, P., R. Chatterton, et al. "The Effects of a Low-Fat/High-Fiber Diet on Sex Hormone Levels and Menstrual Cycling in Premenopausal Women: A 12-Month Randomized Trial (the Diet and Hormone Study)." *Cancer,* vol. 98, iss. 9 (2003): 1870–79.

Garrido, J. "Low-Carbohydrate Diets as Compared with Low-Fat Diets." *N Engl J Med,* vol. 349, iss. 10 (2003): 1000–02; author reply 1000–02.

Goldstein, B. J., and R. Scalia. "Adiponectin: A Novel Adipokine Linking Adipocytes and Vascular Function." *J Clin Endocrinol Metab,* vol. 89, iss. 6 (2004): 2563–68.

Hays, N., R. Starling, et al. "Effects of an Ad Libitum Low-Fat, High-Carbohydrate Diet on Body Weight, Body Composition, and Fat Distribution in Older Men and Women: A Randomized Controlled Trial." *Arch Intern Med,* vol. 164, iss. 2 (2004): 210–17.

Hoffstedt, J., E. Arvidsson, et al. "Adipose Tissue Adiponectin Production and Adiponectin Serum Concentration in Human Obesity and Insulin Resistance." *J Clin Endocrinol Metab,* vol. 89, iss. 3 (2004): 1391–96.

Iso, H., K. Rexrode, et al. "Intake of Fish and Omega-3 Fatty Acids and Risk of Stroke in Women." *JAMA,* vol. 285, iss. 3 (2001): 304–12.

Knight, E. L., M. J. Stampfer, et al. "The Impact of Protein Intake on Renal Function Decline in Women with Normal Renal Function or Mild Renal Insufficiency." *Ann Intern Med,* vol. 138, iss. 6 (2003): 460–67.

Korner, J., and R. L. Leibel. "To Eat or Not to Eat—How the Gut Talks to the Brain." *N Engl J Med,* vol. 349, iss. 10 (2003): 926–28.

Lieberman, H. "Nutrition, Brain Function and Cognitive Performance." *Appetite,* vol. 40, iss. 3 (2003): 245–54.

Lopez-Ridaura, R., W. C. Willett, et al. "Magnesium Intake and Risk of Type 2 Diabetes in Men and Women." *Diabetes Care,* vol. 27, iss. 1 (2004): 134–40.

McDonald, J., B. Zielinska, et al. "Emissions from Charbroiling and Grilling of Chicken and Beef." *J Air Waste Manag Assoc,* vol. 53, iss. 2 (2003): 185–94.

Saiyed, H., A. Dewan, et al. "Effect of Endosulfan on Male Reproductive Development." *Environ Health Perspect,* vol. 111, iss. 16 (2003): 1958–62.

Samaha, F., N. Iqbal, et al. "A Low-Carbohydrate as Compared with a Low-Fat Diet in Severe Obesity." *N Engl J Med,* vol. 348, iss. 21 (2003): 2074–81.

Sandoval, D. A., A. C. Ertl, et al. "Estrogen Blunts Neuroendocrine and Metabolic Responses to Hypoglycemia." *Diabetes,* vol. 52, iss. 7 (2003): 1749–55.

Serafini, M., R. Bugianesi, et al. "Plasma Antioxidants from Chocolate." *Nature,* vol. 424, iss. 6952 (2003): 1013.

Smith, A., S. Kuznesof, et al. "Behavioural, Attitudinal and Dietary Responses to the Consumption of Wholegrain Foods." *Proc Nutr Soc,* vol. 62, iss. 2 (2003): 455–67.

Stein, C., and G. Colditz. "The Epidemic of Obesity." *J Clin Endocrinol Metab,* vol. 89, iss. 6 (2004): 2522–25.

Teff, K., S. Elliott, et al. "Dietary Fructose Reduces Circulating Insulin and Leptin, Attenuates Postprandial Suppression of Ghrelin, and Increases Triglycerides in Women." *J Clin Endocrinol Metab,* vol. 89, iss. 6 (2004): 2963–72.

Thomas, G. N., P. Chook, et al. "Deleterious Impact of 'High Normal' Glucose Levels and Other Metabolic Syndrome Components on Arterial Endothelial Function and Intima-Media Thickness in Apparently Healthy Chinese Subjects: The CATHAY Study." *Arterioscler Thromb Vasc Biol,* vol. 24, iss. 4 (2004): 739–43.

Wansink, B., M. Cheney, et al. "Exploring Comfort Food Preferences Across Age and Gender." *Physiol Behav,* vol. 79, iss. 4–5 (2003): 739–47.

Webster, P. "TOXICOLOGY: Exposure to Flame Retardants on the Rise." *Science,* vol. 304, iss. 5678 (2004): 1730a.

Westerterp-Plantenga, M., V. Rolland, et al. "Satiety Related to 24 H Diet-Induced Thermogenesis During High Protein/Carbohydrate vs. High Fat Diets Measured in a Respiration Chamber." *Eur J Clin Nutr,* vol. 53, iss. 6 (1999): 495–502.

Zellner, D., A. Garriga-Trillo, et al. "Chocolate Craving and the Menstrual Cycle." *Appetite,* vol. 42, iss. 1 (2004): 119–21.

CHAPTER 5

Barger, L., K. Wright, et al. "Daily Exercise Facilitates Phase Delays of Circadian Melatonin Rhythm in Very Dim Light." *Am J Physiol Regul Integr Comp Physiol,* vol. 286, iss. 6 (2004): R1077–84.

Casper, R., E. Reed, et al. "Mood, Its Relationship to Physical Activity and Nutrition." *World Rev Nutr Diet,* vol. 90 (2001): 73–88.

Hansen, C., L. Stevens, et al. "Exercise Duration and Mood State: How Much Is Enough to Feel Better?" *Health Psychol,* vol. 20, iss. 4 (2001): 267–75.

Hu, F., T. Li, et al. "Television Watching and Other Sedentary Behaviors in Relation to Risk of Obesity and Type 2 Diabetes Mellitus in Women." *JAMA,* vol. 289, iss. 14 (2003): 1785–91.

John, E., P. Horn-Ross, et al. "Lifetime Physical Activity and Breast Cancer Risk in a Multi-ethnic Population: The San Francisco Bay Area Breast Cancer Study." *Cancer Epidemiol Biomarkers Prev,* vol. 12, iss. 11, pt. 1 (2003): 1143–52.

Nielsen, S., Z. Guo, et al. "Energy Expenditure, Sex, and Endogenous Fuel Availability in Humans." *J Clin Invest,* vol. 111, iss. 7 (2003): 981–88.

Pittler, M., C. Stevinson, et al. "Chromium Picolinate for Reducing Body Weight: Meta-analysis of Randomized Trials." *Int J Obes Relat Metab Disord,* vol. 27, iss. 4 (2003): 522–29.

Ray, U., S. Mukhopadhyaya, et al. "Effect of Yogic Exercises on Physical and Mental Health of Young Fellowship Course Trainees." *Indian J Physiol Pharmacol,* vol. 45, iss. 1 (2001): 37–53.

Redman, L., and R. Weatherby. "Measuring Performance During the Menstrual Cycle: A Model Using Oral Contraceptives [in process citation]." *Med Sci Sports Exerc,* vol. 36, iss. 1 (2004): 130–36.

Salmon, P. "Effects of Physical Exercise on Anxiety, Depression, and Sensitivity to Stress: A Unifying Theory." *Clin Psychol Rev,* vol. 21, iss. 1 (2001): 33–61.

Sheffield-Moore, M., and R. Urban. "An Overview of the Endocrinology of Skeletal Muscle [in process citation]." *Trends Endocrinol Metab,* vol. 15, iss. 3 (2004): 110–15.

Teixeira, P., S. Going, et al. "Resistance Training in Postmenopausal Women with and without Hormone Therapy." *Med Sci Sports Exerc,* vol. 35, iss. 4 (2003): 555–62.

Wang, C., J. P. Collet, et al. "The Effect of Tai Chi on Health Outcomes in Patients with Chronic Conditions: A Systematic Review." *Arch Intern Med,* vol. 164, iss. 5 (2004): 493–501.

Watkins, L. L., A. Sherwood, et al. "Effects of Exercise and Weight Loss on Cardiac Risk Factors Associated with Syndrome X." *Arch Intern Med,* vol. 163, iss. 16 (2003): 1889–95.

Williams, N. "Lessons from Experimental Disruptions of the Menstrual Cycle in Humans and Monkeys." *Med Sci Sports Exerc,* vol. 35, iss. 9 (2003): 1564–72.

Yarasheski, K. "Exercise, Aging, and Muscle Protein Metabolism." *J Gerontol A Biol Sci Med Sci,* vol. 58, iss. 10 (2003): M918–22.

CHAPTER 6

Barger, L., K. Wright, et al. "Daily Exercise Facilitates Phase Delays of Circadian Melatonin Rhythm in Very Dim Light." *Am J Physiol Regul Integr Comp Physiol,* vol. 286, iss. 6 (2004): R1077–84.

Casper, R., E. Reed, et al. "Mood, Its Relationship to Physical Activity and Nutrition." *World Rev Nutr Diet,* vol. 90 (2001): 73–88.

Hansen, C., L. Stevens, et al. "Exercise Duration and Mood State: How Much Is Enough to Feel Better?" *Health Psychol,* vol. 20, iss. 4 (2001): 267–75.

Hollmann W., H. K. Struder. "Brain Function, Mind, Mood, Nutrition, and Physical Exercise." *Nutrition,* vol. 16, iss. 7/8 (2000): 516–19.

Hu, F., T. Li, et al. "Television Watching and Other Sedentary Behaviors in Relation to Risk of Obesity and Type 2 Diabetes Mellitus in Women." *JAMA,* vol. 289, iss. 14 (2003): 1785–91.

John, E., P. Horn-Ross, et al. "Lifetime Physical Activity and Breast Cancer Risk in a Multi-ethnic Population: The San Francisco Bay Area Breast Cancer Study." *Cancer Epidemiol Biomarkers Prev,* vol. 12, iss. 11, pt. 1 (2003): 1143–52.

Nielsen, S., Z. Guo, et al. "Energy Expenditure, Sex, and Endogenous Fuel Availability in Humans." *J Clin Invest,* vol. 111, iss. 7 (2003): 981–88.

Pittler, M., C. Stevinson, et al. "Chromium Picolinate for Reducing Body Weight: Meta-analysis of Randomized Trials." *Int J Obes Relat Metab Disord,* vol. 27, iss. 4 (2003): 522–29.

Ray, U., S. Mukhopadhyaya, et al. "Effect of Yogic Exercises on Physical and Mental Health of Young Fellowship Course Trainees." *Indian J Physiol Pharmacol,* vol. 45, iss. 1 (2001): 37–53.

Redman, L., and R. Weatherby. "Measuring Performance During the Menstrual Cycle: A Model Using Oral Contraceptives [in process citation]." *Med Sci Sports Exerc,* vol. 36, iss. 1 (2004): 130–36.

Salmon, P. "Effects of Physical Exercise on Anxiety, Depression, and Sensitivity to Stress: A Unifying Theory." *Clin Psychol Rev,* vol. 21, iss. 1 (2001): 33–61.

Sheffield-Moore, M., and R. Urban. "An Overview of the Endocrinology of Skeletal Muscle [in process citation]." *Trends Endocrinol Metab,* vol. 15, iss. 3 (2004): 110–15.

Teixeira, P., S. Going, et al. "Resistance Training in Postmenopausal Women with and without Hormone Therapy." *Med Sci Sports Exerc,* vol. 35, iss. 4 (2003): 555–62.

Wang, C., J. P. Collet, et al. "The Effect of Tai Chi on Health Outcomes in Patients with Chronic Conditions: A Systematic Review." *Arch Intern Med,* vol. 164, iss. 5 (2004): 493–501.

Watkins, L. L., A. Sherwood, et al. "Effects of Exercise and Weight Loss on Cardiac Risk Factors Associated with Syndrome X." *Arch Intern Med,* vol. 163, iss. 16 (2003): 1889–95.

Williams, N. "Lessons from Experimental Disruptions of the Menstrual Cycle in Humans and Monkeys." *Med Sci Sports Exerc,* vol. 35, iss. 9 (2003): 1564–72.

Yarasheski, K. "Exercise, Aging, and Muscle Protein Metabolism." *J Gerontol A Biol Sci Med Sci,* vol. 58, iss. 10 (2003): M918–22.

CHAPTER 7

Burkman, R., J. Collins, et al. "Current Perspectives on Benefits and Risks of Hormone Replacement Therapy." *Am J Obstet Gynecol,* vol. 185, 2 suppl. (2001): S13–23.

Coelingh, B. H. "Are All Estrogens the Same?" *Maturitas,* vol. 47, iss. 4 (2004): 269–75.

Gavaler, J. "Thoughts on Individualizing Hormone Replacement Therapy Based on the Postmenopausal Health Disparities Study Data." *Journal of Women's Health,* vol. 12, iss. 8 (2003): 757–68.

Greene, R., and W. Dixon. "The Role of Reproductive Hormones in Maintaining Cognition." *Obstet Gynecol Clin North Am,* vol. 29, iss. 3 (2002): 437–53.

Greene, R., R. Burkman, and J. Collins. "Current Perspectives on Benefits and Risks of Hormone Replacement Therapy." *Am J Obstet Gynecol,* vol. 185 (2001): S13–23.

Greenlee, A., T. Arbuckle, et al. "Risk Factors for Female Infertility in an Agricultural Region." *Epidemiology,* vol. 14, iss. 4 (2003): 429–36.

Greenlee, A., T. Ellis, et al. "Low-Dose Agrochemicals and Lawn-Care Pesticides Induce Developmental Toxicity in Murine Preimplantation Embryos." *Environ Health Perspect,* vol. 112, iss. 6 (2004): 703–09.

Hampton, T. "Testosterone Trials." *JAMA,* vol. 290, iss. 24 (2003): 3186c.

Kang, J. H., J. Weuve, et al. "Postmenopausal Hormone Therapy and Risk of Cognitive Decline in Community-Dwelling Aging Women." *Neurology,* vol. 63, iss. 1 (2004): 101–07.

Nilsen, J., and R. Brinton. "Impact of Progestins on Estrogen-Induced Neuroprotection: Synergy by Progesterone and 19-Norprogesterone and Antagonism by Medroxyprogesterone Acetate." *Endocrinology,* vol. 143, iss. 1 (2002): 205–12.

Paganini-Hill, A., and L. Clark. "Preliminary Assessment of Cognitive Function in Breast Cancer Patients Treated with Tamoxifen." *Breast Cancer Res Treat,* vol. 64, iss. 2 (2000): 165–76.

Roegge, C., V. Wang, et al. "Motor Impairment in Rats Exposed to PCBs and Methylmercury During Early Development [in process citation]." *Toxicol Sci,* vol. 77, iss. 2 (2004): 315–24.

Sharpe, R., and D. Irvine. "How Strong Is the Evidence of a Link Between Environmental Chemicals and Adverse Effects on Human Reproductive Health?" *BMJ,* vol. 328, iss. 7437 (2004): 447–51.

Sitruk-Ware, R. "Pharmacological Profile of Progestins." *Maturitas,* vol. 47, iss. 4 (2004): 277–83.

Somboonporn, W., and S. R. Davis. "Testosterone Effects on the Breast: Implications for Testosterone Therapy for Women." *Endocr Rev,* vol. 25, iss. 3 (2004): 374–88.

Vasiliu, O., J. Muttineni, et al. "In Utero Exposure to Organochlorines and Age at Menarche [in process citation]." *Hum Reprod,* vol. 19, iss. 7 (2004): 1506–12.

CHAPTER 8

Bachmann, G., and S. Leiblum. "Sexuality in Sexagenarian Women." *Maturitas,* vol. 13, iss. 1 (1991): 43–50.

———. "The Impact of Hormones on Menopausal Sexuality: A Literature Review." *Menopause,* vol. 11, iss. 1 (2004): 120–30.

Basson, R. "Female Sexual Response: The Role of Drugs in the Management of Sexual Dysfunction." *Obstet Gynecol,* vol. 98, iss. 2 (2001): 350–53.

———. "Rethinking Low Sexual Desire in Women." *BJOG,* vol. 109, iss. 4 (2002): 357–63.

Berman, J., S. Adhikari, et al. "Anatomy and Physiology of Female Sexual Function and Dysfunction: Classification, Evaluation and Treatment Options." *Eur Urol,* vol. 38, iss. 1 (2000): 20–29.

Berman, J., L. Berman, et al. "Safety and Efficacy of Sildenafil Citrate for the Treatment of Female Sexual Arousal Disorder: A Double-Blind, Placebo Controlled Study." *J Urol,* vol. 170, iss. 6, pt. 1 (2003): 2333–38.

———. "Clinical Evaluation of Female Sexual Function: Effects of Age and Estrogen Status on Subjective and Physiologic Sexual Responses." *Int J Impot Res,* vol. 11, suppl. 1 (1999): S31–38.

Billups, K., L. Berman, et al. "A New Non-Pharmacological Vacuum Therapy for Female Sexual Dysfunction." *J Sex Marital Ther,* vol. 27, iss. 5 (2001): 435–41.

Exton, M., A. Bindert, et al. "Cardiovascular and Endocrine Alterations After Masturbation-Induced Orgasm in Women." *Psychosom Med,* vol. 61, iss. 3 (1999): 280–89.

Fisher, H., A. Aron, et al. "Defining the Brain Systems of Lust, Romantic Attraction, and Attachment." *Arch Sex Behav,* vol. 31, iss. 5 (2002): 413–19.

Geiss, I., W. Umek, et al. "Prevalence of Female Sexual Dysfunction in Gynecologic and Urogynecologic Patients According to the International Consensus Classification." *Urology,* vol. 62, iss. 3 (2003): 514–18.

Guay, A., J. Jacobson, et al. "Serum Androgen Levels in Healthy Premenopausal Women with and without Sexual Dysfunction: Part B: Reduced Serum Androgen Levels in Healthy Premenopausal Women with Complaints of Sexual Dysfunction [in process citation]." *Int J Impot Res,* vol. 16, iss. 2 (2004): 121–29.

Ito, T., A. Trant, et al. "A Double-Blind Placebo-Controlled Study of ArginMax, a Nutritional Supplement for Enhancement of Female Sexual Function." *J Sex Marital Ther,* vol. 27, iss. 5 (2001): 541–49.

Karama, S., A. Lecours, et al. "Areas of Brain Activation in Males and Females During Viewing of Erotic Film Excerpts." *Hum Brain Mapp,* vol. 16, iss. 1 (2002): 1–13.

Laumann, E. O., A. Paik, et al. "Sexual Dysfunction in the United States: Prevalence and Predictors." *JAMA,* vol. 281, iss. 6 (1999): 537–44.

Maravilla, K., J. Heiman, et al. "Dynamic MR Imaging of the Sexual Arousal Response in Women." *J Sex Marital Ther,* vol. 29, suppl. 1 (2003): 71–76.

Meston, C. "Sympathetic Nervous System Activity and Female Sexual Arousal." *Am J Cardiol,* vol. 86, iss. 2A (2000): 30F–34F.

Ogawa, S., A. Chester, et al. "Abolition of Male Sexual Behaviors in Mice Lacking Estrogen Receptors Alpha and Beta (Alpha Beta ERKO)." *Proc Natl Acad Sci USA,* vol. 97, iss. 26 (2000): 14737–41.

Reed, B., A. Advincula, et al. "Sexual Activities and Attitudes of Women with Vulvar Dysesthesia." *Obstet Gynecol,* vol. 102, iss. 2 (2003): 325–31.

Riley, A., and E. Riley. "Controlled Studies on Women Presenting with Sexual Drive Disorder: I. Endocrine Status." *J Sex Marital Ther,* vol. 26, iss. 3 (2000): 269–83.

Segraves, R., A. Clayton, et al. "Bupropion Sustained Release for the Treatment of Hypoactive Sexual Desire Disorder in Premenopausal Women [in process citation]." *J Clin Psychopharmacol,* vol. 24, iss. 3 (2004): 339–42.

CHAPTER 9

Aikens, J., B. Reed, et al. "Depressive Symptoms Among Women with Vulvar Dysesthesia." *Am J Obstet Gynecol,* vol. 189, iss. 2 (2003): 462–66.

Cepeda, M., and D. Carr. "Women Experience More Pain and Require More Morphine Than Men to Achieve a Similar Degree of Analgesia." *Anesth Analg,* vol. 97, iss. 5 (2003): 1464–68.

Cobellis, L., G. Latini, et al. "High Plasma Concentrations of di-(2-ethylhexyl)-phthalate in Women with Endometriosis." *Hum Reprod,* vol. 18, iss. 7 (2003): 1512–15.

Cronje, W., A. Vashisht, et al. "Hysterectomy and Bilateral Oophorectomy for Severe Premenstrual Syndrome [epub ahead of print] [record supplied by publisher]." *Hum Reprod* (2004).

Engel, P. "New Onset Migraine Associated with Use of Soy Isoflavone Supplements." *Neurology,* vol. 59, iss. 8 (2002): 1289–90.

Giffin, N., L. Ruggiero, et al. "Premonitory Symptoms in Migraine: An Electronic Diary Study." *Neurology,* vol. 60, iss. 6 (2003): 935–40.

Hellstrom, B., and U. Anderberg. "Pain Perception Across the Menstrual Cycle Phases in Women with Chronic Pain." *Percept Mot Skills,* vol. 96, iss. 1 (2003): 201–11.

Hellstrom, B., and U. Lundberg. "Pain Perception to the Cold Pressor Test During the Menstrual Cycle in Relation to Estrogen Levels and a Comparison with Men." *Integr Physiol Behav Sci,* vol. 35, iss. 2 (2000): 132–41.

Jensen, J., K. Wilder, et al. "Quality of Life and Sexual Function After Evaluation and Treatment at a Referral Center for Vulvovaginal Disorders." *Am J Obstet Gynecol,* vol. 188, iss. 6 (2003): 1629–35; discussion 1635–37.

Levin, M. "The Many Causes of Headache: Migraine, Vascular, Drug-Induced, and More." *Postgrad Med,* vol. 112, iss. 6 (2002): 67–68, 71–72, 75–76 *passim.*

Mantyselka, P., J. Turunen, et al. "Chronic Pain and Poor Self-Rated Health." *JAMA,* vol. 290, iss. 18 (2003): 2435–42.

Melton, L. "Aching Atrophy: More Than Unpleasant, Chronic Pain Shrinks the Brain." *Sci Am,* vol. 290, iss. 1 (2004): 22–24.

Parazzini, F., F. Chiaffarino, et al. "Selected Food Intake and Risk of Endometriosis [in process citation]." *Hum Reprod,* vol. 19, iss. 8 (2004): 1755–59.

Reed, B., A. Advincula, et al. "Sexual Activities and Attitudes of Women with Vulvar Dyses-thesia." *Obstet Gynecol,* vol. 102, iss. 2 (2003): 325–31.

Riley, J., M. Robinson, et al. "A Meta-analytic Review of Pain Perception Across the Men-strual Cycle." *Pain,* vol. 81, iss. 3 (1999): 225–35.

Sackett, S., E. Gates, et al. "Psychosexual Aspects of Vulvar Vestibulitis." *J Reprod Med,* vol. 46, iss. 6 (2001): 593–98.

Schwartzman, R. J., J. Grothusen, et al. "Neuropathic Central Pain: Epidemiology, Etiology, and Treatment Options." *Arch Neurol,* vol. 58, iss. 10 (2001): 1547–50.

Smart, O., and A. MacLean. "Vulvodynia." *Curr Opin Obstet Gynecol,* vol. 15, iss. 6 (2003): 497–500.

Solomon, G., and N. Santanello. "Impact of Migraine and Migraine Therapy on Productivity and Quality of Life." *Neurology,* vol. 55, iss. 9, suppl. 2 (2000): S29–35.

Wang, S., J. Fuh, et al. "Migraine Prevalence During Menopausal Transition." *Headache,* vol. 43, iss. 5 (2003): 470–78.

Young, W., M. Hopkins, et al. "Topiramate: A Case Series Study in Migraine Prophylaxis." *Cephalalgia,* vol. 22, iss. 8 (2002): 659–63.

CHAPTER 10

Brown, C., F. Ling, et al. "A New Monophasic Oral Contraceptive Containing Drospirenone: Effect on Premenstrual Symptoms." *J Reprod Med,* vol. 47, iss. 1 (2002): 14–22.

Dolan, R. J. "Emotion, Cognition, and Behavior." *Science,* vol. 298, iss. 5596 (2002): 1191–94.

Freeman, E., R. Kroll, et al. "Evaluation of a Unique Oral Contraceptive in the Treatment of Premenstrual Dysphoric Disorder." *J Women's Health Gend Based Med,* vol. 10, iss. 6 (2001): 561–69.

Girdler, S., P. Straneva, et al. "Allopregnanolone Levels and Reactivity to Mental Stress in Premenstrual Dysphoric Disorder." *Biol Psychiatry,* vol. 49, iss. 9 (2001): 788–97.

Hendrick, V., L. Altshuler, et al. "Hormonal Changes in the Postpartum and Implications for Postpartum Depression." *Psychosomatics,* vol. 39, iss. 2 (1998): 93–101.

Ostlund, H., E. Keller, et al. "Estrogen Receptor Gene Expression in Relation to Neuropsy-chiatric Disorders." *Ann NY Acad Sci,* vol. 1007 (2003): 54–63.

Parry, B. "The Role of Central Serotonergic Dysfunction in the Aetiology of Premenstrual Dysphoric Disorder: Therapeutic Implications." *CNS Drugs,* vol. 15, iss. 4 (2001): 277–85.

Parry, B., D. Sorenson, et al. "Hormonal Basis of Mood and Postpartum disorders." *Curr Women's Health Rep,* vol. 3, iss. 3 (2003): 230–35.

Pies, R. "The Diagnosis and Treatment of Subclinical Hypothyroid States in Depressed Patients." *Gen Hosp Psychiatry,* vol. 19, iss. 5 (1997): 344–54.

Rapkin, A. "A Review of Treatment of Premenstrual Syndrome and Premenstrual Dysphoric Disorder." *Psychoneuroendocrinology,* vol. 28, suppl. 3 (2003): 39–53.

Rasgon, N., M. Thomas, et al. "Menstrual Cycle–Related Brain Metabolite Changes Using 1H Magnetic Resonance Spectroscopy in Premenopausal Women: A Pilot Study." *Psychiatry Res,* vol. 106, iss. 1 (2001): 47–57.

Reiman, E., S. Armstrong, et al. "The Application of Positron Emission Tomography to the Study of the Normal Menstrual Cycle." *Hum Reprod,* vol. 11, iss. 12 (1996): 2799–805.

Soares, C., O. Almeida, et al. "Efficacy of Estradiol for the Treatment of Depressive Disorders in Perimenopausal Women: A Double-Blind, Randomized, Placebo-Controlled Trial." *Arch Gen Psychiatry,* vol. 58, iss. 6 (2001): 529–34.

Wyatt, K., P. Dimmock, et al. "Efficacy of Vitamin B6 in the Treatment of Premenstrual Syndrome: Systematic Review." *BMJ,* vol. 318, iss. 7195 (1999): 1375–81.

Yonkers, K. "Special Issues Related to the Treatment of Depression in Women." *J Clin Psychiatry,* vol. 64, suppl. 18 (2003): 8–13.

CHAPTER 11

Berendsen, H. "The Role of Serotonin in Hot Flushes." *Maturitas,* vol. 36, iss. 3 (2000): 155–64.

Carpenter, J., S. Gautam, et al. "Circadian Rhythm of Objectively Recorded Hot Flashes in Postmenopausal Breast Cancer Survivors." *Menopause,* vol. 8, iss. 3 (2001): 181–88.

Dormire, S., and N. Reame. "Menopausal Hot Flash Frequency Changes in Response to Experimental Manipulation of Blood Glucose." *Nurs Res,* vol. 52, iss. 5 (2003): 338–43.

Greene, R. "Cerebral Blood Flow." *Fertil Steril,* vol. 73, iss. 1 (2000): 143.

———. "Estrogen and Cerebral Blood Flow: A Mechanism to Explain the Impact of Estrogen on the Incidence and Treatment of Alzheimer's Disease." *Int J Fertil Women's Med,* vol. 45, iss. 4 (2000): 253–57.

Hlatky, M., D. Boothroyd, et al. "Quality-of-Life and Depressive Symptoms in Postmenopausal Women After Receiving Hormone Therapy: Results from the Heart and Estrogen/Progestin Replacement Study (HERS) Trial." *JAMA,* vol. 287, iss. 5 (2002): 591–97.

Huntley, A., and E. Ernst. "Soy for the Treatment of Perimenopausal Symptoms: A Systematic Review." *Maturitas,* vol. 47, iss. 1 (2004): 1–9.

Leal, M., J. Diaz, et al. "Hormone Replacement Therapy for Oxidative Stress in Postmenopausal Women with Hot Flushes." *Obstet Gynecol,* vol. 95, iss. 6, pt. 1 (2000): 804–09.

Lindh-Astrand, L., E. Nedstrand, et al. "Vasomotor Symptoms and Quality of Life in Previously Sedentary Postmenopausal Women Randomised to Physical Activity or Estrogen Therapy [in process citation]." *Maturitas,* vol. 48, iss. 2 (2004): 97–105.

Notelovitz, M. "Hot Flashes and Androgens: A Biological Rationale for Clinical Practice." *Mayo Clin Proc,* vol. 79, iss. 4, suppl. (2004): S8–13.

Simon, J., R. Stevens, et al. "Perimenopausal Women in Estrogen Vasomotor Trials: Contribution to Placebo Effect and Efficacy Outcome." *Climacteric,* vol. 4, iss. 1 (2001): 19–27.

CHAPTER 12

Andersen, M., M. Bignotto, et al. "Does Paradoxical Sleep Deprivation and Cocaine Induce Penile Erection and Ejaculation in Old Rats?" *Addict Biol,* vol. 7, iss. 3 (2002): 285–90.

Baker, F., H. Driver, et al. "High Nocturnal Body Temperatures and Disturbed Sleep in Women with Primary Dysmenorrhea." *Am J Physiol,* vol. 277, iss. 6, pt. 1 (1999): E1013–21.

Baker, F., J. Waner, et al. "Sleep and 24-Hour Body Temperatures: A Comparison in Young Men, Naturally Cycling Women and Women Taking Hormonal Contraceptives." *J Physiol,* vol. 530, pt. 3 (2001): 565–74.

Camacho-Arroyo, I., R. Hernandez-Gollas, et al. "Progesterone Microinjections into the Pontine Reticular Formation Modify Sleep in Male and Female Rats." *Neurosci Lett,* vol. 269, iss. 1 (1999): 9–12.

Hays, J., J. Ockene, et al. "Effects of Estrogen Plus Progestin on Health-Related Quality of Life." *N Engl J Med,* vol. 348, iss. 19 (2003): 1839–54.

Jahn, H., F. Kiefer, et al. "Sleep Endocrine Effects of the 11-betahydroxysteroid-dehydrogenase Inhibitor Metyrapone." *Sleep,* vol. 26, iss. 7 (2003): 823–29.

Lancel, M., J. Faulhaber, et al. "The GABA(A) Receptor Antagonist Picrotoxin Attenuates Most Sleep Changes Induced by Progesterone." *Psychopharmacology (Berl),* vol. 141, iss. 2 (1999): 213–19.

Luboshitzky, R., S. Lavi, et al. "The Association Between Melatonin and Sleep Stages in Normal Adults and Hypogonadal Men." *Sleep,* vol. 22, iss. 7 (1999): 867–74.

Manber, R., T. Kuo, et al. "The Effects of Hormone Replacement Therapy on Sleep-Disordered Breathing in Postmenopausal Women: A Pilot Study." *Sleep,* vol. 26, iss. 2 (2003): 163–68.

Marquet, P. "The Role of Sleep in Learning and Memory." *Science,* vol. 294 (2001): 1048–63.

Montplaisir, J., J. Lorrain, et al. "Sleep in Menopause: Differential Effects of Two Forms of Hormone Replacement Therapy." *Menopause,* vol. 8, iss. 1 (2001): 10–16.

Nader, K. "Re-recording Human Memories." *Nature,* vol. 425 (2003): 571–72.

Prinz, P., S. Bailey, et al. "Urinary Free Cortisol and Sleep Under Baseline and Stressed Conditions in Healthy Senior Women: Effects of Estrogen Replacement Therapy." *J Sleep Res,* vol. 10, iss. 1 (2001): 19–26.

Regestein, Q. "Menopausal Progesterone Replacement and Sleep Quality." *Menopause,* vol. 8, iss. 1 (2001): 3–4.

Schüle, C., M. F. di Michele, et al. "Influence of Sleep Deprivation on Neuroactive Steroids in Major Depression." *Neuropsychopharmacology,* vol. 28, iss. 3 (2003): 577–81.

Soderpalm, A., S. Lindsey, et al. "Administration of Progesterone Produces Mild Sedative-like Effects in Men and Women." *Psychoneuroendocrinology,* vol. 29, iss. 3 (2004): 339–54.

Touzet, S., M. Rabilloud, et al. "Relationship Between Sleep and Secretion of Gonadotropin and Ovarian Hormones in Women with Normal Cycles." *Fertil Steril,* vol. 77, iss. 4 (2002): 738–44.

Zhou, X., S. Shahabuddin, et al. "Effect of Gender on the Development of Hypocapnic Apnea/Hypopnea During NREM Sleep." *J Appl Physiol,* vol. 89, iss. 1 (2000): 192–99.

CHAPTER 13

Asthana, S., L. D. Baker, et al. "High-Dose Estradiol Improves Cognition for Women with AD: Results of a Randomized Study." *Neurology,* vol. 57, iss. 4 (2001): 605–12.

Bhavnani, B. "Estrogens and Menopause: Pharmacology of Conjugated Equine Estrogens and Their Potential Role in the Prevention of Neurodegenerative Diseases Such as Alzheimer's." *J Steroid Biochem Mol Biol,* vol. 85, iss. 2–5 (2003): 473–82.

Duka, T., R. Tasker, et al. "The Effects of 3-Week Estrogen Hormone Replacement on Cognition in Elderly Healthy Females." *Psychopharmacology (Berl),* vol. 149, iss. 2 (2000): 129–39.

Greene, R. "Estrogen and Cerebral Blood Flow: A Mechanism to Explain the Impact of Estrogen on the Incidence and Treatment of Alzheimer's Disease." *Int J Fertil Women's Med,* vol. 45, iss. 4 (2000): 253–57.

Johnson-Kozlow, M., D. Kritz-Silverstein, et al. "Coffee Consumption and Cognitive Function Among Older Adults." *Am J Epidemiol,* vol. 156, iss. 9 (2002): 842–50.

Luchsinger, J., M. Tang, et al. "Antioxidant Vitamin Intake and Risk of Alzheimer Disease." *Arch Neurol,* vol. 60, iss. 2 (2003): 203–08.

Maki, P., and S. Resnick. "Longitudinal Effects of Estrogen Replacement Therapy on PET Cerebral Blood Flow and Cognition." *Neurobiol Aging,* vol. 21, iss. 2 (2000): 373–83.

Mayeux, R. "Dissecting the Relative Influences of Genes and the Environment in Alzheimer's Disease." *Ann Neurol,* vol. 55, iss. 2 (2004): 156–58.

Morris, M., D. Evans, et al. "Dietary Fats and the Risk of Incident Alzheimer Disease." *Arch Neurol,* vol. 60, iss. 2 (2003): 194–200.

Onozuka, M., M. Fujita, et al. "Mapping Brain Region Activity During Chewing: A Functional Magnetic Resonance Imaging Study." *J Dent Res,* vol. 81, iss. 11 (2002): 743–46.

———. "Age-Related Changes in Brain Regional Activity During Chewing: A Functional Magnetic Resonance Imaging Study." *J Dent Res,* vol. 82, iss. 8 (2003): 657–60.

Paganini-Hill, A., and L. Clark. "Preliminary Assessment of Cognitive Function in Breast Cancer Patients Treated with Tamoxifen." *Breast Cancer Res Treat,* vol. 64, iss. 2 (2000): 165–76.

Poon, H., V. Calabrese, et al. "Free Radicals: Key to Brain Aging and Heme Oxygenase as a Cellular Response to Oxidative Stress [in process citation]." *J Gerontol A Biol Sci Med Sci,* vol. 59, iss. 5 (2004): M478–93.

Rice, M., A. Graves, et al. "Postmenopausal Estrogen and Estrogen-Progestin Use and 2-Year Rate of Cognitive Change in a Cohort of Older Japanese American Women: The Kame Project." *Arch Intern Med,* vol. 160, iss. 11 (2000): 1641–49.

Robertson, D., T. van Amelsvoort, et al. "Effects of Estrogen Replacement Therapy on Human Brain Aging: An in Vivo 1H MRS Study." *Neurology,* vol. 57, iss. 11 (2001): 2114–17.

Senanarong, V., S. Vannasaeng, et al. "Endogenous Estradiol in Elderly Individuals: Cognitive and Noncognitive Associations." *Arch Neurol,* vol. 59, iss. 3 (2002): 385–89.

Slopien, R., R. Junik, et al. "Influence of Hormonal Replacement Therapy on the Regional Cerebral Blood Flow in Postmenopausal Women." *Maturitas,* vol. 46, iss. 4 (2003): 255–62.

Smith, Y., B. Giordani, et al. "Long-Term Estrogen Replacement Is Associated with Improved Nonverbal Memory and Attentional Measures in Postmenopausal Women." *Fertil Steril,* vol. 76, iss. 6 (2001): 1101–07.

Trojanowski, J. "Tauists, Baptists, Syners, Apostates, and New Data." *Ann Neurol,* vol. 52, iss. 3 (2002): 263–65.

Verghese, J., G. Kuslansky, et al. "Cognitive Performance in Surgically Menopausal Women on Estrogen." *Neurology,* vol. 55, iss. 6 (2000): 872–4.

White, L., H. Petrovitch, et al. "Brain Aging and Midlife Tofu Consumption." *J Am Coll Nutr,* vol. 19, iss. 2 (2000): 242–55.

Yaffe, K., D. Barnes, et al. "A Prospective Study of Physical Activity and Cognitive Decline in Elderly Women: Women Who Walk." *Arch Intern Med,* vol. 161, iss. 14 (2001): 1703–08.

Yaffe, K., L. Lui, et al. "Cognitive Decline in Women in Relation to Non-Protein-Bound Oestradiol Concentrations." *Lancet,* vol. 356, iss. 9231 (2000): 708–12.

Zandi, P., M. Carlson, et al. "Hormone Replacement Therapy and Incidence of Alzheimer Disease in Older Women: The Cache County Study." *JAMA,* vol. 288, iss. 17 (2002): 2123–29.

CHAPTER 14

Abbot, A. "Ageing: Growing Old Gracefully." *Nature,* vol. 428, iss. 6979 (2004): 116–18.

Currie, L., M. Harrison, et al. "Postmenopausal Estrogen Use Affects Risk for Parkinson Disease." *Arch Neurol,* vol. 61, iss. 6 (2004): 886–88.

Hannan, E., J. Magaziner, et al. "Mortality and Locomotion 6 Months After Hospitalization for Hip Fracture: Risk Factors and Risk-Adjusted Hospital Outcomes." *JAMA,* vol. 285, iss. 21 (2001): 2736–42.

Hazeltine, E., and R. B. Ivry. "NEUROSCIENCE: Can We Teach the Cerebellum New Tricks?" *Science,* vol. 296, iss. 5575 (2002): 1979–80.

Liu-Ambrose, T., K. Khan, et al. "Resistance and Agility Training Reduce Fall Risk in Women Aged 75 to 85 with Low Bone Mass: A 6-Month Randomized, Controlled Trial." *J Am Geriatr Soc,* vol. 52, iss. 5 (2004): 657–65.

Lui, L., K. Stone, et al. "Bone Loss Predicts Subsequent Cognitive Decline in Older Women: The Study of Osteoporotic Fractures." *J Am Geriatr Soc,* vol. 51, iss. 1 (2003): 38–43.

Marcell, T. "Sarcopenia: Causes, Consequences, and Preventions." *J Gerontol A Biol Sci Med Sci,* vol. 58, iss. 10 (2003): M911–16.

Moss, F., and J. Milton. "Balancing the Unbalanced." *2003,* vol. 425, iss. 6961 (2003): 911–13.

Naessen, T., B. Lindmark, et al. "Better Postural Balance in Elderly Women Receiving Estrogens." *Am J Obstet Gynecol,* vol. 177, iss. 2 (1997): 412–16.

Shults, C., D. Oakes, et al. "Effects of Coenzyme Q10 in Early Parkinson Disease: Evidence of Slowing of the Functional Decline." *Arch Neurol,* vol. 59, iss. 10 (2002): 1541–50.

Smith, M., L. Adams, et al. "Abnormal Luteal Phase Excitability of the Motor Cortex in Women with Premenstrual Syndrome." *Biol Psychiatry,* vol. 54, iss. 7 (2003): 757–62.

Tsang, K.-L., S.-L. Ho, et al. "Estrogen Improves Motor Disability in Parkinsonian Post-menopausal Women with Motor Fluctuations." *Neurology,* vol. 54, iss. 12 (2000): 2292–98.

CHAPTER 15

Azziz, R. "The Evaluation and Management of Hirsutism." *Obstet Gynecol,* vol. 101, iss. 5, pt. 1 (2003): 995–1007.

Farquhar, C., O. Lee, et al. "Spironolactone Versus Placebo or in Combination with Steroids for Hirsutism and/or Acne." Cochrane Database Syst Rev (2003).

Griffiths, C. "Drug Treatment of Photoaged Skin." *Drugs Aging,* vol. 14, iss. 4 (1999): 289–301.

Koh, J., H. Kang, et al. "Cigarette Smoking Associated with Premature Facial Wrinkling: Image Analysis of Facial Skin Replicas." *Int J Dermatol,* vol. 41, iss. 1 (2002): 21–27.

Moalli, P., L. Talarico, et al. "Impact of Menopause on Collagen Subtypes in the Arcus Tendineous Fasciae Pelvis." *Am J Obstet Gynecol,* vol. 190, iss. 3 (2004): 620–27.

Raine-Fenning, N., M. Brincat, et al. "Skin Aging and Menopause: Implications for Treat-ment." *Am J Clin Dermatol,* vol. 4, iss. 6 (2003): 371–78.

Schindler, A. "Antiandrogenic Progestins for Treatment of Signs of Androgenisation and Hormonal Contraception." *Eur J Obstet Gynecol Reprod Biol,* vol. 112, iss. 2 (2004): 136–41.

Shah, M., and H. Maibach. "Estrogen and Skin: An Overview." *Am J Clin Dermatol,* vol. 2, iss. 3 (2001): 143–50.

Smith, J., S. Vitale, et al. "Dry Eye Signs and Symptoms in Women with Premature Ovarian Failure." *Arch Ophthalmol,* vol. 122, iss. 2 (2004): 151–56.

Thiboutot, D., and W. Chen. "Update and Future of Hormonal Therapy in Acne." *Dermatology,* vol. 206, iss. 1 (2003): 57–67.

Tsukahara, K., S. Moriwaki, et al. "Ovariectomy Accelerates Photoaging of Rat Skin." *Photochem Photobiol,* vol. 73, iss. 5 (2001): 525–31.

van Vloten, W. A., C. W. van Haselen, et al. "The Effect of 2 Combined Oral Contraceptives Containing Either Drospirenone or Cyproterone Acetate on Acne and Seborrhea." *Cutis,* vol. 69, iss. 4 suppl. (2002): 2–15.

Youn, C., O. Kwon, et al. "Effect of Pregnancy and Menopause on Facial Wrinkling in Women." *Acta Derm Venereol,* vol. 83, iss. 6 (2003): 419–24.

CHAPTER 16

Borugian, M., S. Sheps, et al. "Insulin, Macronutrient Intake, and Physical Activity: Are Potential Indicators of Insulin Resistance Associated with Mortality from Breast Cancer [in process citation]?" *Cancer Epidemiol Biomarkers Prev,* vol. 13, iss. 7 (2004): 1163–72.

Calle, E. E., C. Rodriguez, et al. "Overweight, Obesity, and Mortality from Cancer in a Prospectively Studied Cohort of U.S. Adults." *N Engl J Med,* vol. 348, iss. 17 (2003): 1625–38.

Chlebowski, R. T., J. Wactawski-Wende, et al. "Estrogen plus Progestin and Colorectal Cancer in Postmenopausal Women." *N Engl J Med,* vol. 350, iss. 10 (2004): 991–1004.

Czene, K., P. Lichtenstein, et al. "Environmental and Heritable Causes of Cancer Among 9.6 Million Individuals in the Swedish Family-Cancer Database." *Int J Cancer,* vol. 99, iss. 2 (2002): 260–66.

Darbre, P. "Underarm Cosmetics and Breast Cancer." *J Appl Toxicol,* vol. 23, iss. 2 (2003): 89–95.

Darbre, P., A. Aljarrah, et al. "Concentrations of Parabens in Human Breast Tumours [in process citation]." *J Appl Toxicol,* vol. 24, iss. 1 (2004): 5–13.

Darbre, P., J. Byford, et al. "Oestrogenic Activity of Benzylparaben." *J Appl Toxicol,* vol. 23, iss. 1 (2003): 43–51.

Deligeoroglou, E., E. Michailidis, et al. "Oral Contraceptives and Reproductive System Cancer." *Ann N Y Acad Sci,* vol. 997 (2003): 199–208.

Demicheli, R., G. Bonadonna, et al. "Menopausal Status Dependence of Early Mortality Reduction Due to Diagnosis of Smaller Breast Cancers (T1 v T2-T3): Relevance to Screening." *J Clin Oncol,* vol. 22, iss. 1 (2004): 102–07.

Fraser, I., and G. Kovacs. "The Efficacy of Non-Contraceptive Uses for Hormonal Contraceptives." *Med J Aust,* vol. 178, iss. 12 (2003): 621–23.

Hartge, P. "Genes, Hormones, and Pathways to Breast Cancer." *N Engl J Med,* vol. 348, iss. 23 (2003): 2352–54.

Harvey, P. "Parabens, Oestrogenicity, Underarm Cosmetics and Breast Cancer: A Perspective on a Hypothesis." *J Appl Toxicol,* vol. 23, iss. 5 (2003): 285–88.

Holmes, M., and C. Kroenke. "Beyond Treatment: Lifestyle Choices After Breast Cancer to Enhance Quality of Life and Survival." *Women's Health Issues,* vol. 14, iss. 1 (2004): 11–13.

Kozak, K., M. Amneus, et al. "Identification of Biomarkers for Ovarian Cancer Using Strong Anion-Exchange ProteinChips: Potential Use in Diagnosis and Prognosis." *Proc Natl Acad Sci USA,* vol. 100, iss. 21 (2003): 12343–48.

Lee, I. "Physical Activity and Cancer Prevention—Data from Epidemiologic Studies." *Med Sci Sports Exerc,* vol. 35, iss. 11 (2003): 1823–27.

McGrath, K. "An Earlier Age of Breast Cancer Diagnosis Related to More Frequent Use of Antiperspirants/Deodorants and Underarm Shaving." *Eur J Cancer Prev,* vol. 12, iss. 6 (2003): 479–85.

Michels, K., and A. Ekbom. "Caloric Restriction and Incidence of Breast Cancer." *JAMA,* vol. 291, iss. 10 (2004): 1226–30.

Natrajan, P., and R. Gambrell. "Estrogen Replacement Therapy in Patients with Early Breast Cancer." *Am J Obstet Gynecol,* vol. 187, iss. 2 (2002): 289–94; discussion 294–95.

O'Meara, E. S., M. A. Rossing, et al. "Hormone Replacement Therapy After a Diagnosis of Breast Cancer in Relation to Recurrence and Mortality." *J Natl Cancer Inst,* vol. 93, iss. 10 (2001): 754–61.

Partridge, A., P. Wang, et al. "Nonadherence to Adjuvant Tamoxifen Therapy in Women with Primary Breast Cancer." *J Clin Oncol,* vol. 21, iss. 4 (2003): 602–06.

Somboonporn, W., Davis, S. R. "Testosterone Effects on the Breast: Implications for Testosterone Therapy for Women." *Endocrine Reviews,* vol. 25 (2004): 374–388.

Tchen, N., H. Juffs, et al. "Cognitive Function, Fatigue, and Menopausal Symptoms in Women Receiving Adjuvant Chemotherapy for Breast Cancer." *J Clin Oncol,* vol. 21, iss. 22 (2003): 4175–83.

Walker, G., J. Schlesselman, et al. "Family History of Cancer, Oral Contraceptive Use, and Ovarian Cancer Risk." *Am J Obstet Gynecol,* vol. 186, iss. 1 (2002): 8–14.

Wefel, J., R. Lenzi, et al. "'Chemobrain' in Breast Carcinoma?: A prologue [in process citation]." *Cancer,* vol. 101, iss. 3 (2004): 466–75.

INDEX

ABOUT THE AUTHORS

ROBERT A. GREENE received his medical degree from Ohio State University. His internship/residency in obstetrics and gynecology was completed at the University of Louisville, followed by a fellowship at Harbor-UCLA Medical Center for subspecialty training in reproductive endocrinology and infertility. He is board certified in both his specialty and subspecialty. Dr. Greene is an assistant clinical professor at UC Davis School of Medicine and is the founder of Specialty Care for Women in Redding, California, a clinical- and research-based private practice catering to the unique needs of women with hormonal imbalance.

His research has been published in prestigious medical journals, including *Fertility & Sterility, The Female Patient, OB/GYN Clinics of North America,* and *The Aging Male.* Dr. Greene has lectured extensively throughout the United States as well as at international conferences in Europe, Japan, Singapore, and South America. He sits on numerous advisory committees to establish treatment guidelines for sexual dysfunction, hot flashes, migraine headaches, pelvic pain, and epilepsy in women.

Dr. Greene lives in Northern California, where he balances his life with his wife, two dogs, and two cats. If you or your health care provider would like additional information to balance your hormonal problem, check out his website at www.SpecialtyCare4Women.com.

LEAH FELDON is a journalist, TV correspondent, author, and coauthor of the *New York Times* bestseller *The Okinawa Program* as well as *The Okinawa Diet Plan* and *Help Your Baby Talk.* A longtime *People* magazine reporter, her articles have also appeared in *New York Magazine, InStyle, First, Ladies Home Journal, Family Circle, Redbook,* and *Entertainment Weekly.* She currently divides her time between New York and Mexico.